T0309751

ANNALS *of* THE NEW YORK ACADEMY OF SCIENCES

DIRECTOR AND EXECUTIVE EDITOR
Douglas Braaten

ASSISTANT EDITOR
Joseph Abrajano

PROJECT MANAGER
Steven E. Bohall

PROJECT COORDINATOR
Ralph W. Brown

CREATIVE DIRECTOR
Ash Ayman Shairzay

The New York Academy of Sciences
7 World Trade Center
250 Greenwich Street, 40th Floor
New York, NY 10007-2157

annals@nyas.org
www.nyas.org/annals

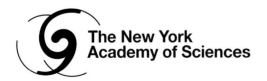
The New York Academy of Sciences

Published by Blackwell Publishing
On behalf of the New York Academy of Sciences

Boston, MA
2010

ANNALS *of* THE NEW YORK ACADEMY OF SCIENCES

VOLUME 1198

ISSUE
Neurons and Networks in the Spinal Cord

ISSUE EDITORS
Lea Ziskind-Conhaim, Joseph R. Fetcho, Shawn Hochman, Amy B. MacDermott, and Paul S.G. Stein

This volume presents manuscripts stemming from the conference entitled "Cellular and Network Functions in the Spinal Cord," held on June 23–26, 2009 at the Pyle Center, University of Wisconsin, Madison, Wisconsin.

TABLE OF CONTENTS

Become a Member Today of the New York Academy of Sciences

The New York Academy of Sciences is dedicated to identifying the next frontiers in science and catalyzing key breakthroughs. As has been the case for 200 years, many of the leading scientific minds of our time rely on the Academy for key meetings and publications that serve as the crucial forum for a global community dedicated to scientific innovation.

 Select one FREE *Annals* volume and up to five volumes for only $40 each.

 Network and exchange ideas with the leaders of academia and industry.

 Broaden your knowledge across many disciplines.

 Gain access to exclusive online content.

Join Online at **www.nyas.org**

Or by phone at **800.344.6902** (516.576.2270 if outside the U.S.).

Dorsal Horn

Development

Injury

Ann. N.Y. Acad. Sci. ISSN 0077-8923

ANNALS OF THE NEW YORK ACADEMY OF SCIENCES
Issue: *Neurons and Networks in the Spinal Cord*

Updating neural representations of objects during walking

Keir Pearson and Rod Gramlich

Department of Physiology, University of Alberta, Edmonton, Alberta, Canada

Address for correspondance: Keir Pearson, Department of Physiology, University of Alberta, Edmonton, AB T6G 2H7, Canada. Voice: (780) 492-5628; fax: (780) 492-8915. keir.pearson@ualberta.ca

In quadrupeds, a unique form of memory is used to guide the hind legs over barriers that have already been stepped over by the forelegs. This memory is very long-lasting (many minutes), incorporates precise information about the size and position of the barrier relative to the hind legs, and is updated as the animal steps sequentially across a barrier. Recent findings from electrophysiological and lesion studies have revealed that neuronal systems in the parietal cortex are necessary for establishing the long-lasting feature of the memory and may be involved in representing the current position of the barrier relative to the moving body. We hypothesize that the latter involves the modulation of activity in neuronal systems in the posterior parietal cortex by efference copy signals of motor commands for stepping and by sensory signals from muscle proprioceptors. We propose that motor pattern generation for walking occurs within a framework of a body schema that constantly informs pattern generating networks about the geometry of the body and the location of near objects relative to the body.

Keywords: walking; body schema; working memory; parietal cortex; object avoidance

Introduction

As we walk we often must avoid obstacles either by navigating around them or stepping over them. These adaptations can be made without conscious thought as, for example, we move through a crowd or step over a culvert while conversing with another person. This ability to automatically avoid obstacles obviously requires mechanisms in the brain for (1) representing the properties of the obstacle (size, orientation, movement, etc.), (2) representing the location of the obstacle relative to the body (egocentric representation), and (3) updating these representations as the body moves. In normal individuals vision is the primary sensory channel for providing information to establish the representations of the properties of an obstacle and the initial location of an obstacle relative to the body. On the other hand, once an obstacle has been visually detected, numerous sensory and central signals could be used for updating the representation of the changing location of the obstacle relative to the body as we move: visual signals, limb and body proprioceptive signals, vestibular signals, and efference copy of the motor command producing the movements. In this article, we review recent investigations on the neuronal mechanisms for tracking and updating the location of obstacles relative to the body, and present some new findings in cats that indicate feedback from muscle proprioceptors has an important role in modulating stepping movements to avoid remembered obstacles that are out of sight.

A role for working memory in guiding leg movements during walking

There is now a substantial literature on the use of vision in guiding locomotor movements to avoid obstacles in humans and quadrupeds (reviewed in references 1–4). One of the important conclusions from studies in humans is that adaptation of leg movement for obstacle avoidance is, to a large extent, produced by feedforward motor commands and not by moment-by-moment visual feedback regulation of the locomotor system. For example, occlusion of vision for a few steps immediately before a subject steps over a barrier has only a modest effect on the trajectory of the leading leg and no influence on the trailing leg.[5] Similarly, walking cats can accurately place their paws for a few steps on remembered targets when vision is occluded.[6] These investigations, and others, clearly demonstrate a role

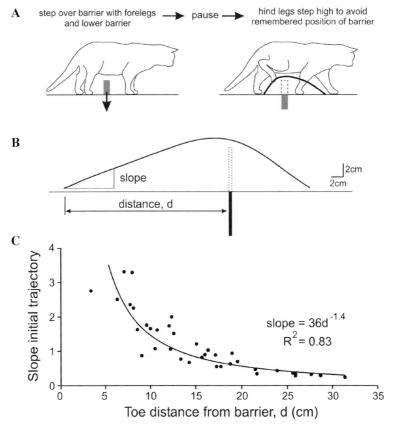

Figure 1. Initial slope of hind toe trajectories in the barrier-memory task. **(A)** Schematic of barrier-memory task. The animal steps over a barrier (*gray rectangle*) with its forelegs and stops walking. The barrier is then lowered, and after a variable interval (pause) the animal walks forward. The hind legs are lifted higher so the toe avoids the remembered position of the barrier (*dotted rectangle*). **(B)** An example of the trajectory of the toe of the leading hind leg and the parameters that were measured. The *dotted* and *filled rectangles* show the position of the remembered and final positions of the barrier, respectively. **(C)** Scatter plot of the relationship between the initial slope of the toe trajectory and the toe distance from the barrier. The relationship was quantified by fitting the data with a power function (*curved line*).

for working memory in guiding leg trajectories in walking mammals. That is, visually derived information about the geometry of the external world is held for a short time in memory and then used to guide stepping movements.

One of the clearest demonstrations of a role for working memory in regulating stepping has come from a series of recent studies from our laboratory on cats.[7–9] These studies were motivated by recognizing that when quadrupeds approach and step over a barrier, they are very unlikely to use vision for directly guiding the trajectories of the hind legs because the visual field of the animal is well ahead of the barrier at the time the hind legs pass over the

barrier. To examine the characteristics of this working memory we devised the protocol illustrated in Figure 1A. Cats were enticed with food to step over a barrier with their forelegs and then to stop walking so they stood with their forelegs on one side of the barrier and their hind legs on the other side. While standing in this manner, the barrier was removed to eliminate any possibility that vision of the barrier could be used for controlling any subsequent movements. After a variable delay (ranging from seconds to minutes) the animals were again enticed by food to move forward and the movement of the hind legs was observed. The clear and consistent result of this procedure was that the hind paws were lifted higher as if avoiding the remembered position of the removed barrier. A unique feature of this working memory is that it lasts for many minutes with little or no decrement. The longest delay we have observed for the maintenance of the memory was 10 min, and we have been unable to document any decline in the retention of the memory of the barrier (investigating delays of this magnitude and longer is difficult because of the reluctance of animals to remain standing in one position for these long durations). However, in a recent study in horses using a similar procedure[10] the memory of the barrier was found to be maintained for 15 min (the longest interval tested), but there was clearly some loss in memory at this interval when compared to the memory at intervals of a few minutes.

Two other characteristics of the memory for obstacle location in cats are noteworthy. The first is that stepping of the forelegs over the barrier is required to establish the long-lasting feature of the memory,[8] and the second is that it can very accurately guide the trajectories of the hind paws. The precision of the memory for guiding the hind paws over the barrier was revealed by the precise modifications of the toe trajectories midway through the swing phase to avoid the remembered position of the removed barrier[7] and by a lawful inverse relationship between the initial slope of the toe trajectories and the distance of the paw from the barrier at the onset of the step (Fig. 1C).

Recently, we identified another significant characteristic of this memory system, namely the capacity to be updated during the delay period when a hind leg is repositioned during the delay period. When an animal is standing and straddling the removed barrier it will often take a small step either forward or backward thus changing the location of the paw relative to the barrier (Fig. 2, *inset at top left*). When this occurs the initial slope of the toe trajectory when the hind leg eventually steps over the remembered barrier (Fig. 1B) corresponds closely to the slope expected for the updated location of the paw relative to the barrier (Fig. 2). This occurs regardless of whether the small step during the delay period is toward or away from the remembered barrier. The filled circles in the plot in Figure 2 show data for updated forward steps from a mean initial position of about 21 cm from the barrier, while the curve shows the relationship between the initial slope and toe distance from the barrier in control trials when

there was no updating (control data and best fitting power function are shown in Fig. 1B). Note that the slopes of the updated steps increase relative to what would have been expected had there been no updating. The data points are also scattered around the control curve thus indicating that the updating of the toe trajectory was quite precise. Similar results to those shown in Figure 2 were obtained when backward steps occurred during the delay period from initial toe positions located relatively close to the barrier (mean initial distance from barrier was 7.8 cm). In these cases the slopes of the toe trajectories over the remembered barrier were reduced from those expected had the step been initiated from the initial position.

The fact that memory of the barrier location can be updated during the delay period when small forward or backward steps are taken during the delay period, raises the obvious question of what information is used to update the memory? There are two distinct possibilities: the first is that it arises from an efference copy of the motor command producing the additional step, and the second is that it originates from proprioceptors in the moved leg (with perhaps information from other proprioceptors due to shifts in weight distribution). Another signal that could potentially contribute to the updating is from the vestibular system, although we consider this very unlikely because on most trials updating occurred without any forward movement of the body and head. In an attempt to distinguish between the two main possibilities, we examined the effect of *passively* moving the paw either forward or backward during the delay period, thus eliminating any contribution from an efference copy signal. To do this, we placed a thin (1.5 mm) plate on the right-hand side of the walkway surface. The plate could be moved manually either toward or away from the barrier (*insets* Fig. 3). A similar plate was placed on the left-hand side of the walkway surface but was not moveable so as to match surface texture for the two hind legs. The initial position of the moveable plate was set so that the right hind paw was placed on this plate when the animal was paused straddling the barrier. The barrier was then lowered and after a variable delay (5–10 sec) the plate supporting the right hind leg was moved either toward or away from the barrier. About 10 sec later the animal was induced to move forward and step over the remembered barrier. On all trials the trajectory

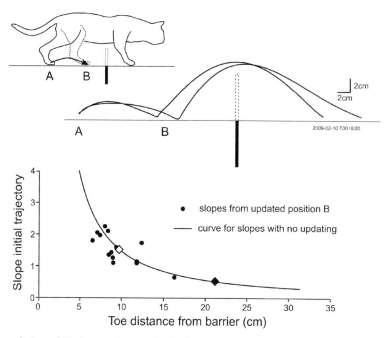

Figure 2. Active updating of hind toe trajectory in the barrier-memory task. Active updating occurs when a hind leg steps forward while straddling the remembered position of the barrier (*schematic, top left*). The *middle panel* shows two examples of the toe trajectory of the leading hind leg when the step over the remembered barrier (*dotted rectangle*) was preceded by a step that shifted the toe from position A to position B (also labeled in schematic of the cat). The *bottom panel* shows a scatter plot of the initial slope of actively updated trajectories versus toe distance from the barrier for the step over the remembered barrier (*filled circles*). The curve shows the slope–distance relationship for trials with no updating (see Fig. 1B). The *filled diamond* indicated the expected means of the initial slope and the initial toe position A if the updating step had not occurred. The *open diamond* shows the means of the initial slope and toe position of the updated steps. Note the mean slope of updated steps was increased, and that the means lie on the curve fitted to data from trials with no updating.

of the right toe was always close to that expected from the updated position and not the original position (Fig. 3). Thus passive movements of a hind leg can update the memory of the location of the barrier with respect to the leg. The strong implication of these observations is that input from leg proprioceptors has a major role in updating the egocentric representation of near objects with respect to the body. This finding does not exclude the possibility that efference copy signals could also contribute to the updating, but in this situation they may be of minor importance.

The concept of "body schema" in locomotion

Our recent observations on walking cats, summarized in the preceding section, have clearly demonstrated that hind leg movements when stepping over barriers depend on a stored representation (working memory) of the obstacle height and its location relative to the body. In addition, this representation can be updated by movements of the hind legs prior to stepping, and updating is primarily dependent on proprioceptive signals from the legs. These observations force us to consider whether current concepts for describing the neuronal control of walking are sufficient to account for these new data. We believe they are inadequate. The main reason is that contemporary concepts on the neurobiology of walking are primarily focused on segmental mechanisms in the spinal cord derived from reduced preparations, thus completely ignoring mechanisms that might function when animals move naturally through complex and unpredictable environments. Contemporary concepts, such as central pattern

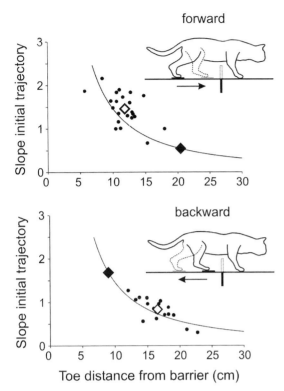

Figure 3. Passive updating of hind toe trajectory in the barrier-memory task. Passive updating occurs when a hind leg is shifted either forward (*top*) or backward (*bottom*) while straddling the remembered position of the barrier (*schematics above plots*). The scatter plots show the relationship between initial slope of passively updated trajectories versus toe distance from the barrier for the step over the remembered barrier (*filled circles*). The curves in each plot show the slope–distance relationship for trials with no updating (see Fig. 1B). The *filled diamonds* indicated the expected means of the initial slopes and the initial toe positions if the updating steps had not occurred. The *open diamonds* show the means of the initial slopes and toe positions of the updated steps. Note the mean slope of passively updated steps was increased when the foot was moved forward, and decreased when the foot was moved backwards. Note that the means lie close to curve fitted to data from trials with no updating.

generation, sensory feedback modulation of central pattern generators, and descending brain-stem command systems cannot account for our recent finding that working memory and dynamic updating of objects in the external world have important roles in regulating stepping. It should be noted,

however, that a series of studies on cats stepping over barriers by Trevor Drew and his colleagues have extended our conceptual framework to include a role of the motor cortex in issuing commands via descending corticospinal neurons to selectively modify burst activity in different groups of motoneurons via spinal pattern generating networks.[3,11] The question of how visual signals function to modify the commands in corticospinal neurons remains unanswered, but it likely depends on visual-motor transformations via the posterior parietal cortex.[12]

How then might we conceptualize our recent findings? An attractive possibility is to view them within the framework of a *body schema*. The concept of body schema was first proposed almost a century ago by Head and Holmes[13] in part to explain the deficits in the ability of patients with cortical lesions to recognize the postural configuration of their body and the location of a stimulus on the skin. They postulated that past sensory impressions form organized internal models of themselves that they termed "schemata" (p. 189). Today, the general notion of body schema is that sensory signals establish a neural representation of the state of the body, and that this representation is updated automatically as we move and in doing so provides a dynamic framework for the production of motor commands appropriate for the current state of the body. Although there is no precise definition of body schema, most definitions include the idea that the representation and updating of body configuration in humans, and presumably in animals, occurs more-or-less unconsciously. A definition we feel could be slightly extended to incorporate our findings in the walking cat is as follows from Graziano and Botvinick,[14] with our addition bolded at the end:

"... *an implicit knowledge structure that encodes the body's form, the constraints on how the body's own parts can be configured, and the consequences of this configuration on touch, vision and movements **that include interactions of the body with near objects***"

Despite being almost a century old, the concept of body schema has only been discussed seriously in the neuroscience community during the past 20 years, mainly in the context of posture control[15] and reaching and tool use.[14,16–18] The concept of body schema has been almost completely ignored by investigators interested in the neurobiology of

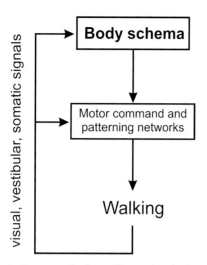

visual, vestibular, somatic signals

Body schema

Motor command and patterning networks

Walking

Figure 4. Conceptual scheme illustrating the hierarchical regulation of command and pattern generating networks for walking by a body schema. Visual, vestibular, and somatic sensory systems provide important information to establish the body schema and to directly influence command and pattern generating networks.

walking. The only publication we are aware of that considers the concept of body schema in walking is a recent investigation on the effects of modifying the body geometry by leg extension.[19] Decreases in the accuracy of path integration by leg extension were interpreted within the framework of a mismatch between the new body geometry and the old body schema.

Figure 4 illustrates one possibility for how a body schema could be viewed in relation to pattern generating networks for walking; the latter could include neurons in many regions of the nervous system, such as the motor cortex, in addition to neuronal networks in the spinal cord. The hierarchical arrangement illustrated in Figure 4 easily accounts for two necessary requirements for the neuronal system controlling walking: (1) constant monitoring of the geometry of the limb and body and the geometrical arrangement of the body with respect to external objects and (2) precise regulation of the neuronal networks generating the motor patterns for walking to produce limb and body movements appropriate for the current state of the body and the state of the external world with respect to the body. This hierarchical scheme is unquestionably overly simplistic, but it does at least provide a conceptual framework

to begin to address the neurobiology of high-level control of walking.

If the concept of body schema is accepted for the moment, then one obvious question is how is the body schema represented in the central nervous system? Another is how does this representation control neuronal networks that are more directly involved in the generation of motor commands? Currently these questions cannot be answered, but hints have come from studies on humans, monkeys, cats, and frogs. First, it is very likely that the neuronal representation of the state of the body is distributed throughout the central nervous system, including the spinal cord. Evidence implicating the spinal cord comes from the observation that the trajectory of the wiping reflex of a hind leg in spinal frogs is strongly dependent upon the position of the stimulated foreleg.[20] A role for subcortical networks in representing information about the state of the body also comes from the fact that cats raised without cerebral hemispheres display a remarkable capacity for a wide range of complex behaviors, including walking through mazes.[21] However, high-level control of behavior involving detailed visual processing and the memories of objects almost certainly requires neuronal systems in the cerebral hemispheres. One cortical region that appears especially important for this level of control is the posterior parietal cortex. Damage of the posterior parietal cortex in humans can drastically alter the awareness of the position of the arms[22,23] and awareness of the spatial relationships between body parts,[24,25] and in monkeys inactivation of the lateral intraparietal area produces inaccurate eye movements directed to remembered locations of visual targets.[26] Moreover, electrophysiological recordings from neurons in different regions of the posterior parietal cortex in behaving monkeys have revealed that different groups of neurons have activity patterns correlated with high-level aspects of motor control, such as planning movements,[27] updating sensory representations during movement,[28,29] representing the remembered location of external objects,[30–32] and integrating visual and proprioceptive information.[33]

There is also some evidence that the posterior parietal cortex has an essential role in the high-level regulation of motor behavior in cats. For example, lesions in this region result in inaccurate reaching movements to moving objects[34] and a decrease in the ability to step accurately over a visually perceived moving barrier.[12] Moreover, a recent study from our laboratory found that small lesions in area 5 of the posterior parietal cortex severely reduced the ability of adult cats to remember the height of a barrier over which the forelegs had stepped.[9] Recordings from single neurons in the same region have revealed that different groups of neurons become selectively active as an animal approaches and steps over a barrier; one group becoming increasingly active as an animal approaches the barrier and another group active as the barrier passes under the animal.[3] A preliminary study also found that the latter group remains active when the animal is paused during walking after the forelegs, but not the hind legs, have stepped over the barrier.[35] These recent findings strongly indicate that neuronal systems in the posterior parietal cortex are involved in storing and representing information about the location of external objects with respect to the body, and that these systems form part of the animal's body schema in so far as this schema includes knowledge of the location of near objects. Based on these observations it is conceivable that different groups of neurons in area 5 of the posterior parietal cortex represent different locations of the barrier relative to the legs, and that activity in each group functions to maintain a working memory for a specific motor action that follows the action leading to the activation of the group. For example, the group of neurons that becomes tonically active after the forelegs have stepped over the barrier[3,35] could be elements in the working memory system for controlling the subsequent stepping of the hind legs over the barrier (see McVea et al.[9] for a discussion of this idea). Thus the sequential activation of different groups of neurons would be a neural correlate of the updating of knowledge of barrier locations with respect to the position of the legs.

Our conclusion that neuronal systems in the posterior parietal cortex of walking cats have roles in representing the location of objects close to the body and in updating the egocentric representations of near objects is quite consistent with studies on reaching and tool-use in monkeys. First, many neurons in area 5 of monkeys are tonically active prior to reaching towards a remembered target.[36] Second, the visual receptive fields of many neurons in the area 5 of monkeys are confined to locations that are reachable,[37] and a functional magnetic resonance imaging (fMRI) study has shown that there

is more activity in the posterior parietal cortex when subjects are viewing reachable targets compared to viewing targets out of reach.[38] Finally, neurons of the posterior parietal cortex have been found that have visual receptive fields located close to the location of a hand, shift with movements of the hand, and elongated when a monkey uses a tool, an observation that has been interpreted as a modification of the body schema by tool use.[17,39] It should be noted, however, that the representation of the body schema in cortical regions is not necessarily confined to neuronal systems in the posterior parietal cortex. Especially important may be systems in the ventral premotor cortex that have been found to be involved in the monitoring of the location of objects close to the body and eliciting motor responses to avoid these objects.[40,41] The extent to which neuronal systems in the premotor cortex of cats are involved in object avoidance is unknown (due to the absence of any recordings from this region in behaving cats), but based on the monkey data this possibility must be considered likely.

Conclusions

Recent observations on walking quadrupeds (cats and horses) have demonstrated that these animals use working memory to precisely guide the stepping of their hind legs over barriers. Lesion and electrophysiological recording studies have strongly indicated that neuronal systems in area 5 of the posterior parietal cortex have an essential role in the maintenance of this working memory. We propose that these systems form part of a body schema that provides a representation of the geometry of the body with respect to external objects close to the body and that this representation is progressively updated as the body moves relative to the objects. Sensory information from muscle proprioceptors likely contributes to the updating process. We conclude that the current conceptual framework for describing the neurobiology of walking must be extended to account for new observations on the complex, high-level regulation of stepping in mammals.

Acknowledgments

We thank Andrew Taylor for his comments on a draft of this article. Supported by the Canadian Institutes of Health Research.

Conflicts of interest

The authors declare no conflicts of interest.

References

1. Patla, A.E. 1997. Understanding the roles of vision in the control of human locomotion. *Gait Posture* **5:** 54–69.

2. Marigold, D.S. 2008. Role of peripheral visual cues in online visual guidance of locomotion. *Exer. Sport. Sci. Rev.* **36:** 145–151.

3. Drew, T., J.-E. Andujar, K. Lajoie, *et al.* 2008. Cortical mechanisms involved in visuomotor coordination during precision walking. *Brain Res. Rev.* **57:** 199–211.

4. Mcvea, D.A. & K.G. Pearson. 2009. Object avoidance during locomotion. *Adv. Exp. Med. Biol.* **629:** 293–316.

5. Mohagheghi, A.A., R. Moraes & A.E. Patla. 2004. The effects of distant and on-line visual information on the control of approach phase and step over an obstacle during locomotion. *Exp. Brain Res.* **155:** 459–468.

6. Wilkinson, E.J. & H.A. Sherk. 2005. The use of visual information for planning accurate steps in a cluttered environment. *Behav. Brain Res.* **164:** 270–274.

7. Mcvea, D.A. & K.G. Pearson. 2006. Long-lasting memories of obstacles guide leg movements in the walking cat. *J. Neurosci.* **26:** 1175–1178.

8. Mcvea, D.A. & K.G. Pearson. 2007. Stepping of the forelegs over obstacles establishes long-lasting memories in cats. *Curr. Biol.* **17:** R621–R623.

9. Mcvea, D.A., A.J. Taylor & K.G. Pearson. 2009. Long-lasting working memories of obstacles established by foreleg stepping in walking cats require area 5 of the posterior parietal cortex. *J. Neurosci.* **29:** 9396–9404.

10. Whishaw, I.Q., L.-A.R. Sacrey & B. Gorny. 2009. Hind limb stepping over obstacles in the horse guided by place-object memory. *Behav. Brain Res.* **198:** 372–379.

11. Drew, T., W. Jiang & W. Widajewicz. 2002. Contribution of the motor cortex to the control of hindlimbs during locomotion in the cat. *Brain Res. Rev.* **40:** 178–191.

12. Lajoie, K. & T. Drew. 2007. Lesions in area 5 of the posterior parietal cortex in the cat produce errors in the accuracy of paw placement during visually-guided locomotion. *J. Neurophysiol.* **97:** 2339–2354.

13. Head, H. & G. Holmes. 1911. Sensory disturbances from cerebral lesions. *Brain* **34:** 102–254.

14. Graziano, M.S.A. & M.M. Botvinick. 2002. How the brain represents the body: insights from neurophysiology and psychology. *Attention Perform.* **19:** 136–157.

15. Gurfinkel, V.S. & Y.S. Levik. 1991. Perceptual and automatic aspects of the postural body scheme. In *Brain and Space.* J. Paillard, Ed.: 112–132. Oxford University Press. Oxford.

16. Maravita, A., C. Spence & J. Driver. 2003. Multisensory integration and body schema: close to hand and within reach. *Curr. Biol.* **13:** R531–R539.

17. Maravita, A. & A. Iriki. 2004. Tools for the body (schema). *Trends Neurosci.* **8:** 79–86.

18. Cardinali, L., F. Frassinetti, C. Brozzoli, *et al.* 2009. Tool-use induces morphological updating of body schema. *Curr. Biol.* **19:** R478–R479.

19. Dominici, N., E. Daprati, D. Nico, *et al.* 2009. Changes in limb kinematics and walking-distance estimation after shank elongation: evidence for a locomotor body schema? *J. Neurophysiol.* **101:** 1419–1429.

20. Fukson, O.I., M.B. Berkinblit & A.G. Feldman. 1980. The spinal frog takes into account the scheme of its body during the wiping reflex. *Science* **209:** 1261–1263.

21. Bjursten, L.-M., K. Norrsell & U. Norrsell. 1976. Behavioural repertory of cats without cerebral cortex from infancy. *Exp. Brain Res.* **25:** 115–130.

22. Wolpert, D.M., S.J. Goodbody & M. Husain. 1998. Maintaining internal representations: the role of the human superior parietal lobe. *Nat. Neurosci.* **1:** 529–533.

23. Caminiti, R., S. Ferraina & P.B. Johbson. 1996. The sources of visual information to the primate frontal lobe: a novel role for the superior parietal cortex. *Cereb. Cortex* **6:** 319–328.

24. Corradi-Del'Acqua, C., M.D. Hesse, R.I. Rumiati, *et al.* 2008. Where is a nose with respect to the foot? The left posterior parietal cortex processes spatial relationships among body parts. *Cereb. Cortex* **18:** 2879–2890.

25. Corradi-Del'Acqua, C., B. Tomasino & G.R. Fink. 2009. What is the position of an arm relative to the body? Neural correlates of body schema and body structural description. *J. Neurosci.* **29:** 4162–4171.

26. Li, C.-S.R., P. Mazzoni & R.A. Andersen. 1999. Effect of reversible inactivation of macaque lateral intraparietal area on visual and memory saccades. *J. Neurophysiol.* **81:** 1827–1838.

27. Buneo, C.A. & R.A. Andersen. 2006. The posterior parietal cortex: sensorimotor interface for the planning and online control of visually guided movements. *Neuropsychologia* **44:** 2594–2606.

28. Duhamel, J.-R., C.L. Colby & M.E. Goldberg. 1992. The updating of the representation of visual space in parietal cortex by intended eye movements. *Science* **255:** 90–92.

29. Colby, C.L. 1998. Action-orientated spatial reference frames in cortex. *Neuron* **20:** 15–24.

30. Gnadt, J.W. & R.A. Andersen. 1988. Memory related motor planning activity in posterior parietal cortex of macaque. *Exp. Brain Res.* **70:** 216–220.

31. Xing, J. & R.A. Andersen. 2000. Memory activity of LIP neurons for sequential eye movements simulated with neural networks. *J. Neurophysiol.* **84:** 651–665.

32. Baldauf, D., H. CUI & R.A. Andersen. 2008. The posterior parietal cortex encodes in parallel both goals for double-reach sequences. *J. Neurosci.* **28:** 10081–10089.

33. Graziano, M.S.A., D.F. Cooke & C.S.R. Taylor. 2000. Coding the location of the arm by sight. *Science* **290:** 1782–1786.

34. Fabre, M. & P. Buser. 1981. Effects of lesioning the anterior suprasylvian cortex on visuo-motor guidance performance in the cat. *Exp. Brain Res.* **41:** 81–88.

35. Lajoie, K., J. Andujar, K.G. Pearson, *et al.* 2007. Persistent neuronal activity in posterior parietal cortex area 5 related to long-lasting memories of obstacles in walking cats. *Neurosci. Abst.* **37:** 397–398.

36. Kalaska, J.F. 1996. Parietal cotex area 5 and visuomotor behavior. *Can. J. Physiol. Pharmacol.* **74:** 483–498.

37. Mountcastle, V.B., J.C. Lynch, A.P. Georgopoulos, *et al.* 1975. Posterior parietal association cortex of the monkey: command functions for operations with extrapersonal space. *J. Neurophysiol.* **38:** 871–908.

38. Gallivan, J.P., C. Cavina-Pratesi & J.C. Culham. 2009. Is that within reach? fMRI reveals that the human superior parieto-occipital cortex encodes objects reachable by the hand. *J. Neurosci.* **29:** 4381–4391.

39. Iriki, A., M. Tanaka & Y. Iwamura. 1996. Coding of modified body schema during tool use by macaque postcentral neurones. *Neuroreport* **7:** 2325–2330.

40. Graziano, M.S.A., X.T. Hu & C.G. Gross. 1997. Visuospatial properties of ventral premotor cortex. *J. Neurophysiol.* **77:** 2268–2292.

41. Graziano, M.S.A. & D.F. Cooke. 2006. Parieto-frontal interactions, personal space, and defensive behavior. *Neuropsychologia* **44:** 845–859.

Ann. N.Y. Acad. Sci. ISSN 0077-8923

ANNALS OF THE NEW YORK ACADEMY OF SCIENCES
Issue: *Neurons and Networks in the Spinal Cord*

Afferent inputs to mid- and lower-lumbar spinal segments are necessary for stepping in spinal cats

Jonathan A. Norton[1,3] and Vivian K. Mushahwar[2,3]

[1]Departments of Surgery, Faculty of Medicine and Dentistry, University of Alberta, Edmonton, Alberta, Canada. [2]Cell Biology Faculty of Medicine and Dentistry, University of Alberta, Edmonton, Alberta, Canada. [3]Centre for Neuroscience, Faculty of Medicine and Dentistry, University of Alberta, Edmonton, Alberta, Canada

Address for correspondence: Dr. Vivian Mushahwar, Department of Cell Biology and Centre for Neuroscience, 5005 Katz Building, University of Alberta, Edmonton, Alberta T6G 2E1, Canada. vivian.mushahwar@ualberta.ca

Afferent inputs are known to modulate the activity of locomotor central pattern generators, but their role in the *generation* of locomotor patterns remains uncertain. This study sought to investigate the importance of afferent input for producing bilateral, coordinated hindlimb stepping in adult cats. Following complete spinal transection, animals were trained to step on the moving belt of a treadmill until proficient, weight-bearing stepping of the hindlimbs was established. Selective dorsal rhizotomies of roots reaching various segments of the lumbosacral enlargement were then conducted, and hindlimb stepping capacity was reassessed. Depending on the deafferented lumbosacral segments, stepping was either abolished or unaffected. Deafferentation of mid-lumbar (L3/L4) or lower-lumbar (L5-S1) segments abolished locomotion. Locomotor capacity in these animals could not be restored with the administration of serotonergic or adrenergic agonists. Deafferentation of L3, L6, or S1 had mild effects on locomotion. This suggested that critical afferent inputs pertaining to hip position (mid-lumbar) and limb loading (lower-lumbar) play an important role in the *generation* of locomotor patterns after spinal cord injury.

Keywords: central pattern generation; hip position; limb loading; afferent input; locomotion

Introduction

The interplay between the locomotor central pattern generator (CPG) and afferent inputs in the formation of locomotor patterns remains a topic of debate. The ability to train an adult spinal cat to step on a moving treadmill belt has been known for many years,[1,2] yet the underlying mechanisms are uncertain. The works of Sherrington[3] and Brown[4] provide two opposing views in explaining these observations: that the activity seen is reflex-driven or is the result of intrinsic properties of the spinal cord, respectively. The latter view has dominated our thinking in recent years and the intrinsic factors are now known as the CPG.[5,6]

Evidence in favor of a CPG comes from studies in which the spinal cord is isolated from descending and/or peripheral connections, either anatomically or pharmacologically.[7] In these preparations, no motor activity is observed in the absence of stimulation. The application of excitatory neurotransmitters such as L-DOPA or serotonin leads to a pattern of reciprocal activity in flexor and extensor nerves.[8,9] This activity is also reciprocal across the spinal cord so that ipsilateral flexors and contralateral extensors are activated simultaneously.[10] The similarity of this pattern to that observed in walking has led to the view that these patterns are the output of the locomotor CPG.[11,12]

Treadmill stepping patterns in the awake, spinalized animal, nevertheless, are very different from the patterns seen in fictive preparations. Stepping on a moving treadmill belt provides sensory inputs to the spinal cord, which play a major role in phase transitions.[13] For example, transitions from stance (extensor phase) to swing (flexor phase) occur only when sensory information pertaining to hip position and limb loading is permissive. Stretch of the flexor muscles resets the locomotor pattern in decerebrate cats,[14] and hindrance of hip extension delays

doi: 10.1111/j.1749-6632.2010.05540.x
Ann. N.Y. Acad. Sci. 1198 (2010) 10–20 © 2010 New York Academy of Sciences.

or prevents the initiation of swing while prolonging stance.[14] Hip position is also important for the swing to stance transition.[15]

The locomotor activity patterns in the presence of sensory inputs are also more robust, involving shorter flexor than extensor bursts and a period of double stance.[16] Importantly, they also contain a distinct burst of activity in the semitendinosus muscle of the hindlimbs that appears before the onset of stance and is not seen in fictive preparations.[17] It therefore appears that sensory inputs not only modulate the timing and intensity of CPG generated motor patterns and adapt them to the environment,[18–20] but also contribute to the generation of locomotor bursts.[17–21]

Further insights regarding the interplay between the CPG and afferent inputs in locomotion are gained from neuromechanical models. Yakovenko et al.[22] showed that in instances with low central drive (i.e., a weak CPG) the contribution of the stretch reflex is crucial in maintaining stable gait patterns. Ekeberg and Pearson[23] further demonstrated that gait can be established through sensory inputs and independently of a CPG. They also examined the relative importance of hip position and limb loading for locomotion, and were able to generate a stable gait using either a combination of hip angle (relayed through inputs to mid-lumbar segments) and ankle force (relayed through inputs to lower-lumbar segments), or ankle force alone.[23]

The goal of the present study was to assess directly the role of afferent inputs in locomotor pattern generation. We specifically asked the question: could a chronically spinalized cat, previously trained to step on a moving treadmill belt, cope with sensory disturbances? Stepping capacity was evaluated after removal of sensory inputs reaching various spinal segments. We found that sensory information *is a necessary component for locomotor pattern generation*. Afferent inputs pertaining to hip position and limb loading are both critically needed for stepping in the chronically spinalized cat. The findings further demonstrate that the mid-lumbar segments in cats (equivalent to L1/L2 upper-lumbar segments in rodents) are incapable of producing a potent locomotor pattern in the absence of afferent inputs.

Some of this work was previously presented in abstract form.[24]

General methods

Experiments were performed on nine adult cats (1 male) weighing 2.8–4.5 kg. All experiments were approved by the University of Alberta Animal Welfare Committee.

Spinalization

A laminectomy was performed at the T11 vertebral level under isoflourane anaesthesia and aseptic surgical conditions. The dura mater was opened and the spinal cord exposed. A complete transection of the spinal cord was made under microscope vision using micro-dissection scissors, and the completeness of the lesion verified visually. The lesion space was filled with absorbable haemostat (Surgicel) and the dura mater, muscle, and skin sutured shut in layers. Analgesia (Ketoprofen) and antibiotics (Cefazolin) were administered. Following recovery from surgery, animals were transferred to individual cages and attended twice daily for bladder expression. Antibiotics and analgesics were continued as required.

Treadmill training

Treadmill training was initiated on the third postoperative day. The animals were placed in a harness suspended over a custom-made, split-belt treadmill with independent force plates under each belt. The forelimbs were supported on a stationary platform and the hindlimbs were placed over the moving belts. A plexiglass divider prevented excessive limb adduction. Training intensity increased to three 10 min sessions a day over the first week. The treadmill belts were set at a speed of 0.25 ms^{-1}. Training involved manual placement of the hindlimbs and perineal stimulation until weight bearing and toe clearance were achieved. Initially, training was also supplemented with quipazine (0.5 mg/kg i.p.), a non-specific serotonergic precursor. Subsequently, only perineal stimulation and later the moving treadmill belts alone were needed to stimulate a stepping behavior.

Deafferentation

Once stable, proficient stepping was achieved (typically after 3 months of training) a baseline record of the stepping was obtained (see Testing section). In a subsequent surgical procedure the dura mater was opened to expose the dorsal rootlets innervating various lumbosacral spinal segments. Dorsal rootlets to: (1) S1, (2) L6 and the rostral third of L7 (hereafter referred to as L6), (3) L4, (4) L3, L4 and the rostral third of L5 (hereafter referred to as L3/4), or (5) L5-S1 were identified, tied with suture, and cut bilaterally. The size of the rhizotomy in the L3/4 and the L6 deafferentations was approximately the same. The dura mater, muscle layers, and skin were then sutured and the animal recovered as previously described.

Two days after surgery training recommenced on the treadmill at the same speed and intensity as before. Perineal stimulation was applied as needed to facilitate stepping.

Testing

A total of three testing sessions were performed for each cat. Two, full-length tests were performed prior to the deafferentation and two weeks after the deafferentation, and one shorter test was conducted one week postdeafferentation. The ability of the cat to stand and to step spontaneously at a variety of treadmill speeds ranging from 0.1 to 0.6 m/s and the cat's pawshake and flexor withdrawal reflexes were assessed. Kinematic, kinetic, and electromyographical (EMG) recordings were acquired to quantify the hindlimb responses of the cat. To quantify the kinematics, reflective markers were bilaterally placed on the iliac crest, hip, knee, ankle, and metatarsophalengeal joints and the tip of the third toe. The limbs were then filmed using two high-speed, digital camcorders placed orthogonally to the sagittal plane of each limb. To record EMG activity, pairs of fine wires (9-strand stainless steel Cooner wire AS 362, insulated except for 2–3 mm at the tip; Cooner Wire, Chatsworth, California) were transcutaneously inserted into the major hip, knee, and ankle flexor and extensor muscles under isoflourane anaesthesia prior to the testing session. After the acquisition of a complete set of data, quipazine (0.5 mg/kg i.p.) was administered and the tests repeated 20 min later. Clonidine (an α_2 noradrenergic agonist) was then administered (75 μg/kg i.p.) and the tests repeated when the paw shake reflex had disappeared, typically 15–20 min following administration of the drug. The time from the administration of the quipazine to the completion of the clonidine and quipazine testing was less than 1 h.

One week after the deafferentation a shorter test was conducted in which kinematic, kinetic, and EMG data were recorded but no pharmacological agents were administered.

Data acquisition and analysis

The EMG recordings were band-pass filtered (30–1000 Hz) and amplified 1000× using custom-built amplifiers and a Neurolog system (Digitimer, Welyen Garden City, UK). Data were sampled (4000 samples/sec) using a CED 1401Power analog-to-digital card and Signal2 or Spike2 software (Cambridge Electronic Design, Cambridge, UK). Video clips of the hindlimbs (120 frames/sec) were transferred to a computer and limb movements were extracted using MotionTracker2D (Dr. Douglas Webber, University of Pittsburgh). Data analyses were performed in the MATLAB environment (Mathworks, Natick, Massachusetts) using custom-written routines.

Ground reaction forces (GRFs) generated during stepping in each testing session were normalized to the amount of force generated by each leg during periods of full weight-bearing standing obtained in the predeafferentation testing session for each animal. A 95% confidence level was deemed to be significant.

Results

Following 2–4 months of intensive treadmill training all spinal cats were able to step independently on the moving treadmill belt with only lateral, balance support provided, and without the need for pharmacological or perineal stimulation. Animals were able to step at a wide variety of speeds and under "taxing" circumstances in which the split belts were set to different speeds. Once the animals stepped proficiently, no instances of double flexion were encountered, that is, at least one hindlimb provided weight-support at any one time during stepping.

The location of the deafferentation dramatically affected spinal stepping. Reconstructed stick figures representing the spontaneous stepping of the hindlimbs on a moving treadmill belt at 0.25 m/s from a spinalized, but sensory intact animal and one example animal from each of the rhizotomized groups are shown in Figure 1. Also shown are the generated GRFs averaged over all the steps (mean ± standard deviation, 50 ± 15 steps) taken by the animal in each condition. Rhizotomies of single spinal segments (L4, L6, or S1) had little effect on the stepping pattern. In stark contrast, the

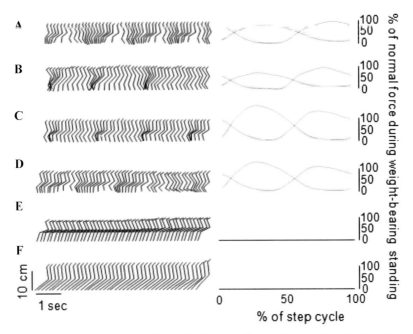

Figure 1. Stick figure representation of the effect of various deafferentations on hindlimb walking movements in the completely spinalized cat. (**A**) No deafferentation, (**B**) S1 rhizotomy, (**C**) L6 rhizotomy, (**D**) L4 rhizotomy, (**E**) L3/4 rhizotomy, and (**F**) L5-S1 rhizotomy. To the right of the stick figures are the GRFs averaged over a step cycle and normalized to the full load taken by the hindlimb during full weight-bearing standing. The upper four plots are qualitatively similar indicating a lack of major effect of the deafferentation on the evoked stepping pattern. The L3/4 and L5-S1 rhizotomies abolished spontaneous stepping activity of the hindlimbs as evidenced by the lack of modulation of joint angles in the stick figures and the flat GRF traces.

L3/4 and L5-S1 deafferentations removed the ability of the animal to step spontaneously on the moving treadmill belt.

The effects of the L3/4 and L5-S1 deafferentations, which led to the loss of sensory information pertaining to hip position and limb loading, respectively, are further exemplified in Figures 2 and 3. Stick figure representations from one cat in each group and joint angles averaged over a step cycle (35 ± 12 steps) are presented for three stepping conditions. With no stimulation other than the moving treadmill belt, neither the L3/4 nor L5-S1 deafferented cat could spontaneously step (Figs. 2A and 3A, respectively). Addition of the serotonergic and noradrenergic agonists quipazine and clonidine, failed to elicit a functional stepping pattern on the moving treadmill belt (Figs. 2B and 3B). In both deafferentations the addition of the pharmacological agents led to some increase in the phasic modulation of load force (Figs. 2D-2F and 3D-3F). Perineal stimulation in both cases restored some semblance

of rhythmic oscillations in the legs (Figs. 2C and 3C); however, neither pharmacological nor perineal stimulation was capable of eliciting a stepping behavior similar to that obtained with intact sensory inputs (Fig. 1A), and significant abnormalities were noted. Moreover, the effects of the L3/4 and L5-S1 deafferentations were not the same.

The range of angles that the hip traversed during a step following the deafferentation compared to pre-deafferentation ranges provided an indicator of the deficit generated by the loss of the sensory information. The S1, L6, and L4 deafferentations produced a small, non-significant decrease in the range of hip motion (a decrease of ~5%). The L5-S1 deafferentation also produced only a small decrease in the range of hip angle that was not statistically significant during perineal stimulation. In contrast, the L3/4 deafferentation significantly reduced the range of hip angle by 45% ($P < 0.05$, paired t-test).

The differences in hindlimb stepping in cats with L3/4 and L5-S1 deafferentations are further

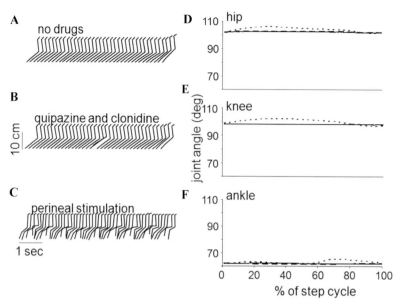

Figure 2. Stick figure representations and joint angle plots of the stepping evoked with various forms of stimulation in a cat with an *L3/4 deafferentation*. A shows the stepping on a moving treadmill belt with no pharmacological or perineal stimulation, and (**B**) with the addition of quipazine followed by clonidine. No appreciable stepping is demonstrated in each of these plots. In C, perineal stimulation is applied to an animal with no pharmacological agents. In this case, rhythmic oscillations in the hindlimbs are evoked. Joint angle modulations are shown on the right for the hip (**D**), knee (**E**), and ankle (**F**). The solid line corresponds to no stimulation, the dashed to the quipazine followed by clonidine, and the dotted to the perineal stimulation. Note that in all cases, the hips only traversed a comparatively small range of angles and the hindlimb is not placed forward of the hip.

highlighted in Figure 4 in which the best stepping trials obtained in these animals are shown. Stick figure representations along with EMG activity are shown in which stepping was evoked by a combination of the moving treadmill belt, perineal stimulation, quipazine and clonidine. The L3/4 cat was unable to bring the leg forward of the hip, the stepping movements were rapid and limb placement was on the dorsum of the paw. In contrast, the L5-S1 cat performed each phase of the step cycle and placed the foot on the plantar surface of the paw, but exhibited deficits in the transitions between the phases of the step cycle.

A summary of the average peak GRFs (loading) produced by the hindlimbs during stepping following each deafferentation is shown in Figure 5A. Data are normalized to each cat's GRF produced during weight-bearing standing prior to the deafferentation. On average, the L3/4 and L5-S1 deafferentations significantly reduced the GRF to ∼10% of baseline values (Fig. 5A black bars; $P < 0.05$,

ANOVA, Tukey HSD *post hoc* comparisons). All other deafferentations produced changes of less than 10%.

Clonidine significantly decreased GRF in animals with intact sensory inputs as well as in those with L6 and L4 rhizotomies (Fig. 5A hashed bars; $P < 0.05$, ANOVA, Tukey HSD *post hoc* comparisons). While clonidine had no effect on GRF in animals with L3/4 or L5-S1 deafferentations, quipazine significantly increased GRF in animals with L3/4 deafferentation relative to pre-drug levels (Fig. 5A gray bars). The effects of clonidine, the α2-noradrenergic agonist, are not surprising in light of its inhibitory actions. Clonidine is used as an antispasmodic agent in individuals with spinal cord injury,[25] and the hallmark indicator of its action in spinal cats is the loss of the paw shake reflex. The effectiveness of clonidine in facilitating locomotor-like patterns in spinal cats has been attributed to the localization of its receptors to the mid-lumbar segments of the cord, segments previously thought to contain the locomotor CPG

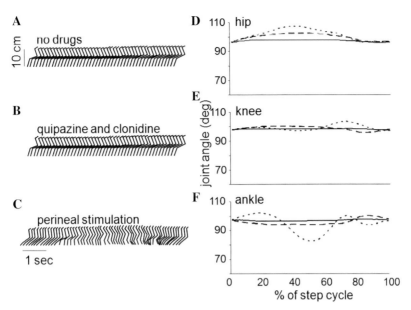

Figure 3. Stick figure representations and joint angle plots of the stepping evoked with various forms of stimulation in a cat with an *L5-S1 deafferentation.* **A** shows the stepping on a moving treadmill belt with no pharmacological or perineal stimulation, and (**B**) with the addition of quipazine followed by clonidine. No appreciable stepping is demonstrated in each of these plots. In **C**, perineal stimulation is applied to an animal with no pharmacological agents. In this case, disorganized elements of a locomotor pattern are evoked. Joint angle modulations are shown on the right for the hip (**D**), knee (**E**), and ankle (**F**). The solid line corresponds to no stimulation, the dashed to the quipazine followed by clonidine, and the dotted to the perineal stimulation.

networks.[26] In this study, clonidine was ineffective in producing locomotor-like stepping patterns in the absence of sensory inputs to the L3/4 or L5-S1 segments, and significantly reduced the level of GRF produced during stepping. In contrast to clonidine, receptors for the serotonergic agonist, quipazine, are widely distributed throughout the spinal cord.[45] Because quipazine enhances the excitability of spinal motoneurons,[27,28] its effects on increasing GRF were anticipated. Interestingly, however, quipazine had no effect on GRF after the L5-S1 deafferentation, suggesting that its effects may be primarily presynaptic.[29]

Representative GRF traces averaged over a step cycle from a spinal, sensory-intact animal, and an animal in each of the L3/4, L5-S1, and S1 deafferentation groups are shown in Figure 5B. Whereas the sensory-intact and S1 deafferented cats showed a normal pattern of modulation of step force during all stimulation conditions (less with clonidine), there was little or no modulation in the GRF generated in the cats with the L3/4 or L5-S1 deafferentations.

Discussion

The ability of the spinal cat to step on a moving treadmill belt under a variety of conditions is remarkable. Devoid of descending supraspinal control, and with only sensory inputs, the cord is able to generate a motor pattern that adapts to changing and novel environmental demands. Moreover, proficient spinal stepping continues to be "safe," in that at least one leg is always in contact with the ground, bearing the weight of the hindquarters. The present study demonstrated that the spinal cord is also able to adapt to changes in sensory inputs. Removal of the sensory inputs to an entire spinal segment had only minor consequences on the motor output. This would suggest that after learning to walk, the disconnected spinal cord retains plastic capacity even after some sensory disruption. Carrier and colleagues examined the effect of neuroectomy on the locomotion of spinal cats.[30] They demonstrated that spinal animals that underwent a neuroectomy after learning to walk were able to maintain a symmetrical locomotor pattern, despite

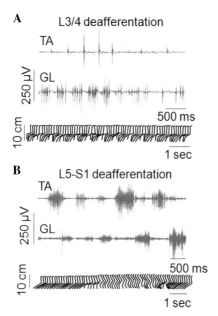

A L3/4 deafferentation

TA

250 µV

GL

500 ms

10 cm

1 sec

B L5-S1 deafferentation

TA

250 µV

GL

500 ms

10 cm

1 sec

Figure 4. Evoked stepping during a *prolonged period of perineal stimulation* in an L3/4 and an L5-S1 deafferentated cat that had received quipazine and clonidine. Differences in the locomotor deficits associated with each of the deafferentations are illustrated. (**A**) Alternating, rhythmic-like stepping movements of the hindlimbs could be elicited following the L3/4 deafferentation, but with deficits in limb placement in space: the paw was not placed in front of the hip and the cat stepped on the dorsum of the paw. (**B**) Normal range of limb placement could be achieved with proper stepping on the plantar surface of the paw following the L5-S1 deafferentation; however, the hindlimbs were unable to switch regularly between the swing and stance phases and pauses occurred at these transition points.

a unilateral absence of dorsiflexion, again suggesting that the spinal cord is able to make further plastic changes after learning how to generate spinal locomotion.

Both hip angle and load information are necessary for spinal stepping

Throughout this study successful stepping consisted of both weight-bearing of the hindquarters through the hindlimbs and forward movement of the limbs with paw placement occurring in front of the hip. The most striking finding is the effect of both the L3/4 and the L5-S1 deafferentations in abolishing

the treadmill-evoked stepping behavior in the spinal cats. Removal of the sensory inputs to the L3/4 spinal segments removes the information concerning the hip position whilst the L5-S1 deafferentation leaves those inputs intact but removes all of the load information. The "rules" of locomotion as outlined by Prochazka[13] and with experimental evidence from Pearson and coworkers[14,15,31] indicate that the phase transitions within the stepping pattern rely upon hip position or load information. In this study we demonstrated that both of these components are required for the generation of spinal stepping. This is somewhat in contrast to the recent modeling result from Ekeburg and Pearson[23] who showed that only loading information was required to generate adequate stepping in their coupled hindlimb model of a cat. An earlier model by Yakovenko et al.[22] highlighted the role of sensory feedback (stretch reflexes) in the presence of weak central drive. However, this is the first study that experimentally examined the role of bilateral sensory feedback to spinal locomotion. The results herein will further refine studies focused on modeling the neural control of locomotion.

Differences between mid-lumbar and lower-lumbar deafferentations

The L3/4 and the L5-S1 deafferentations abolished the spinal cats' ability to step spontaneously on a moving treadmill belt. In both conditions additional stimulation (primarily perineal) generated some oscillations in the hindlimbs but the patterns were missing critical elements that define locomotion. Moreover, the evoked oscillations were characteristically different in the two deafferentations. The animals without information concerning the position of their hip (L3/4 rhizotomy) were unable to bring their paws forward of their hips, even when the spinal circuits were activated through several forms of stimulation. This suggests that the hip sensory information is critical for enabling proper activation of the flexor muscles and in turn, forward placement of the leg in space. In contrast, the removal of all load information (L5-S1) did not alter the placement of the limb during each individual phase of the gait cycle. Rather, the primary deficit was in the switching between the phases. The animal was unable to switch easily and fluidly from the stance to swing phase with either leg. Presumably, this is a result of the lack of loading information

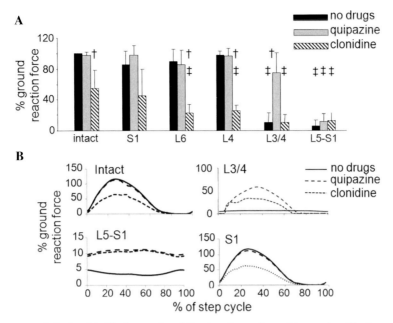

Figure 5. GRF generated during hindlimb stepping following the various rhizotomies. The forces are normalized to the load carried by the limb during full weight-bearing standing prior to the deafferentation. (A) Mean GRF and standard deviation bars are shown for all animals in the study. No decreases in force were seen with the S1, L6, and L4 deafferentations relative to predeafferentation levels (*black bars*), while large decreases were seen following the L3/4 and L5-S1 deafferentations. Quipazine generally increased the peak GRF, especially following the L3/4 deafferentation (*gray bars*), while clonidine generally decreased it (*hashed bars*). Cross symbols (†) indicate the significant changes in GRF induced by the application of pharmacological agents within a condition (sensory intact or a particular deafferentation). Double cross symbols (‡) indicate the significant changes in GRF relative to predeafferentation levels. (B) GRF averaged over a step cycle for a spinal animal with intact dorsal roots, an animal with L3/4, L5-S1, or S1 rhizotomy. In each plot the no-drugs (*solid*), quipazine (*dashed*), and clonidine (*dotted*) traces are shown. Note that the *y*-axis range is different for the different rhizotomy conditions.

leading to uncertainty about whether it is "safe" to take one leg off the ground. Furthermore, the amount of loading produced by the legs was severely reduced.

Deficits in stepping induced by deafferentation of a single spinal segment were comparatively minor, even when the same size deafferentations as the L3/4 rhizotomies was performed in another part of the spinal cord (e.g., the L6 deafferentation). This leads us to believe that the effects we see from the L3/4 and L5-S1 rhizotomies are not due to the size of the sensory disruption, but to the nature of the sensory inputs removed. In the L4, L6, and S1 deafferentations, adequate information pertaining to hip position and limb loading was preserved, allowing for proper generation of the locomotor pattern.

Comparison with fictive and *in vitro* preparations

Previous studies in fictive preparations demonstrated that in the absence of any sensory feedback, the spinal cord is capable of generating a rhythmic, locomotor-like pattern. In the present study we showed that removal of sensory information concerning just one of the primary inputs for spinal locomotion disrupts and inhibits the stepping ability of the chronically spinalized cat. It is likely that the rhythmic oscillations induced via a combination of stimuli (treadmill belt, pharmacological agents, and perineal stimulation) were produced by the CPG networks in the spinal cord. Such oscillations may represent the patterns seen during fictive locomotion that is commonly induced by pharmacological agents or electrical stimulation of the mesencephalic locomotor center or the dorsal columns. However, this study demonstrates that such oscillations are inadequate for locomotion in spinal animals.

Interestingly, the application of perineal stimulation was much more efficacious in eliciting alternating oscillations of the hindlimbs following the L3/4 and L5-S1 rhizotomies than the serotonergic and noradrenergic agonists.[32] This suggests a more prominent role for lower segments of the lumbar enlargement in the production of locomotion than previously suggested.[33,34]

Previous *in vitro* studies in neonatal preparations of rodent spinal cords suggested that the CPG networks involved in locomotion reside within the lumbar segments of the spinal cord.[35,36] Similarly, studies in adult cat preparations[33,37–39] highlighted the importance of the lumbar segments for the generation of stepping-like locomotor patterns. However, findings from both the rodent and cat preparations have diverged in their interpretation of the organization and distribution of these CPG networks. While some studies suggest that the locomotor CPG is localized to the upper- and mid-lumbar segments in rodents,[35] and cats[38] respectively, others demonstrated that the CPG networks are more distributed throughout the lumbar cord.[33,36,37,39] Furthermore, some researchers within the latter camp proposed that the locomotor rhythmogenic capacity of the lumbar segments decreases caudally (i.e., within the lower-lumbar segments).[36,39]

The findings from this study do not address the distribution or organization of the CPG locomotor networks. Nonetheless, they strongly highlight the importance of sensory inputs to pattern generation. Most importantly, the findings demonstrate that the L3/4 segments in the spinal cats are incapable of generating stepping locomotor patterns in the absence of sensory information pertaining to hip position. Similarly, these same segments are incapable of generating appropriate stepping patterns in the absence of loading information relayed to lower-lumbar segments. Furthermore, lower-lumbar segments with intact sensory inputs are incapable of generating full locomotor patterns in the absence of sensory information pertaining to hip position relayed to the mid-lumbar segments. Therefore, the concepts of localized or distributed CPG with a rhythmogenic gradient in the lumbar cord do not appear to be prominent in the absence of sensory inputs to either the L3/L4 or L5-S1 segments. After chronic spinalization, sensory inputs pertaining to hip position and limb loading appear to play a primary role in the rhythmogenesis of locomotor stepping.

Functional implications

This study demonstrated the importance of the previously hypothesized rules for locomotion (Prochazka[13]), which depend on hip position and limb loading. Indeed these rules not only appear to safeguard against unsafe stepping, but are a prerequisite for the initiation and maintenance of stepping in the adult spinalized cat. The results present sensory inputs as critical components for locomotor pattern *generation* in the spinalized cat.

On the basis of the present findings, which demonstrated the critical dependence of the CPG on sensory inputs, one may refute the argument that the locomotor CPG is a necessary element for stepping. However, previous work from our laboratory and the laboratory of others strongly suggests that both the CPG and sensory inputs are necessary for stepping, and each alone is incapable of producing robust locomotion.[40,41]

Therefore, when developing rehabilitation programs or control paradigms for devices to restore stepping after spinal cord injury in humans, it may be advantageous to utilize spinal CPG and sensory-driven rules of locomotion as guidelines.[40,42–44]

Conclusions

In this study we demonstrated the critical importance of both hip position and limb loading for the generation of locomotor patterns that enable spinal stepping. Removal of either leads to an inability to step spontaneously on a moving treadmill belt. With additional stimulation animals with either sensory loss can produce rhythmic oscillations; however, these oscillations are incomplete locomotor patterns. Both the CPG and afferent inputs are *necessary for locomotor pattern generation.*

Acknowledgments

We wish to express our sincere appreciation to Enid Pehowich, Lisa Stirling, Roger Calixto, and Bernice Lau for their assistance with this study, and the Health Sciences Laboratory Animal Services at the University of Alberta for their excellent care of the animals. This study was funded by the Alberta

Heritage Foundation for Medical Research (AHFMR), the Canadian Institutes for Health Research (CIHR), and the National Institute of Health (NIH).

Conflicts of interest

The authors declare no conflicts of interest.

References

1. Barbeau, H. & S. Rossignol. 1987. Recovery of locomotion after chronic spinalization in the adult cat. *Brain Res.* **412:** 84–95.

2. Shurrager, P.S. & R.A. Dykman. 1951. Walking spinal carnivores. *J. Comp. Physiol. Psychol.* **44:** 252–262.

3. Sherrington, C.S. 1898. On the spinal animal and the nature of spinal reflex activity. *Phil. Trans. R. Soc. Lond. (B)* **190:** 45–186.

4. Brown, T.G. 1911. The intrinsic factors in the act of progression in the mammal. *Proc. R. Soc. Lond.* **84:** 308–319.

5. Grillner, S. & P. Zangger. 1979. On the central generation of locomotion in the low spinal cat. *Exp. Brain Res.* **34:** 241–261.

6. Kiehn, O. & P.S. Katz. 1999. Making circuits dance: neuromodulation of motor systems. In *Beyond Neurotransmission, Neuromodulation.* Oxford University Press. Oxford.

7. Duysens, J. & H.W.A.A. van de Crommert. 1998. Neural control of locomotion. Part 1. The central pattern generator from cats to humans. *Gait Posture* **7:** 131–141.

8. Jankowska, E., M.G.M. Jukes, S. Lund & A. Lundberg. 1967. The effect of DOPA on the spinal cord. 6. Half-centre organization of interneurones transmitting effects from the flexor reflex afferents. *Acta Physiol. Scand.* **70:** 389–402.

9. Jankowska, E., M.G.M. Jukes, S. Lund & A. Lundberg. 1967. The effect of DOPA on the spinal cord. 5. Reciprocal organization of pathways transmitting excitatory action to alpha motoneurones of flexors and extensors. *Acta Physiol. Scand.* **70:** 369–388.

10. Kiehn, O. 2006. Locomotor circuits in the mammalian spinal cord. *Annu. Rev. Neurosci.* **29:** 279–306.

11. Kremer, E. & A. Lev-Tov. 1997. Localization of the spinal network associated with generation of hindlimb locomotion in the neonatal rat and organization of its transverse coupling system. *J. Neurophysiol.* **77:** 1155–1170.

12. Burke, R.E., M. Degtyarenko & E.S. Simon. 2001. Patterns of locomotor drive to motoneurons and last-order

13. Prochazka, A. 1996. Proprioceptive feedback and movement regulation. In *Neural Control of Movement.* 89–127. Plenum Press. New York.

14. Hiebert, G.W., P.J. Whelan, A. Prochazka & K.G. Pearson. 1996. Contribution of hind limb flexor muscle afferents to the timing of phase transitions in the cat step cycle. *J. Neurophysiol.* **75:** 1126–1137.

15. McVea, D.A., J.M. Donelan, A. Tachibana & K.G. Pearson. 2005. A role for hip position in initiating the swing-to-stance transition in walking cats. *J. Neurophysiol.* **94:** 3497–3508.

16. S. Yakovenko, D.A. McCrea, K. Stecina & A. Prochazka. 2005. Control of locomotor cycle durations. *J. Neurophysiol.* **94:** 1057–1065.

17. Smith, J.L., S,H. Chung & R.F. Zernicke. 1993. Gait-related motor patterns and hindlimb kinetics for the cat trot and gallop. *Exp. Brain Res.* **94:** 308–322.

18. van de Crommert, H.W.A.A., T. Mulder & J. Duysens. 1998. Neural control of locomtion. Part 2. Sensory control of the central pattern generator and its relation to treadmill training. *Gait Posture* **7:** 251–263.

19. Buschges, A. & A. El Manira. 1998. Sensory pathways and their modulation in the control of locomotion. *Curr. Opin. Neurobiol.* **8:** 733–739.

20. Pearson, K.G. 2004. Generating the walking gait: role of sensory feedback. *Progr. Brain Res.* **143:** 123–129.

21. Samuel, A.D.T. & P. Sengupta. 2005. Sensorimotor integration: locating locomotion in neural circuits. *Curr. Biol.* **15:** 341–343.

22. Yakovenko, S., V. Gritsenko & A. Prochazka. 2004. Contribution of stretch reflexes to locomotor control: a modelling study. *Biol. Cybern.* **90:** 146–155.

23. Ekeberg, O. & K.G. Pearson. 2005. Computer simulation of stepping in the hind legs of the cat: an examination of mechanisms regulating the stance-to-swing transition. *J. Neurophysiol.* **94:** 4256–4268.

24. Norton, J.A., L. Guevremont & V.K. Mushahwar. 2005. Significance of segmental sensory input for stepping in the adult chronically spinalised cat. *Soc. Neurosci. Abstract 630.5.* **93:** 3442–3452.

25. Barbeau, H. & K.E. Norman. 2003. The effect of noradrenergic drugs on the recovery of walking after spinal cord injury. *Spinal Cord* **41:** 137–143.

26. Chau, C.W., N. Giroux, J. Senecal, *et al.* 2001. Topology and coupling of alpha-2-adrenergic receptors in cat lumbo-sacral spinal cord following complete lesions. In *Spinal Cord Trauma; Neural Repair and Functional Recovery.* Faculty of Medicine, Universite de Montreal.

interneurons: clues to the structure of the CPG. *J. Neurophysiol.* **86:** 447–462.

27. Jackson, D.A. & S.R. White. 1990. Receptor subtypes mediating facilitation by serotonin of excitability of spinal motoneurons. *Neuropharmacology* **29:** 787–797.

28. Myslinki, N.R. & E.G. Anderson. 1983. The effect of serotonin precursors on Alpha- and Gamma-motoneuron activity. *J. Pharmacol. Exp. Ther.* **204:** 19–26.

29. Curtins, D.R., J.D. Leah & M.J. Peet. 1983. Effects of noradrenaline and 5-hydroxytryptamine on spinal Ia afferent terminations. *Brain Res.* **258:** 328–332.

30. Carrier, L., E. Brustein & S. Rossignol. 1997. Locomotion of the hindlimbs after neurectomy of ankle flexors in intact and spinal cats: model for the study of locomotor plasticity. *J. Neurophysiol.* **77:** 1979–1993.

31. Lam, T. & K.G. Pearson. 2001. Proprioceptive modulation of hip flexor activity during the swing phase of locomotion in decerebrate cats. *J. Neurophysiol.* **86:** 1321–1332.

32. Barbeau, H., C. Chau & S. Rossignol. 1993. Noradrenergic agonists and locomotor training affect locomotor recovery after cord transection in adult cats. *Brain Res. Bull.* **30:** 387–393.

33. Guevremont, L., C. Renzi, J.A. Norton, *et al.* 2006. Locomotor-related networks in the lumbosacral enlargement of the adult spinal cat: activation through intraspinal microstimulation. *IEEE Trans. Neural Syst. Rehabil. Eng.* **14:** 266–272.

34. Strauss, I. & A. Lev-Tov. 2003. Neural pathways between sacrocaudal afferents and lumbar pattern generators in neonatal rats. *J. Neurophysiol.* **89:** 773–784.

35. Cazalets, J-R., M. Borde & F. Clarac. 1995. Localization and organization of the central pattern generator for hindlimb locomotion in newborn rat. *J. Neurosci.* **15:** 4943–4951.

36. Kjaerulff, O. & O. Kiehn. 1996. Distribution of networks generating and coordinating locomotor activity in the neonatal rat spinal cord *in vitro*: a lesion study. *J. Neurosci.* **16:** 5777–5794.

37. Dai, X., B.R. Noga, J.R. Douglas & L.M. Jordan. 2005. Localisation of spinal neurons activated during locomotion using the C-fos immunohistochemical method. *J. Neurophysiol* **93:** 3442–3452.

38. Langlet, C., H. Leblond & S. Rossignol. 2005. The mid-lumbar segments are needed for the expression of locomotion in chronic spinal cats. *J. Neurophysiol.* **93:** 2474–2488.

39. Deliagina, T.G., G.N. Orlovsky & G.A. Pavlova. 1983. The capacity for generation of rhythmic oscillations is distributed in the lumbosacral spinal cord of the cat. *Exp. Brain Res.* **53:** 81–90.

40. Guevremont, L., J.A. Norton & V.K. Mushahwar. 2007. A physiologically-based controller for generating overground locomotion using functional electrical stimulation. *J. Neurophysiol.* **97:** 2499–2510.

41. Musienko, P.E., I.N. Bogacheva & Y.P Gerasimenko. 2007. Significance of peripheral feedback in the generation of stepping movements during epidural stimulation of the spinal cord. *Neurosci. Behav. Physiol.* **37:** 181–190.

42. Guevremont, L., J.A. Norton, B. Lau & V.K Mushahwar. 2005. An open- and closed-loop control system for generating over-ground locomotion using functional electrical stimulation. NIH Neural Prosthesis Workshop, Bethesda, Maryland.

43. Veltnik, P.H., W. de Vries, H. Hermens, *et al.* 1990. A comprehensive FES control system for mobility restoration in paraplegics. In *Neuroprosthetics; from Basic Research to Clinical Applications.* A. Pedotti, M. Ferrarin, J. Quintern & R. Riener, Eds. Springer, New York.

44. Courtine, G., Y.P. Gerasimenko, R. Van Den Brand, *et al.* 2009. Transformation of nonfunctional spinal circuits into functional states after the loss of brain input. *Nat. Neurosci.* **12:** 1333–1342.

45. Cowley, K.C. & B. J. Schmidt. 1995. Effects of inhibitory amino acid antagonists on reciprocal inhibitory interactions during rhythmic motor activity in the in vitro neonatal rat spinal cord. *J. Neurophysiol.* **74:** 1109–1117.

Ann. N.Y. Acad. Sci. ISSN 0077-8923

ANNALS OF THE NEW YORK ACADEMY OF SCIENCES

Issue: *Neurons and Networks in the Spinal Cord*

Afferent control of locomotor CPG: insights from a simple neuromechanical model

Sergey N. Markin,[1] Alexander N. Klishko,[2] Natalia A. Shevtsova,[1] Michel A. Lemay,[1] Boris I. Prilutsky,[2] and Ilya A. Rybak[1]

[1]Department of Neurobiology and Anatomy, Drexel University College of Medicine, Philadelphia, Pennsylvania. [2]Center for Human Movement Studies, School of Applied Physiology, Georgia Institute of Technology, Atlanta, Georgia

Address for correspondence: Dr. Ilya A. Rybak, Department of Neurobiology and Anatomy, Drexel University College of Medicine, 2900 Queen Lane, Philadelphia, PA 19129. rybak@drexel.edu

A simple neuromechanical model has been developed that describes a spinal central pattern generator (CPG) controlling the locomotor movement of a single-joint limb via activation of two antagonist (flexor and extensor) muscles. The limb performs rhythmic movements under control of the muscular, gravitational and ground reaction forces. Muscle afferents provide length-dependent (types Ia and II) and force-dependent (type Ib from the extensor) feedback to the CPG. We show that afferent feedback adjusts CPG operation to the kinematics and dynamics of the limb providing stable "locomotion." Increasing the supraspinal drive to the CPG increases locomotion speed by reducing the duration of stance phase. We show that such asymmetric, extensor-dominated control of locomotor speed (with relatively constant swing duration) is provided by afferent feedback independent of the asymmetric rhythmic pattern generated by the CPG alone (in "fictive locomotion" conditions). Finally, we demonstrate the possibility of reestablishing stable locomotion after removal of the supraspinal drive (associated with spinal cord injury) by increasing the weights of afferent inputs to the CPG, which is thought to occur following locomotor training.

Keywords: locomotion; central pattern generator; afferent control; spinal cord injury; recovery of locomotor function; modeling

Introduction

The mammalian spinal cord can generate locomotor activity in the absence of rhythmic inputs from higher brain centers and sensory feedback.[1] These observations led to the concept of the locomotor central pattern generator (CPG) that is located in the spinal cord and generates a primary locomotor rhythm and alternating pattern of motoneuron activations.[2–5] Substantial evidence for this concept came from studies of "fictive locomotion," in which sustained stimulation of the brain stem mesencephalic locomotor region in decerebrate, immobilized cats can evoke rhythmic locomotor activity with flexor-extensor and left-right alternations specific for locomotion.[3–9] Fictive locomotion studies have also demonstrated that electrical stimulation of flexor and extensor afferents can modulate the fictive locomotor pattern, change the timing of lo-

comotor phase transitions (and hence the durations of locomotor phases), control locomotor speed (i.e., overall step cycle duration), and produce various types of rhythm resetting.[10–13] Although the spinal CPG can generate locomotor rhythm in the absence of sensory feedback, during normal overground locomotion it operates under feedback control. The latter plays a critical role in stabilizing the locomotor movement, contributes to weight support during stance phase, and adjusts the locomotor pattern to the biomechanical characteristics of limbs and body and the characteristics of the environment (terrain, obstacles, etc.).[14,15]

An important feature of normal overground locomotion in mammals, including cats,[16,17] rats,[18,19] and humans,[20] is that the speed of locomotion normally changes due to a shortening of the stance (extensor) phase duration while the swing (flexor) phase duration remains relatively constant, which

doi: 10.1111/j.1749-6632.2010.05435.x

represents the so-called "extensor (or stance) phase dominance" in control of locomotion speed. In principle, the physiological basis for this extensor-dominated locomotion could derive from one (or combination) of the following[21]: (1) an extensor/flexor asymmetry in the organization of CPG *per se*,[22,23] (2) an asymmetry in the descending drive from the brainstem to the flexor and extensor half-centers,[24–26] or (3) afferent control of the CPG.[21,27–31] Despite extensive studies in different animals and experimental preparations, this issue remains unresolved and is continuously debated in the literature.[21,26,30]

Another important issue is the potential role of afferent feedback in the recovery of locomotor function after spinal cord injury (SCI). Complete SCI results in the loss of descending propriospinal inputs from above the level of transection as well as supraspinal (cortical and brainstem) inputs to the CPG, which is expected to interrupt the normal CPG operation and hence to stop generation of locomotor oscillations.[32–34] At the same time, many studies have provided evidence that locomotor function can be recovered by locomotor training alone or in combination with afferent stimulation or pharmacological treatment.[4,15,35–39] It is commonly accepted that the recovery of locomotor function after SCI by locomotor training occurs, at least in part, due to an increase in the strength of afferent inputs to the CPG which re-enforces its operation despite the loss of supraspinal drive.[4,15,35,36,38] However, the feasibility of such re-enforcement of the spinal CPG and locomotor pattern generation by afferent feedback after removal of supraspinal drive has never been theoretically investigated.

In this study, we have developed a simple neuro-mechanical model that describes a locomotor CPG controlling the movement of a simple biomechanical system and used this model to investigate the possible role of afferent feedback from flexor and extensor muscles in the control of locomotor oscillations, including the extensor-dominated control of locomotor speed, and in the recovery of locomotor function after the loss of supraspinal drive to the CPG (to model SCI conditions).

Model description

The model schematic is shown in Figure 1. The two-level half-center CPG represents a simplified version

of a previous model[6,7] and consists of a half-center rhythm generator (RG, containing flexor, RG-F, and extensor, RG-F, half-centers/neurons), pattern formation (PF) circuits (represented by PF-F and PF-E neurons) and inhibitory interneurons (In-F and In-E) which mediate reciprocal inhibition between flexor and extensor half-centers. The CPG receives tonic "supraspinal" drive and generates a basic "locomotor" rhythm providing alternating activation of flexor and extensor neurons within the CPG and alternating activation of flexor and extensor motoneurons (Mn-F and Mn-E). The controlled biomechanical system represents a simplified model of a single-joint limb described as a pendulum. The forces acting at the limb include: (1) forces of two antagonistic muscles (flexor, F, and extensor, E, activated by Mn-F and Mn-E, respectively), (2) gravitational force, and (3) ground reaction force, whose moment (M_{GR}) is applied during the "stance phase" when the limb moves counterclockwise (i.e., with angular velocity $\dot{q} > 0$). Muscle afferents provide the length-dependent (type Ia from both muscles and type II from the flexor) and force-dependent (Ib from the extensor) feedback to the CPG through additional excitation to the homonymous (F or E) interneurons of the CPG. This afferent feedback affects motoneuron activity through the CPG by controlling the timing of phase transitions at the RG level and the excitability of the PF circuits. Sensory feedback from the extensor muscle also accesses an additional circuit (In and Inab-E) providing disynaptic excitation of Mn-E during extension.[40,41]

Biomechanical model of single-joint limb

The biomechanical model of a single-joint limb consists of a rigid segment of mass m and length l_s connected to a stationary rigid base by a hinge joint (see Fig. 1). The segment oscillates in the sagittal plane by rotating around the suspension point under control of two muscles, flexor (F) and extensor (E). The muscles are attached to the segment and the stationary base. Motion of the segment is described by a second order differential equation:

$$I \cdot \ddot{q} = 0.5 \cdot m \cdot g \cdot l_s \cdot \cos q$$
$$- b \cdot \dot{q} + F_F(q, \dot{q}, t) \cdot h_F(q) \qquad (1)$$
$$- F_E(\pi - q, -\dot{q}, t) \cdot h_E(q) + M_{GR}(q),$$

where q is the generalized coordinate (joint angle); I is the moment of inertia of the segment with

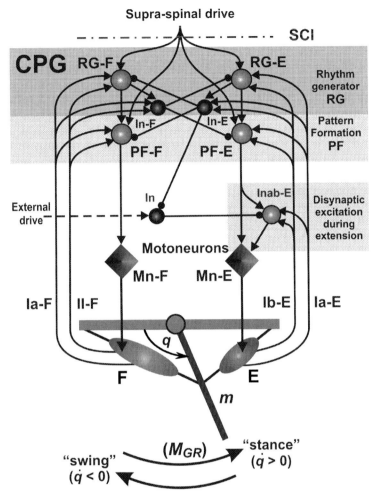

Figure 1. Model schematics. The two-level spinal CPG consists of a half-center rhythm generator (RG, containing flexor, RG-F, and extensor, RG-E, half-centers), pattern formation (PF) circuits (PF-F and PF-E neurons) and inhibitory interneurons (In-F and In-E), which mediate reciprocal inhibition between flexor and extensor sides of the CPG. The CPG receives tonic "supraspinal" drive and generates a basic "locomotor" rhythm providing alternating activation of all flexor and extensor CPG neurons and corresponding flexor and extensor motoneurons (Mn-F and Mn-E). An additional circuit including In and Inab-E interneurons is incorporated to provide disynaptic excitation of Mn-E by extensor afferents during extension (see text for details). All interneurons are represented by spheres: *light* spheres are excitatory, and *dark* spheres are inhibitory interneurons. Motoneurons are represented by *diamonds*. Excitatory and inhibitory synaptic connections are shown by *arrows* and *small circles*, respectively. The biomechanical system represents a simplified model of a single-joint limb that is forced to oscillate by the forces of two antagonistic muscles (flexor, F, and extensor, E, activated by Mn-F and Mn-E, respectively). Muscle afferents provide length-dependent (Ia type from both muscles, and type II type from the flexor muscle) and force-dependent (Ib from the extensor) feedback to the CPG providing excitation to the homonymous (F or E) interneurons of the CPG (see text for details).

respect to the suspension point ($I = m \cdot l_s^2/3$); b is the angular viscosity in the hinge joint; F_F is the flexor muscle force; F_E is the extensor muscle force; h_F is the flexor muscle moment arm; and h_E is the extensor muscle moment arm. The generalized force on the right side of equation (1) consists of moment of gravitational force, moment of friction force in hinge joint, moments of muscle forces, and moment of external forces (M_{GR}) emulating the effect of ground reaction forces during "stance." Contracting the flexor muscle produces negative moment while contracting the extensor muscle produces positive moment applied to the segment. The following parameters were used in our simulations: $m = 300$ g; $l_s = 300$ mm; $b = 0.002$ g $\cdot$ mm^2/(ms $\cdot$ rad).

Length of muscles (L) is calculated as the distance from origin to attachment point, and the moment arm (h) is calculated as the shortest distance from the muscle to the joint. For the flexor muscle:

$$L = \sqrt{a_1^2 + a_2^2 - 2a_1 \cdot a_2 \cdot \cos q};$$
$$h = \frac{a_1 \cdot a_2 \cdot \sin q}{L}, \tag{2}$$

where a_1 is the distance between suspension point and muscle origin, ($a_1 = 60$ mm) and a_2 is the distance between suspension point and muscle attachment to the segment ($a_2 = 7$ mm). For the extensor muscle, the same description (2) was used by substituting q with $\pi - q$.

Muscle velocities are defined as:

$$v_F = \dot{q} \cdot h_F; v_E = -\dot{q} \cdot h_E, \tag{3}$$

where $\dot{q}$ is the segment angular velocity and h is the moment arm of the corresponding muscle.

Calculation of muscle forces is based on the Hill-type model proposed by Harischandra and Ekeberg.[42] The total force F in each muscle (F_F and F_E) is defined by the normalized length- (F_l) and velocity- (F_v) dependent variables describing the muscle contractile component and the passive parallel component F_p as follows:

$$F = F_{max} \cdot (f(V) \cdot F_l \cdot F_v + F_p), \tag{4}$$

where $f(V)$ is the neural activation (output activity of the corresponding motoneuron, Mn-F or Mn-E, respectively, see Fig. 1 and neuron description below; $0 \leq f(V) < 1$) and F_{max} is the maximal isometric force of the corresponding muscle (F_{max} for the flexor and extensor muscles was set to 72.5 and 37.7 N, respectively).

Muscle lengths (L) are normalized with respect to L_{opt} (the length of muscle for which $F_l = 1$; $L_{opt} = 68$ mm for both muscles); the normalized muscle lengths $l = L/L_{opt}$.

The force–length dependence F_l in (4) is given by:

$$F_l = \exp\left(-\left|\frac{l \cdot \beta - 1}{\omega}\right|^\rho\right) \tag{5}$$

with parameters $\beta = 2.3$, $\omega = 1.26$, and $\rho = 1.62$.[42]

The force–velocity dependence F_v in (4) is calculated as:

$$F_v = \begin{cases} \dfrac{b_1 - c_1 \cdot v}{v + b_1}, & \text{if } v < 0; \\ \dfrac{b_2 - c_2(l) \cdot v}{v + b_2}, & \text{if } v \geq 0, \end{cases} \tag{6}$$

where v is muscle velocity; $c_1 = 0.17$, $b_1 = -0.69$, $c_2(l) = -5.34 \cdot l^2 + 8.41 \cdot l - 4.7$, and $b_2 = 0.18$. Negative velocities correspond to shortening of the muscles.

The passive force F_p in (4) is calculated as follows[42]:

$$F_p = 3.5 \cdot \ln(\exp((l - 1.4)/0.005) + 1.0)$$
$$-0.02 \cdot \exp(-18.7 \cdot (l - 0.79)) - 1.0). \tag{7}$$

To simulate the effect of the ground, we assumed that increasing segment angle q (in counterclockwise direction of movement in Fig. 1) corresponds to the stance phase, and decreasing q (in clockwise direction) corresponds to the flexion phase. The moment of ground reaction forces is described as:

$$M_{GR}(q) = \begin{cases} -M_{GRmax} \cdot \cos q, & \text{if } \dot{q} \geq 0 \ (stance); \\ 0, & \text{if } \dot{q} < 0 \ (swing), \end{cases} \tag{8}$$

where $M_{GRmax} > 0$ is a constant ($M_{GRmax} = 585$ N $\cdot$ mm).

Activity of muscle afferents

Only length-dependent feedback from the flexor muscle (primary Ia-F and secondary II-F) and primary length- and force-dependent afferents from the extensor muscle (Ia-E and Ib-E) have been considered (see Fig. 1). The descriptions of muscle afferent activities are derived and modified from the formulas suggested by Prochazka[43,44]:

$$Ia = k_v \cdot v_{norm}^{p_v} + k_{dI} \cdot d_{norm} + k_{nI} \cdot f(V) + const_I;$$
$$Ib = k_F \cdot F_{norm};$$
$$II = k_{dII} \cdot d_{norm} + k_{nII} \cdot f(V) + const_{II}, \tag{9}$$

where v_{norm} is the normalized muscle velocity ($v_{norm} = v/L_{th}$); $p_v = 0.6$; d_{norm} is the normalized muscle lengthening ($d_{norm} = (L - L_{th})/L_{th}$, if $L \geq L_{th}$, and 0 otherwise); L_{th} is the minimal muscle length evoking afferent activation; $f(V)$ is the output activity of the corresponding (flexor or extensor) motoneuron; $const_I$ and $const_{II}$

are constant components; F_{norm} is the normalized muscle force ($F_{norm} = (F - F_{th})/F_{max}$, if $F \geq F_{th}$, and 0 otherwise); k_v, k_{dI}, k_{nI}, k_F, k_{dII}, and k_{nII} are coefficients ($L_{th} = 59$ mm; $F_{th} = 3.38$ N; $k_v = 6.2$; $k_{dI} = 2$; $k_{dII} = 1.5$; $k_{nI} = k_{nII} = 0.06$; $k_F = 1$).

Modeling neurons and the CPG

The CPG model is a simplified version of a previous model[6,7] and includes a half-center rhythm generator that receives tonic supraspinal drive and generates the locomotor rhythm producing alternating activation of flexor and extensor motoneurons. Because our major focus was on the afferent control of the CPG, the classical reflex circuits and low-level interactions involving Ia interneurons and Renshaw cells have not been included in the model. We however incorporated circuits simulating disynaptic excitation of extensors by group I extensor afferents (In and Inab-E interneurons in Fig. 1, see details in Rybak *et al.*[7]).

Each neuron in the model represents a neural population and is described by an activity-based neuron model, in which the dependent variable V represents the average membrane voltage of neurons within the population, and the output activity $f(V)$ represents the average or integrated population activity. At the same time, the neuron model was formulated to include an explicit representation of some voltage-gated ionic currents such as potassium rectifier (I_K) and persistent sodium (I_{NaP}) currents. These currents in RG-F and RG-E neurons in combination with reciprocal inhibition between these neurons define the rhythm-generation mechanism in RG.[6,45] Specifically, the membrane potential of CPG neurons (RG-F, RG-E, PF-F, and PF-E) and motoneurons (Mn-F and Mn-E) is described by the following differential equation:

$$C \cdot \frac{dV}{dt} = -I_{NaP} - I_K - I_{Leak} - I_{SynE} - I_{SynI}. \tag{10}$$

The membrane potential of all other neurons (In-E, In-F, Inab-E, and In) is described as follows:

$$C \cdot \frac{dV}{dt} = -I_{Leak} - I_{SynE} - I_{SynI}. \tag{11}$$

In the above equations, C is the neuronal capacitance, I_{Leak} is the leakage current, I_{SynE} and I_{SynI} are the excitatory and inhibitory synaptic currents, respectively. The ionic currents are described as follows:

$$I_{NaP} = \bar{g}_{NaP} \cdot m_{NaP} \cdot h_{NaP} \cdot (V - E_{Na});$$

$$I_K = \bar{g}_K \cdot m_K^4 \cdot (V - E_K);$$

$$I_{Leak} = \bar{g}_{Leak} \cdot (V - E_{Leak});$$

$$I_{SynE,i} = \bar{g}_{SynE} \cdot (V_i - E_{SynE})$$
$$\cdot \left(\sum_j a_{ji} \cdot f(V_j) + \sum_m c_{mi} \cdot d_m \tag{12} \right.$$
$$\left. + \sum_k w_{ki} \cdot fb_k \right);$$

$$I_{SynI,i} = \bar{g}_{SynI} \cdot (V_i - E_{SynI}) \cdot \sum_j b_{ji} \cdot f(V_j),$$

where $\bar{g}_{NaP}$, $\bar{g}_K$, $\bar{g}_{Leak}$, $\bar{g}_{SynE}$, and $\bar{g}_{SynI}$ are the maximal conductances of the corresponding ionic channels; E_{Na}, E_K, E_{Leak}, and E_{SynI} are the corresponding reversal potentials; a_{ji} defines the weight of the excitatory synaptic input from neuron j to neuron i; b_{ji} defines the weight of the inhibitory input from neuron j to neuron i; c_{mi} defines the weight of the excitatory drive d_m to neuron i; w_{ki} defines the synaptic weight of afferent feedback fb_k to neuron i (see Fig. 1).

The nonlinear function $f(V)$ defines the output activity of each neuron:

$$f(V) = \begin{cases} 1/(1 + \exp(-(V - V_{1/2})/k)), & \text{if } V \geq V_{th}; \\ 0, & \text{if } V < V_{th}, \end{cases} \tag{13}$$

where $V_{1/2}$ is the half-activation voltage, k defines the slope of the output function and V_{th} is the threshold for each neuron.

Activation of the potassium rectifier and persistent sodium currents is considered instantaneous. Voltage dependent activation and inactivation variables and time constants for the potassium rectifier and persistent sodium channels are described as follows[6]:

$$m_K = 1/(1 + \exp(-(V + 44.5)/5)),$$

$$m_{NaP} = 1/(1 + \exp(-(V + 47.1)/3.1)),$$

$$\tau_{hNaP} \cdot \frac{d}{dt} h_{NaP} = h_{\infty NaP} - h_{NaP}, \tag{14}$$

$$h_{\infty NaP} = 1/(1 + \exp((V + 51)/4)),$$

$$\tau_{hNaP} = \tau_{hNaP\,max}/\cosh((V + 51)/8).$$

The following values of neuronal parameters were used: $C = 20$ pF; $E_{Na} = 55$ mV, $E_K = -80$ mV,

Table 1. Weights of synaptic connections in the model

Source	Target neuron									
	RG-F	RG-E	In-F	In-E	PF-F	PF-E	In	Inab-E	Mn-F	Mn-E
Connections from drives, c_{mi}										
Supraspinal drive, d_1	0.08	0.08			0.4	0.4				
External drive, $d_2 = 1$							0.18			
Excitatory connections, a_{ji}										
RG-F			0.41		0.7					
RG-E				0.41		0.7				
PF-F									1.95	
PF-E								0.35		1.30
Inab-E										0.82
Inhibitory connections, b_{ji}										
In-F		2.2				6.6				
In-E	2.2				6.6		2.8			
In								0.55		
Afferent feedback connections, w_{ki}										
Ia-F	0.06		0.27		0.19					
II-F	0.0348		0.1566		0.1102					
Ia-E		0.06		0.44		0.10		0.16		
Ib-E		0.066		0.484		0.11		0.176		

$E_{SynE} = -10$ mV, $E_{SynI} = -70$ mV, $E_{Leak} = -64$ mV for RG and PF neurons and motoneurons and -60 mV for all other neurons; $\bar{g}_K = 4.5$ nS, $\bar{g}_{Leak} = 1.60$ nS, $\bar{g}_{SynE} = \bar{g}_{SynI} = 10.0$ nS, $\bar{g}_{NaP} = 3.5$ nS for RG neurons, 0.5 nS for PF neurons, and 0.3 nS for motoneurons; $\tau_{hNaP\,max} = 600$ mS. Parameters of $f(V)$ function were $V_{1/2} = -30$ mV, $V_{th} = -50$ mV, and $k = 3$ mV for motoneurons and 8 mV for other neurons.

The weights of the synaptic connections are shown in Table 1. To change the rate of oscillations (locomotion speed) in the model, we change the supraspinal drive (d_1) in the range of 0.7–3.6. The values of afferent feedback connections in Table 1 correspond to "intact case." To simulate the loss of supraspinal drive after spinal cord injury, we set $d_1 = 0$. To simulate the effects of training on locomotor recovery, the weights of all length-dependent afferent connections (Ia-F, II-F, and Ia-E) to all target neurons were increased by 31%, and the weights from Ib-E to all target neurons were increased fivefold, which "recovered" stable locomotor oscillations in the absence of a supraspinal drive.

The model was implemented using Matlab 7.5.0. Differential equations were solved using a variable order multistep differential equation solver ode15s available in Matlab.

Results and discussion

Model performance under normal conditions

Generation of the locomotor rhythm in the model is performed by the half-center rhythm generator comprised of RG-F and RG-E neurons reciprocally inhibiting each other via In-F and In-E inhibitory interneurons, respectively (see Fig. 1). The generation of this rhythm relies on the dynamics of the persistent sodium current (I_{NaP}) in RG-F and RG-F neurons and the mutual inhibition between them.[6,45] The generation of this rhythm in the "intact" case requires tonic ("supraspinal") drive to the CPG (see Fig. 1) but does not require afferent feedback. The afferent feedback, however, controls the performance of the CPG and modifies the locomotor pattern generated, adjusting the latter to the behavior of the controlled biomechanical system.

Changes in the major characteristics of the biomechanical system during locomotion are shown in Figure 2A. The two top traces in this figure show alternating activity of motoneurons Mn-F

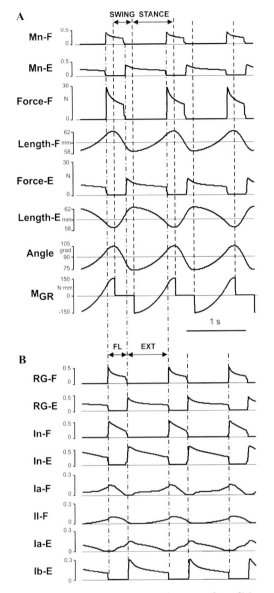

and Mn-E, which activate flexor (F) and extensor (E) muscles, respectively. The next four traces represent the corresponding changes in forces and lengths of F and E muscles. The next trace represents changes in the ("hip") angle (q), and the bottom trace shows changes in the moment of ground reaction forces (M_{GR}) acting during the "stance" phase (when $\dot{q} > 0$). Figure 2B represents the activity of RG neurons (RG-F and RG-E) and corresponding inhibitory interneurons (four top traces) and the activity of all four muscle afferents controlling the RG in the model (see Fig. 1). One important feature of the locomotor oscillations in the model is the existence of a delay (about 100 ms, which slightly changes with the rate of oscillations) between the onsets of flexion (FL) and extension (EXT) (defined by the onset of the corresponding RG neurons and motoneurons) and the onsets of the stance (STANCE) and swing (SWING) phases (defined by the "interaction with the ground," see M_{GR} trace in Fig. 2A). This simulation result exactly reproduces the delay between the onsets of EMG bursts in flexor and extensor muscles and the corresponding onsets of the swing and stance phases (defined by the timing of limb's touch-down and lift-off) observed during real locomotion.[4,5,15,34,37]

The locomotor oscillations produced by the model can be represented by a limit cycle in a 2D diagram (q, $\dot{q}$) (see Fig. 3). Our analysis has shown that the produced locomotor oscillations are stable with respect to both the initial conditions (initial limb position and velocity, e.g., see examples in Figs. 3A and B) and external perturbations (additional moments of force applied in different phases of the step cycle (see examples in Figs. 3C and D)). Stability of these oscillations in the model is provided by afferent control of the CPG. Specifically, the activity of the force-dependent extensor afferents (Ib-E), that provide positive feedback to the extensor motoneuron via both the CPG (PF-E) and disynaptic excitation (Inab-E), plays a major role in compensating for the ground reaction forces and effects of external perturbations during stance.

Control of locomotor speed

An increase in the supraspinal drive to the CPG in the model (Fig. 1) increases the speed of locomotion (rate of oscillation), so that the step cycle duration decreases due to the shortening of the stance phase with a relatively constant swing phase

Figure 2. Model performance under normal conditions. (**A**) Changes in limb biomechanical output during locomotor movement (see text for details). (**B**) Rhythmic activity of RG neurons (RG-F and RG-E) and corresponding inhibitory interneurons (*four top traces*) and the activity of all four afferents controlling the RG (see text for details). The activity of all neurons in (**A**) and (**B**) represent changes of output neural variable of each neuron $f(V)$. The *vertical dashed lines* in (**A**) separate the swing and stance phases (defined by the changes in the moment of ground reaction forces (M_{GR})); the vertical *dash–dotted lines* in (**A**) and (**B**) separate the flexor (FL) and extensor (EXT) phases defined by the onset of activity of RG-F and RG-E neurons.

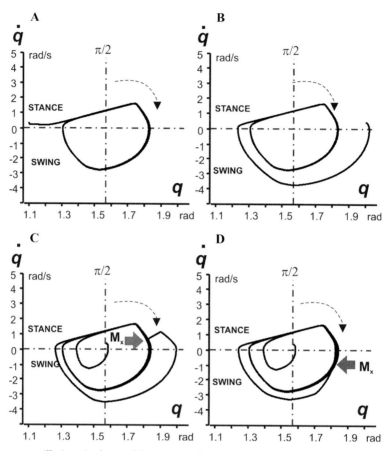

Figure 3. Locomotor oscillations in the model represented as 2D $(q, \dot{q})$ diagrams. In each diagram, the horizontal *dash–dotted line* at $\dot{q} = 0$ splits trajectory into the stance (*top*) and swing (*bottom*) parts; the vertical *dash–dotted line* corresponds to the vertical position of the limb $(q = \pi/2)$; *the arrows* show the direction of movement. In diagrams (**A**) and (**B**), oscillations started from different initial angles $(q_0$ at t = 0). (**C**) and (**D**) show the effect of disturbances, a moment of external force $M_x = 150$ N · mm applied for 100 ms in different phases of the step cycle (during stance in (**C**) and swing in (**D**)).

duration (Figs. 4A and C). Hence, the model with afferent feedback produces an extensor-dominated locomotor pattern (Fig. 4C), which fits the experimental observations in cats[16,17] (see Fig. 4D), rats,[18,19] and humans.[20] Interestingly, an increase of locomotor speed is also accompanied by a symmetrical increase in the amplitude of angular limb deviation from the midpoint vertical position $(q = \pi/2)$ which is kept almost constant (Fig. 4B).

It has been proposed that the physiological basis for the extensor-dominated locomotion may result from an asymmetry in the organization of the CPG *per se*,[22,23] or an asymmetry in the descending drive to the flexor and extensor CPG half-centers.[24–26] To investigate this possibility we have comparatively

investigated the generation of locomotor pattern by the CPG with and without afferent feedback. The latter may be considered as a "fictive locomotion" state. Our simulations have demonstrated that in the symmetrical case (when both half-centers of the RG received the same supraspinal drive), both flexor and extensor phases were equally shortened by an increase of the drive (Fig. 4E). In an asymmetrical case, both flexor-dominated and extensor-dominated "fictive" pattern could be obtained by applying different drives to the RG half-centers.[6,40] For example, Figure 4F shows the case when the drive to RG-E was kept constant, whereas the drive to RG-F was progressively varied, producing gradual transition from an extensor-dominated to a

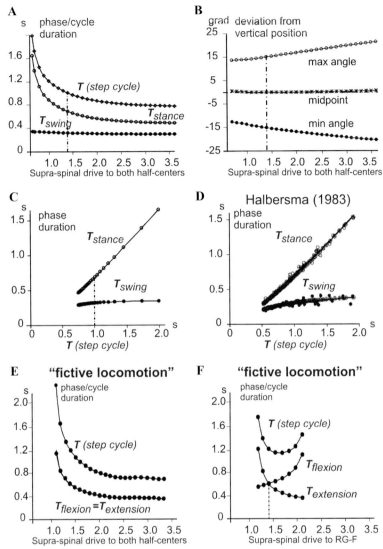

Figure 4. Control of the locomotor speed. (**A**) Changes in the durations of the swing and stance phases and the overall step cycle in the intact model with an increase in the supraspinal drive to the CPG (both half-centers receive the same drive). (**B**) Changes in the amplitude of the angular deviation from the midpoint (vertical limb position at $q = \pi/2$) with an increase in the supraspinal drive to the CPG. (**C**) The durations of simulated swing and stance phases plotted against the step-cycle period, the same data as in A. The vertical *dash-dot lines* in A–C indicate the drive value of 1.4 which was used in all simulations shown in Figures 2 and 3. (**D**) The durations of simulated flexor and extensor phases in the model plotted against the step-cycle period for treadmill locomotion in intact cats (from Halbertsma[17]). (**E**) Changes in the durations of flexor and extensor phases and the overall step cycle in the CPG pattern generated in the absence of afferent feedback ("fictive locomotion" state) when both half-centers receive the same drive. (**F**) Changes in the durations of flexor and extensor phases and the overall step cycle in the CPG pattern generated in the absence of afferent feedback ("fictive locomotion" state), when the drive to RG-E was kept constant (1.4, marked by a *dashed line*), whereas the drive to RG-F was varied from 1.1 to 2.1.

flexor-dominated "fictive" locomotor pattern. Two of the patterns generated during "fictive locomotion" (with no afferent feedback) by different drives to RG-F, one flexor-dominated and one extensor-dominated, are shown in Figures 5(A1 and B1) and (A2 and B2), respectively. However, as seen in Figures 5C1 and C2, incorporating afferent feedback changed both patterns to "normal" extensor-dominated patterns with a relatively constant duration of the flexor phase. Moreover, to provide stable oscillations, afferent feedback prolonged the extensor phase in the first case (Fig. 5C1) and shortened it in the second case (Fig. 5C2).

In summary, our simulations show that afferent feedback can adjust and maintain an asymmetric, extensor-dominated pattern during normal locomotion relatively independent of the pattern (flexor- or extensor-dominated) expressed in the "fictive locomotion" case (without afferent feedback). Specifically, the timing of extension-flexion transition in the CPG is controlled by both the reduction of Ib-E activity (unloading of Mn-E) and the increase in length-dependent flexor (Ia-F and II-F) afferent activity (see Fig. 2B), which make the duration of stance dependent on the locomotor speed. In contrast, the timing of flexion-extension transition in the CPG is mainly controlled by the length- (and velocity-) dependent extensor afferent activity (Ia-E) which adjusts the duration of flexion to limb kinematics during swing, keeping the duration of swing relatively constant. Hence our simulations support the suggestion of Juvin *et al.*[21] and Hayes *et al.*[30] regarding the critical role of afferent feedback in shaping and maintaining the extensor-dominated asymmetry observed during normal locomotion.

Role of afferent feedback in locomotor recovery after loss of supraspinal drive

During the last decade, many studies have provided evidence that after SCI (which removes supraspinal inputs to the spinal CPG) locomotor function can be recovered by locomotor training alone or by various combinations of locomotor training with pharmacological treatment and/or afferent stimulation. It is believed that locomotor training (and other successful treatments) restores locomotor function by an increase of proprioceptive input to the CPG.[4,15,35,36,38] This possibility, however, has not been theoretically investigated with the models. Therefore, as a part of this study, we address the

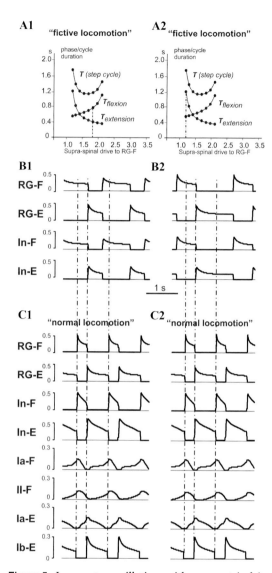

Figure 5. Locomotor oscillations with asymmetric drive to CPG half-centers. (**A1**) and (**A2**) repeat the diagram shown in Figure 4F, with vertical *dash-dot line* indicating drives used in simulations shown in (**B1**) and (**B2**), respectively. (**B1**) An example of a flexion-dominated "fictive locomotion" pattern generated by the CPG (with no afferent feedback) with drive to RG-E set to 1.4, and drive to RG-F set to 1.8 (see in (**A1**)). (**B2**) An example of an extensor-dominated "fictive locomotion" pattern generated by the CPG with drive to RG-E set to 1.4, and drive to RG-F set to 1.2 (see in (**A2**)). (**C1**) and (**C2**) The extensor-dominated pattern of "normal locomotion" with the same values of drives as in (**B1**) and (**B2**), respectively, with afferent feedback intact. Note that feedback prolongs the extensor phase in (**C1**) and shortens it in (**C2**).

question of whether an augmentation of afferent feedback to the CPG (which supposedly simulates the effect of locomotor training) can reestablish locomotor rhythm generation and stable locomotor movement after the loss of the supraspinal drive (emulating the effect of SCI).

Removal of the supraspinal drive in the model (Fig. 1) stopped the generation of the locomotor rhythm. To simulate the proposed effect of locomotor training, we proportionally increased the weights of flexor and extensor length-dependent (Ia and II) and force-dependent (Ib) afferents to all target neurons in the model. We found that progressive increase of these weights can quickly reestablish the generation of locomotor oscillations by the CPG. However, the locomotor movements of the limb remained unstable (the limb simply "fell" during either stance of swing phase in the first step or after a few steps) until the weights of the extensor Ib-E afferents were increased fivefold, and the weights of Ia and II afferents (Ia-F, Ia-E, and II-F) were increased by 31%. After that, the model was able to demonstrate stable locomotor movements without "falling" (see Figs. 6 and 7). The locomotor movement after recovery, however, was less stable in respect to initial conditions and applied perturbations. An additional analysis has shown that a dramatic increase in weights of the force-dependent extensor (Ib-E) afferent inputs to CPG is critical for "locomotor recovery" after supraspinal drive removal.

Figure 6A shows the changes in the biomechanical output of the model during locomotor movement after "locomotor recovery" (compare with Fig. 2A), and Fig. 6B represents, correspondingly, the activity of RG neurons (RG-F and RG-E), inhibitory interneurons, and all 4 afferents controlling the RG (compare with Fig. 2B). Comparison with the intact model (Figs. 2A and B) shows that after removal of the supraspinal drive and "recovery": (a) the delay between the onsets of flexion and extension and the corresponding onsets of stance and swing phases was reduced; (b) the ratio of flexor phase duration to the step cycle was increased; (c) the angle changes during stance became more linear; and (d) a dramatic increase in extensor motoneuron (Mn-E) activity occurred at the beginning of extension preceding the onset of stance. Interestingly, all these features appear (at first glance) to fit the changes of

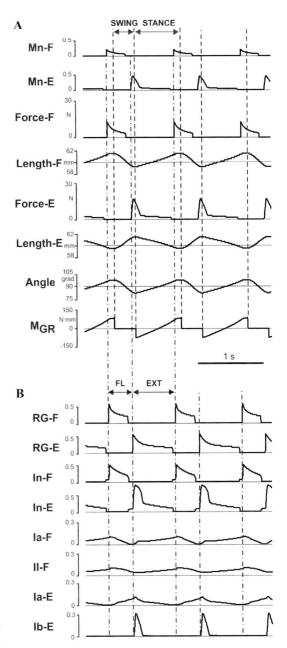

Figure 6. Model performance after removal of supraspinal drive and recovery. (**A**) Changes in the limb biomechanical output during locomotor movement. (**B**) Rhythmic activity of RG neurons (RG-F and RG-E) and corresponding inhibitory interneurons (four *top traces*) and the activity of all four afferents controlling the RG. For the meaning of the *dashed* and *dash–dotted lines* see Figures 2A and B.

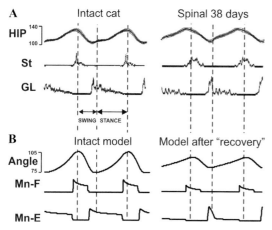

Figure 7. Comparison of simulation results to data obtained during cat locomotion on a treadmill. (A) Changes in hip angle and activity (EMG) of semitendinosus (St) and gastrocnemius lateralis (GL) muscles during locomotion on a treadmill (0.3 m/s) in the intact cat (*left*) and in the same spinal cat after locomotor training (*right*) (adapted from Rossignol and Bouyer[37]). (B) Changes of limb angle and flexor and extensor motoneuron activity produced by the model during normal conditions (*left*, from Figs. 2A and B) and after recovery (*right*, from Figs. 6A and B).

these characteristics observed in intact versus spinal cats after locomotor training (see Fig. 7A).

Conclusions

In this study, a simple neuromechanical model was used to investigate the role of afferent feedback in the control of the locomotor CPG. Despite the simplicity of the model, it may provide important insights into afferent control of locomotion. Specifically, our simulations have demonstrated the essential role of afferent feedback for the adjustment of CPG operation and the locomotor pattern generated to the biomechanical characteristics of the limb and its interactions with the ground. We have also shown that afferent feedback can provide asymmetric, extensor-dominated control of locomotor speed (with a relatively constant swing phase duration) independent of the asymmetric pattern (flexor- or extensor-dominated) generated by the CPG alone (in "fictive locomotion" conditions). Finally, we have demonstrated the possibility of re-establishing stable locomotion after removal of the supraspinal drive by increasing the weights of afferent inputs to the CPG,

which supposedly occurs with locomotor training. These findings will be further investigated using a more detailed and realistic model of neural control of locomotion. The simplified model described in this study has not considered the possible effects of SCI and locomotor recovery on the intrinsic properties of motoneurons and interneurons as well as on the circuits of various spinal reflexes, which will be incorporated and considered in future models.

Acknowledgments

This study was supported by the NINDS/NIH Bioengineering Research Partnership grant R01 NS048844 and NIH Program grants P01 NS055976 and P01 HD032571.

Conflicts of interest

The authors declare no conflicts of interest; NIH funded.

References

1. Brown, T.G. 1911. The intrinsic factors in the act of progression in the mammal. *Proc. R. Soc. Lond. B Biol. Sci.* **84:** 308–319.
2. Brown, T.G. 1914. On the fundamental activity of the nervous centres: together with an analysis of the conditioning of rhythmic activity in progression, and a theory of the evolution of function in the nervous system. *J. Physiol. (London)* **48:** 18–41.
3. Grillner, S. 1981. Control of locomotion in bipeds, tetrapods, and fish. In *Handbook of Physiology. Sect. 1. The Nervous System: Motor Control.* Vol. II, Pt. 2, V.B. Brooks, Ed.: 1179–1236. American Physiological Society. Bethesda, MD.
4. Rossignol, S. 1996. Neural control of stereotypic limb movements. In *Handbook of Physiology. Sect. 12. Exercise: Regulation and Integration of Multiple Systems.* L.B. Rowell & J.T. Sheperd, Eds.: 173–216. American Physiological Society. Oxford, UK.
5. Orlovsky, G.N., T.G. Deliagina & S. Grillner. 1999. *Neuronal Control of Locomotion: From Mollusc to Man.* Oxford University Press. New York, NY.
6. Rybak, I.A., N.A. Shevtsova, M. Lafreniere-Roula & D.A. McCrea. 2006. Modelling spinal circuitry involved in locomotor pattern generation: insights from deletions during fictive locomotion. *J. Physiol. (London)* **577:** 617–639.
7. Rybak, I.A., K. Stecina, N.A. Shevtsova & D.A. McCrea. 2006. Modelling spinal circuitry involved in locomotor

pattern generation: insights from the effects of afferent stimulation. *J. Physiol. (London)* **577**: 641–658.

8. McCrea, D.A. & I.A. Rybak. 2007. Modeling the mammalian locomotor CPG: insights from mistakes and perturbations. *Prog. Brain Res.* **165**: 235–253.

9. McCrea, D.A. & I.A. Rybak. 2008. Organization of mammalian locomotor rhythm and pattern generation. *Brain Res. Rev.* **57**: 134–146.

10. McCrea, D.A. 2001. Spinal circuitry of sensorimotor control of locomotion. *J. Physiol. (London)* **533**: 41–50.

11. Guertin, P., M. Angel, M.C. Perreault & D.A. McCrea. 1995. Ankle extensor group I afferents excite extensors throughout the hindlimb during MLR-evoked fictive locomotion in the cat. *J. Physiol. (London)* **487**: 197–209.

12. Perreault, M.C., M. Enriquez-Denton & H. Hultborn. 1999. Proprioceptive control of extensor activity during fictive scratching and weight support compared to fictive locomotion. *J. Neurosci.* **19**: 10966–10976.

13. Stecina, K., J. Quevedo & D.A. McCrea. 2005. Parallel reflex pathways from flexor muscle afferents evoking resetting and flexion enhancement during fictive locomotion and scratch in the cat. *J. Physiol. (London)* **569**: 275–290.

14. Pearson, K.G. 2004. Generating the walking gait: role of sensory feedback. *Prog. Brain Res.* **143**: 123–129.

15. Rossignol, S., R. Dubuc & J.P. Gossard. 2006. Dynamic sensorimotor interactions in locomotion. *Physiol. Rev.* **86**: 89–154.

16. Goslow, G.E., R.M. Reinking & D.G. Stuart. 1973. The cat step cycle: hind limb joint angles and muscle lengths during unrestrained locomotion. *J. Morph.* **141**: 1–41.

17. Halbertsma, J.M. 1983. The stride cycle of the cat: the modelling of locomotion by computerized analysis of automatic recordings. *Acta Physiol. Scand. Suppl.* **521**: 1–75.

18. Navarrete, R., U. Slawinska & G. Vrbova. 2002. Electromyographic activity patterns of ankle flexor and extensor muscles during spontaneous and L-DOPA-induced locomotion in freely moving neonatal rats. *Exp. Neurol.* **173**: 256–265.

19. Slawinska, U., H. Majczynski & R. Djavadian. 2000. Recovery of hindlimb motor functions after spinal cord transection is enhanced by grafts of the embryonic raphe nuclei. *Exp. Brain Res.* **132**: 27–38.

20. Grillner, S., J. Halbertsma, J. Nilsson & A. Thortensson. 1979. The adaptation to speed in human locomotion. *Brain Res.* **165**: 177–182.

21. Juvin, L., J. Simmers & D. Morin. 2007. Locomotor rhythmogenesis in the isolated rat spinal cord: a phase-coupled set of symmetrical flexion–extension oscillators. *J. Physiol. (London)* **583**: 115–128.

22. Dubuc, R., J.M. Cabelguen & S. Rossignol. 1988. Rhythmic fluctuations of dorsal root potentials and antidromic discharges of primary afferents during fictive locomotion in the cat. *J. Neurophysiol.* **60**: 2014–2036.

23. Grillner, S. & R. Dubuc. 1988. Control of locomotion in vertebrates: spinal and supraspinal mechanisms. *Adv. Neurol.* **47**: 425–453.

24. Armstrong, D.M. 1988. The supraspinal control of mammalian locomotion. *J. Physiol. (London)* **405**: 1–37.

25. Leblond, H. & J.P. Gossard. 1997. Supraspinal and segmental signals can be transmitted through separate spinal cord pathways to enhance locomotor activity in extensor muscles in the cat. *Exp. Brain Res.* **114**: 188–192.

26. Frigon, A. & J.P. Gossard. 2009. Asymmetric control of cycle period by the spinal locomotor rhythm generator in the adult cat. *J. Physiol. (London)* **587**: 4617–4628.

27. Engberg, I. & A. Lundberg. 1969. An electromyographic analysis of muscular activity in the hindlimb of the cat during unrestrained locomotion. *Acta Physiol. Scand.* **75**: 614–630.

28. Barbeau, H. & S. Rossignol. 1987. Recovery of locomotion after chronic spinalization in the adult cat. *Brain Res.* **412**: 84–95.

29. Pearson, K.G. 1995. Proprioceptive regulation of locomotion. *Curr. Opin. Neurobiol.* **5**: 786–791.

30. Hayes, H.B., Y-H. Chang & S. Hochman. 2009. An *in vitro* spinal cord-hindlimb preparation for studying behaviorally relevant rat locomotor function. *J. Neurophysiol.* **101**: 1114–1122.

31. Yakovenko, S., D.A. McCrea, K. Stecina & A. Prochazka. 2005. Control of locomotor cycle durations. *J. Neurophysiol.* **94**: 1057–1065.

32. Jiang, W. & T. Drew. 1996. Effects of bilateral lesions of the dorsolateral funiculi and dorsal columns at the level of the low thoracic spinal cord on the control of locomotion in the adult cat: I. Treadmill walking. *J. Neurophysiol.* **76**: 849–866.

33. Brustein, E. & S. Rossignol. 1998. Recovery of treadmill locomotion after bilateral chronic ventral and ventrolateral spinal lesions in the adult cat. I. Deficits and adaptive mechanisms. *J. Neurophysiol.* **80**: 1245–1267.

34. Rossignol, S., T. Drew, E. Brustein & W. Jiang. 1999. Locomotor performance and adaptation after partial or complete spinal cord lesions in the cat. In *Peripheral and Spinal Mechanisms in the Neural Control of Movement*. M.D. Binder, Ed.: 349–365. Elsevier. Amsterdam, The Netherlands.

35. Barbeau, H. *et al.* 1999. Tapping into spinal circuits to restore motor function. *Brain Res. Rev.* **30**: 27–51.

36. Rossignol, S., L. Bouyer, D. Barthelemy, C. Langlet & H. Leblond. 2002. Recovery of locomotion in the cat following spinal cord lesions. *Brain Res. Rev.* **40:** 257–266.

37. Rossignol, S. & L. Bouyer. 2004. Adaptive mechanisms of spinal locomotion in cats. *Integr. Comp. Biol.* **44:** 71–79.

38. Edgerton, V.R., N.J. Tillakaratne, A.J. Bigbee, *et al.* 2004. Plasticity of the spinal circuitry after injury. *Ann. Rev. Neurosci.* **27:** 145–167.

39. Boyce, V. S., M. Tumolo, I. Fischer, *et al.* 2007. Neurotrophic factors promote and enhance locomotor recovery in untrained spinalized cats. *J. Neurophysiol.* **98:** 1988–1996.

40. Angel, M.J., P. Guertin, I. Jiminez & D.A. McCrea. 1996. Group I extensor afferents evoke disynaptic EPSPs in cat hindlimb extensor motoneurones during fictive locomotion. *J. Physiol. (London)* **494:** 851–861.

41. Angel, M.J., E. Jankowska & D.A. McCrea. 2005. Candidate interneurones mediating group I disynaptic EPSPs in extensor motoneurones during fictive locomotion in the cat. *J. Physiol. (London)* **563:** 597–610.

42. Harischandra, N. & O. Ekeberg. 2008. System identification of muscle-joint interactions of the cat hind limb during locomotion. *Biol. Cybern.* **99:** 125–138.

43. Prochazka, A. & M. Gorassini. 1998. Models of ensemble firing of muscle spindle afferents recorded during normal locomotion in cats. *J. Physiol. (London)* **507:** 277–291.

44. Prochazka, A. 1999. Quantifying proprioception. *Prog. Brain Res.* **123:** 133–142.

45. Daun, S., J.E. Rubin & I.A. Rybak. 2009. Control of oscillation periods and phase durations in half-center central pattern generators: a comparative mechanistic analysis. *J. Comput. Neurosci.* **27:** 3–36.

Ann. N.Y. Acad. Sci. ISSN 0077-8923

Interactions between focused synaptic inputs and diffuse neuromodulation in the spinal cord

M.D. Johnson[1] and C.J. Heckman[2]

[1]Department of Physiology and [2]Department of Physiology, Physical Medicine & Rehabilitation, Northwestern University Medical School, Chicago, Illinois

Address for correspondence: Michael Johnson, Department of Physiology, Northwestern University Medical School, W5-295, 303 E. Chicago Avenue, Chicago, IL 60611. Voice: 312-503-2164; fax: 312-503-5101. m-johnson16@northwestern.edu

Spinal motoneurons (MNs) amplify synaptic inputs by producing strong dendritic persistent inward currents (PICs), which allow the MN to generate the firing rates and forces necessary for normal behaviors. However, PICs prolong MN depolarization after the initial excitation is removed, tend to "wind-up" with repeated activation and are regulated by a diffuse neuromodulatory system that affects all motor pools. We have shown that PICs are very sensitive to reciprocal inhibition from Ia afferents of antagonist muscles and as a result PIC amplification is related to limb configuration. Because reciprocal inhibition is tightly focused, shared only between strict anatomical antagonists, this system opposes the diffuse effects of the descending neuromodulation that facilitates PICs. Because inhibition appears necessary for PIC control, we hypothesize that Ia inhibition interacts with Ia excitation in a "push–pull" fashion, in which a baseline of simultaneous excitation and inhibition allows depolarization to occur via both excitation and disinhibition (and vice versa for hyperpolarization). Push–pull control appears to mitigate the undesirable affects associated with the PIC while still taking full advantage of PIC amplification.

Keywords: PIC; neuromodulation; push–pull; motoneuron

Introduction

Neuromodulation of motoneurons (MNs) by the monoamines serotonin (5HT) and norepinephrine (NE) greatly influences the way MNs receive, process, and transform synaptic inputs into meaningful motor outputs. While ionotropic inputs mediate the fast EPSPs and IPSPs, neuromodulatory inputs work by regulating the overall excitability of MNs and serve as a gain control for ionotropic synaptic inputs.[1] The G-protein coupled receptors associated with neuromodulators activate complex intracellular pathways that ultimately result in amplifying incoming signals. In the case of spinal MNs, this amplification occurs mainly through interactions between incoming synaptic inputs and voltage-activated channels present on the dendrites. Thus, dendrites are now realized to be active processors of synaptic inputs.[2]

However, in voltage clamp experiments performed on mammalian spinal MNs in anesthetized animals, neuromodulation is believed to be greatly attenuated.[3] Such experiments have revealed much about the MN's passive state electrical properties, but to understand fully normal MN behavior, neuromodulatory effects must also be considered. For example, summing all ionotropic synaptic inputs in the absence of neuromodulation results in less than 50% of the drive MNs need to produce maximum firing frequencies and muscle forces.[4] The monoamines 5-HT and NE are the main neuromodulators of motoneuronal activity.[5,6] It has been shown in the decerebrate animal that the areas of the brainstem from which the noradrenergic and serotonergic innervation of the spinal cord arise (i.e., the locus coeruleus and the medulary raphe nuclei) are released from the inhibitory effects of anesthetics, approximating the neuromodulatory state of an awake behaving subject. The decerebrate mammalian preparation is thus both important and unique in that it allows us to study the MN with its full complement of both ionotropic and neuromodulatory inputs intact.

doi: 10.1111/j.1749-6632.2010.05430.x

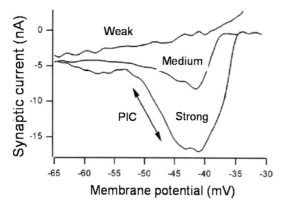

Figure 1. The relative amount of neuromodulatory drive sets the potential amplitude of the PIC and hence the amount of synaptic amplification. With weak monoaminergic drive, the PIC amplitude is small; synaptic current decreases as the cell is depolarized. As monoaminergic drive increases to medium and then strong, a progressively larger PIC and greater amplification of synaptic currents results. Inward (depolarizing) currents are downward.

Neuromodulators have many effects on the MN. They hyperpolarize spike threshold,[7,8] depolarize the resting membrane potential, and reduce the AHP.[9] Perhaps the most profound effect neuromodulators have on MNs is the generation of a persistent inward current.[10,11] The G-protein pathways coupled to 5HT-2 and NE alpha-1 produce a depolarizing current, primarily via dendritic CaV 1.3[12] channels, which can amplify synaptic inputs by as much as fivefold.[13,14] The large differences in firing rate evoked by synaptic inputs in the anesthetized versus unanesthetized decerebrate preparations can be accounted for by the amplification provided by PICs. The effect of monoamines on MNs is thus profound. In fact, even motor behaviors requiring small to moderate forces would be virtually impossible to achieve without substantial monoaminergic drive.

The amount of amplification of synaptic input is dependent on the amplitude of the PIC, which is proportional to the amount of neuromodulatory drive from the brainstem (Fig. 1).[15] The output from the brainstem monoaminergic nuclei is not constant, but varies with different behaviors, is correlated with speed of locomotion,[16] and state of arousal.[17] Thus, neuromodulation, via the PIC, serves as a variable gain controller and has a truly transformative effect on MN behavior that provides a remarkable degree of flexibility for motor commands. Its presence is in fact an essential part of normal MN function.

As critical as PICs are to the generation of normal motor outputs, they also present some potential problems. One of the initial effects that PICs were found to produce was bistability (Fig. 2).[15] Cells with strong PICs tend to display plateau potentials in voltage clamp and prolonged firing in current clamp well after the cessation of excitatory input. Both can be terminated by a short pulse of inhibition.[18,19] Although bistable behavior is probably essential for some normal behaviors, such as maintenance of posture,[20–22] it is easy to see how prolongation of transient inputs would be undesirable for other motor tasks by possibly inducing errors during dynamic changes in motor commands and preventing MNs from accurately tracking any dynamically varying inputs. Another potential problem is the tendency for PICs to display "wind-up." With repeated activation, PICs tend to progressively grow larger,[23] especially in the absence of inhibition.[24] This could cause undesirable, excessive, and uncontrolled motor output. PICs can also show quite a bit of variability in their activation, making them

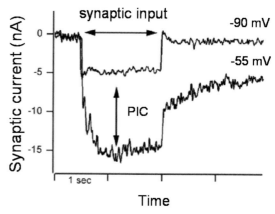

Figure 2. When the MN is held at a hyperpolarized level (*top trace*, −90 mV), a brief excitatory input results in a depolarizing synaptic current with a sharp onset and offset that lasts for the duration of the input. At a more depolarized level (*bottom trace*, −55 mV), the same brief excitatory input results in an amplified depolarizing current that persists (*tail current*) after the excitation is removed. Both the amplification and prolongation can be attributed to the PIC. Baseline current removed.

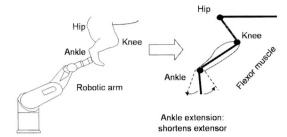

Figure 3. Experimental setup: A six degree-of-freedom robotic arm was used for passively rotating the ankle, knee, and hip joints.

inconsistent amplifiers of synaptic input.[25] In addition, the monoaminergic projections to the spinal cord are highly diffuse.[26] They innervate many motor pools thus simultaneously spreading both the beneficial and undesirable effects of PICs and potentially locking joints or even an entire limb into prolonged states of high excitability.

Results

It is gradually becoming apparent that the nervous system has mechanisms in place to exploit the benefits of the PIC while minimizing these potential problems. Previous work in our lab, as well as others, has shown that the PIC is very sensitive to inhibition[13,27] and that inhibition may be able to compensate for some of the problems associated with the PIC. In recordings from ankle extensor MNs in the decerebrate cat preparation, we have demonstrated that inhibition, in this case tonic inhibition from electrically stimulating nerves to antagonist muscles, reduces the magnitude of the PIC in a linear fashion.[27] Although the interaction between the PIC and synaptic excitation is strong and results in a great deal of amplification of the synaptic input, excitatory inputs only serve to shift the activation threshold of the PIC and have no effect on its amplitude.

In other recent work in the decerebrate feline, we have shown how the Ia reciprocal inhibition system interacts with the PIC.[24] In these experiments, the PIC amplitude and activation voltage were closely related to joint angle. We used a robotic arm and a paralyzed preparation to demonstrate that the PIC amplitude in ankle extensor MNs was extremely sensitive to joint position (Fig. 3). While triceps surae MNs were voltage clamped, the robot alternately

held the ankle in a flexed and then extended position. Ankle extension shortens the triceps surae and lengthens the antagonist flexor muscles (tibialis anterior and extensor digitorum longus; TA/EDL). Ankle flexion has the opposite effect, stretching the triceps and shortening TA/EDL. The dendritic PIC was assessed by linearly increasing voltage ramps applied as the ankle was held steady at three different joint angles: midpoint (defined as the tibia at 90° with the bones of the foot), extended and flexed. We saw significant reduction in PIC amplitude with just 10° of extension of the ankle (Figs. 4 and 5).[24] This further emphasizes the exquisite sensitivity of the PIC to inhibitory inputs, as small changes in the joint angle had a potent effect on the PIC amplitude. The source of inhibition is most likely from muscle spindle Ia afferents that generate reciprocal inhibition from the antagonist muscles, as denervation of cutaneous afferents did not alter this effect. The potent effect of joint angle probably occurs in dendritic regions of the cell, where the synaptic inputs interact with the PIC, because the voltage clamp prevented any changes in the behavior of somatic voltage-sensitive channels. Because the amplitude of the PIC determines the magnitude of synaptic amplification, active

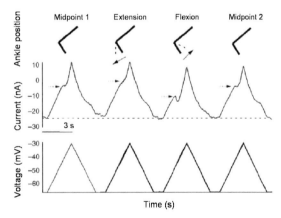

Figure 4. A voltage ramp applied to a tricep surae MN at ankle position midpoint 1 results in the presence of a PIC (*arrow* on current trace). When the same ramp is applied with the hindlimb in the extension position there is a reduction in PIC amplitude. This reduction is due to the interaction between reciprocal inhibition from antagonist muscles and the PIC. At the flexion position, PIC activation is shifted (hyperpolarized). Midpoint 2 conditions are identical to midpoint 1.

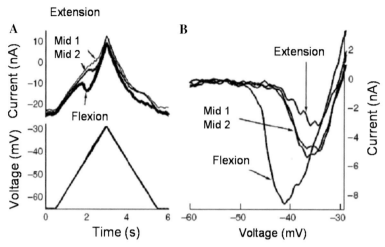

Figure 5. (A) Single cell recording. The overlapping current traces demonstrate the differences in PIC amplitude at the different ankle positions. (B) Same cell as in A, following leak subtraction, with the ankle in the flexion position, synaptic amplification is greatest. At midpoints 1 and 2, the PIC amplitude is fairly similar and decreased from the flexion position. At the extension position, the PIC amplitude and synaptic amplification is smallest. Current traces are leak-subtracted.

synaptic integration in MN dendrites depends on limb configuration.

As mentioned earlier, the neuromodulatory system of the brainstem/spinal cord is diffuse. Axons originating from the locus coeruleus and medullary raphe nuclei, the source of spinal NE and 5HT, innervate all segments and laminae of the entire spinal cord.[28] This diffuse innervation has the potential to spread the benefits as well as the deficits associated with the PIC to all the motor pools. Recently, we studied how the focused nature of the Ia system interacts with the diffuse nature of descending neuromodulation. We used our robotic arm to impose movements about the various joints of the feline hindlimb while voltage clamping ankle extensor MNs. The robot imposed passive flexion and extension of the ankle, knee, and hip individually and then generated combined ankle, knee, and hip rotation to produce a whole limb movement. PIC amplification of sensory inputs associated with the rotations converging onto ankle extensor MNs was restricted to synaptic inputs coming from muscle pairs acting at the ankle joint and not to inputs from the knee or hip (Fig. 6).[29] Studies involving electrical stimulation of muscle, cutaneous, and joint nerves have demonstrated polysynaptic pathways that cross multiple spinal segments. These contribute to whole limb coordination, especially in acutely spinalized prepa-

rations.[30,31] Despite this, inputs from other muscles at other joints only produced weak synaptic currents in the ankle extensor MNs. After spinalization, not only was amplification via the PIC eliminated, but sensory inputs from other joints affected the ankle extensor MNs, effectively broadening their receptive field. The mechanism of this broadening is not clear, but presumably reflects the loss of descending inhibition of spinal circuits.

Discussion

Both Ia monosynaptic excitation and Ia disynaptic reciprocal inhibition are tightly focused pathways.[32] Because of the high sensitivity of the PIC amplitude to Ia reciprocal inhibition, it is likely that Ia reciprocal inhibition helps sculpt individual joint motions from a background of diffuse excitatory neuromodulation (Fig. 7). At present, we assume that this is an example of a diffuse neuromodulatory input interacting with a specific and local ionotropic input. How Ia reciprocal inhibition reduces PICs remains, however, to be fully explained.[33,34] Although Ia reciprocal inhibition certainly involves ionotropic actions of the neurotransmitter glycine,[35] it is possible that there may also be an inhibitory neuromodulatory component mediated through GABAb receptors as well.[36]

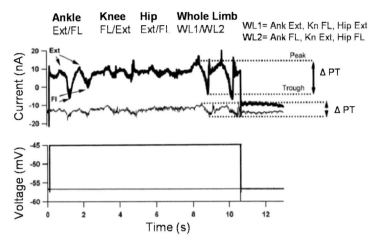

Figure 6. Effective synaptic current in the tricep surae MN was recorded as the ankle, knee, and hip were flexed and extended individually and then in concert. The darker, thicker trace was a result of movements performed at a depolarized voltage, so that the PIC was activated. The thinner trace was a result of movements performed at a hyperpolarized voltage, below the threshold for activation of the PIC. In both voltage conditions it is apparent that the individual ankle and whole limb movements produce the largest amplitude compared to rotations of the knee or hip. This illustrates the focused nature of the cells receptive field.

It seems likely that reciprocal inhibition from muscle stretch is particularly important for the transition from agonist to antagonist activation: as the agonist shortens it would receive reciprocal inhibition from the antagonist, whereas the antagonist reciprocal inhibition from the agonist would be reduced.[24] Our premise here is that the inhibition needed for this compensation should be linked to excitation in a push–pull fashion. In this sense, push–pull control requires a steady background of excitation and inhibition and maximum MN depolarization is the result of disinhibition coupled with excitation instead of excitation alone. Similarly, hyperpolarization is the result of disfacilitation coupled with inhibition instead of inhibition alone (Fig. 8). One potential advantage of push–pull is that net input–output gain is increased because reciprocal changes in two inputs occur simultaneously, as suggested by recent studies in cortical neurons.[37,38] Another potential advantage involves temporal dynamics. Although the tendency of the PIC to prolong excitatory inputs by inducing a plateau potential and self-sustained firing may be an advantage for posture, input prolongation could seriously distort inputs. An obvious example is locomotion, where prolongation of the stance phase by a PIC would be a substantial problem. Ia interneurons are rhythmically active during locomotion[39,40]

and thus the central pattern generator for locomotion may also be organized in a push–pull fashion. We are presently initiating studies of this question

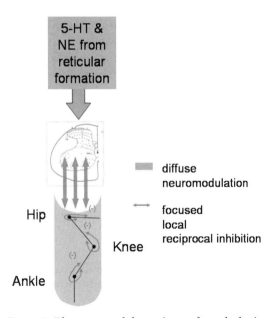

Figure 7. The neuromodulatory inputs from the brainstem are diffuse involving all segments and laminae of the spinal cord. The Ia reciprocal inhibitory system is focused and helps "sculpt" movements out of a background of excitation.

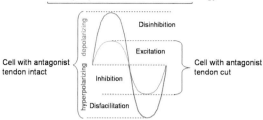

Push-pull predicted results and terminology

Figure 8. When tonic levels of excitation and inhibition are present maximum depolarization (and maximum firing frequencies) are achieved when disinhibition is coupled with excitation. Similarly, maximum hyperpolarization is achieved by the coupling of disfacilitation with inhibition. In our experiments, this is achieved by having either an intact Ia reciprocal inhibition system or disrupting reciprocal inhibition by cutting the tendons to antagonist muscles.

in our lab. A push–pull organization for excitation and inhibition would provide PIC deactivation during the inhibitory/disfacilitation phases and yet still allow strong PIC amplification during the excitatory/disinhibition phases. Thus, push–pull might allow PIC amplification to be combined with accurate tracking of dynamic inputs.

Our recent studies show that extensor MNs in the decerebrate preparation receive a steady inhibitory background drive that is likely to be mainly due to Ia interneurons.[24] We believe that the Ia reciprocal inhibition between antagonist muscle groups provides the inhibitory background needed to interact with excitation and constitute the push–pull relationship. Through this relationship, we propose that the desirable effects of the PIC can be preserved and the undesirable effects minimized. Studies are presently underway to test this hypothesis using voltage clamp in MNs and reflex measurements in muscles to test the hypothesis that passive sensory input to MNs is organized in a push–pull fashion.

Conflicts of interest

The authors declare no conflicts of interest.

References

1. Cushing, S., T. Bui & P.K. Rose. 2005. Effect of nonlinear summation of synaptic currents on the input-output properties of spinal motoneurons. *J. Neurophysiol.* **94:** 3465–3478.

2. Sjostrom, P.J., E.A. Rancz, A. Roth & M. Hausser. 2008. Dendritic excitability and synaptic plasticity. *Physiol. Rev.* **88:** 769–840.

3. Baldissera, F., H. Hultborn & M. Illert. 1981. Integration in spinal neuronal systems. In *Handbook of Physiology. Section 1: The Nervous System.* Vol. 2: Motor Control, part 1. V.B. Brooks, Ed.: 509–595. American Physiological Society. Bethesda.

4. Binder, M.D., C.J. Heckman & C.K. Powers. 2002. Relative strengths and distributions of different sources pf synaptic input to the motoneurone pool: implications for motor unit recruitment. *Adv. Exp. Med. Biol.* **508:** 207–212.

5. Heckman, C.J., R.H. Lee & R.M. Brownstone. 2003. Hyperexcitable dendrites in motoneurons and their neuromodulatory control during motor behavior. *Trends Neurosci.* **26:** 688–695.

6. Hultborn, H., R.B. Brownstone, T.I. Toth & J.P. Gossard. 2004. Key mechanisms for setting the input-output gain across the motoneuron pool. *Prog. Brain Res.* **143:** 77–95.

7. Krawitz, S., B. Fedirchuk, Y. Dai, *et al.* 2001. State-dependent hyperpolarization of voltage threshold enhances motoneurone excitability during fictive locomotion in the cat. *J. Physiol.* **532:** 271–281.

8. Fedirchuk, B. & Y. Dai. 2004. Monoamines increase the excitability of spinal neurones in the neonatal rat by hyperpolarizing the threshold for action potential production. *J. Physiol.* **557:** 355–361.

9. Powers, R.K. & M.D. Binder. 2001. Input-output functions of mammalian motoneurons. *Rev. Physiol. Biochem. Pharmacol.* **143:** 137–263.

10. Rekling, J.C., G.D. Funk, D.A. Bayliss, *et al.* 2000. Synaptic control of motoneuronal excitability. *Physiol. Rev.* **80:** 767–852.

11. Powers, R.K. & M.D. Binder. 2001. Input-output functions of mammalian motoneurons. *Rev. Physiol. Biochem. Pharmacol.* **143:** 137–263.

12. Carlin, K.P., K.E. Jones, Z. Jiang, *et al.* 2000. Dendritic L-typecalcium currents in mouse spinal motoneurons: implications for bistability. *Eur. J. Neurosci.* **12:** 1635–1646.

13. Hultborn, H., M.E. Denton, J. Wienecke & J.B. Nielsen. 2003. Variable amplification of synaptic input to cat spinal motoneurones by dendritic persistent inward current. *J. Physiol.* **552:** 945–952.

14. Lee, R.H. & C.J. Heckman. 2000. Adjustable amplification of synaptic input in the dendrites of spinal motoneurons in vivo. *J. Neurosci.* **20:** 6734–6740.

15. Heckman, C.J., A.S. Hyngstrom & M.D. Johnson. 2008. Active properties of motoneurone dendrites: diffuse

descending neuromodulation, focused local inhibition. *J. Physiol.* **586:** 1225–1231.

16. Jacobs, B.L., F.J. Martin-Cora & C.A. Fornal. 2002. Activity of medullary serotonergic neurons in freely moving animals. *Brain Res. Brain Res. Rev.* **40:** 45–52.

17. Aston-Jones, G., S. Chen, Y. Zhu & M.L. Oshinsky. 2001. A neural circuit for circadian regulation of arousal. *Nat. Neurosci.* **4:** 732–738.

18. Schwindt, P.C. & W.E. Crill. 1980. Properties of a persistent inward current in normal and TEA-injected motoneurons. *J. Neurophysiol.* **43:** 1700–1724.

19. Schwindt, P.C. & W.E. Crill. 1980. Role of a persistent inward current in motoneuron bursting during spinal seizures. *J. Neurophysiol.* **43:** 1296–1318.

20. Hounsgaard, J., H. Hultborn, B. Jespersen & O. Kiehn. 1988. Bistability of alpha-motoneurones in the decerebrate cat and in the acute spinal cat after intravenous 5-hydroxytryptophan. *J. Physiol.* **405:** 345–367.

21. Lee, R.H. & C.J. Heckman. 1998. Bistability in spinal motoneurons in vivo: systematic variations in persistent inward currents. *J. Neurophysiol.* **80:** 583–593.

22. Lee, R.H. & C.J. Heckman. 1998. Bistability in spinal motoneurons in vivo: systematic variations in rhythmic firing patterns. *J. Neurophysiol.* **80:** 572–582.

23. Bennett, D.J., H. Hultborn, B. Fedirchuk & M. Gorassini. 1998. Short-term plasticity in hindlimb motoneurons of decerebrate cats. *J. Neurophysiol.* **80:** 2038–2045.

24. Hyngstrom, A.S., M.D. Johnson, J.F. Miller & C.J. Heckman. 2007. Intrinsic electrical properties of spinal motoneurons vary with joint angle. *Nat. Neurosci.* **10:** 363–369.

25. Lee, R.H., J.J. Kuo, M.C. Jiang & C.J. Heckman. 2003. Influence of active dendritic currents on input-output processing in spinal motoneurons *in vivo*. *J. Neurophysiol.* **89:** 27–39.

26. Björklund, A. & G. Skagerberg. 1982. Descending monoaminergic projections to the spinal cord. In *Brain Stem Control of Spinal Mechanisms*. B. Sjolund & A. Bjorklund, Eds.: 55–88. Elsevier Biomedical Press. Amsterdam.

27. Kuo, J.J., R.H. Lee, M.D. Johnson, *et al.* 2003. Active dendritic integration of inhibitory synaptic inputs in vivo. *J. Neurophysiol.* **90:** 3617–3624.

28. Holstege, J.C. & H.G. Kuypers. 1987. Brainstem projections to spinal motoneurons: an update. *Neuroscience* **23:** 809–821.

29. Hyngstrom, A., M. Johnson, J. Schuster & C.J. Heckman. 2008. Movement-related receptive fields of spinal motoneurones with active dendrites. *J. Physiol.* **586:** 1581–1593.

30. Eccles, R.M. & A. Lundberg. 1958. Integrative pattern of Ia synaptic actions on motoneurones of hip and knee muscles. *J. Physiol.* **144:** 271–298.

31. Lundberg, A. 1987. Reflex pathways from group II muscle afferents 1. Distribution and linkage of reflex actions to alpha-motoneurons. *Exp. Brain Res.* **65:** 271–281.

32. Nichols, T.R. & T.C. Cope. 2001. The organization of distributed proprioceptive feedback in the chronic spinal cat. In *Motor Neurobiology of the Spinal Cord*. T.C. Cope, Ed.: 305–326. CRC Press. London.

33. Bui, T.V., G. Grande & P.K. Rose. 2008. Multiple modes of amplification of synaptic inhibition to motoneurons by persistent inward currents. *J Neurophysiol* **99:** 571–582.

34. Bui, T.V., G. Grande & P.K. Rose. 2008. Relative location of inhibitory synapses and persistent inward currents determines the magnitude and mode of synaptic amplification in motoneurons. *J Neurophysiol* **99:** 583–594.

35. Curtis, D.R. & G. Lacey. 1998. Prolonged GABAB receptor-mediated synaptic inhibition in the cat spinal cord: an in vivo study. *Exp. Brain Res.* **121:** 319–333.

36. Ruscheweyh, R. & J. Sandkuhler. 2002. Lamina-specific membrane and discharge properties of rat spinal dorsal horn neurones in vitro. *J. Physiol.* **541:** 231–244.

37. Steriade, M. 2001. Impact of network activities on neuronal properties in corticothalamic systems. *J. Neurophysiol.* **86:** 1–39.

38. Destexhe, A., M. Rudolph & D. Pare. 2003. The high-conductance state of neocortical neurons in vivo. *Nat. Rev. Neurosci.* **4:** 739–751.

39. Feldman, A.G. & G.N. Orlovsky. 1975. Activity of interneurons mediating reciprocal Ia inhibition during locomotion. *Brain Res.* **84:** 181–194.

40. Deliagina, T.G. & G.N. Orlovsky. 1980. Activity of Ia inhibitory interneurons during fictitious scratch reflex in the cat. *Brain Res.* **193:** 439–447.

Ann. N.Y. Acad. Sci. ISSN 0077-8923

Propriospinal transmission of the locomotor command signal in the neonatal rat

Kristine C. Cowley,[1] Eugene Zaporozhets,[1] and Brian J. Schmidt[1,2]

[1]Department of Physiology, Faculty of Medicine, University of Manitoba, Winnipeg, Canada. [2]Department of Internal Medicine, Section of Neurology, Faculty of Medicine, University of Manitoba, Winnipeg, Canada

Address for correspondance: Brian J. Schmidt, Department of Physiology, Faculty of Medicine, University of Manitoba, 745 Bannatyne Avenue, 406 BMSB, Winnipeg, Manitoba, Canada R3E 0J9. Voice: 204-789-3263; fax: 204-789-3930. brian@scrc.umanitoba.ca

Long direct bulbospinal projections are known to convey descending activation of locomotor networks. Less is understood about the role, if any, of propriospinal mechanisms in this function. Here we review our recent studies on propriospinal neurons in the *in vitro* neonatal rat brainstem-spinal cord preparation. Neurochemical suppression of synaptic activity in the cervicothoracic spinal cord blocked locomotor-like activity, suggesting synaptic relays make a critical contribution to descending transmission of the locomotor signal. Staggered contralateral hemisections in the cervicothoracic region, intended to eliminate all long direct bulbospinal transmission, failed to suppress locomotion, suggesting the propriospinal system alone is sufficient. Midsagittal lesion experiments showed that locomotor-related commissural components are required for rhythm generation in response to electrical stimulation of the brainstem and are redundantly distributed. No single segment was essential, although a bi-directional gradient was noted, centered on the thoracolumbar junction. These results strongly favor a role for propriospinal mechanisms in the activation of locomotion and suggest that propriospinal neurons are a logical target for interventions to restore locomotor function after spinal cord injury.

Keywords: locomotion; central pattern generator; spinal cord; commissural; functional recovery

It has long been known that locomotion in experimental animals is generated and coordinated by endogenous spinal cord circuitry[1,2] that theoretically remains intact below the level of a spinal cord lesion. There is evidence that this is also the case for humans.[3–5] Locomotor circuitry is normally activated by relatively simple un-modulated input from supraspinal and/or peripheral afferent sources.[6] Thus attempts to find ways of re-establishing transmission across spinal cord lesions such that the locomotor network can be recruited under voluntary control from supraspinal centers represents an attractive research challenge with important clinical implications. Obviously this requires identification, as well as characterization, of the anatomy, physiology, and transmitter chemistry of descending locomotor command pathways.

Jordan and colleagues, using brainstem-stimulated decerebrated cats with *acute* spinal cord lesions, demonstrated that bulbospinal projections originating in the medial reticular formation and

coursing through the ventrolateral funiculus (VLF) were essential for the activation of locomotion.[7] Some reports on chronic spinalized cats,[8,9] monkeys,[10] and rats[11–14] also support the hypothesis that preservation of at least some bulbospinal fibres in the VLF is critical for activation of locomotion. However, other investigators have clearly shown that cats with *chronically* lesioned ventrolateral quadrants are, in fact, capable of recovering voluntary hindlimb locomotion.[15,16] Thus, when plasticity and training effects are taken into consideration, no specific region of the spinal cord contains projections essential for eliciting locomotion.[17]

The results of the aforementioned studies implicate long-direct descending projections, such as the reticulospinal system. However, the contribution of propriospinal relays versus long bulbospinal projections cannot be determined from lesion experiments alone. Like reticulospinal projections, propriospinal pathways are widely dispersed in the spinal cord. If

doi: 10.1111/j.1749-6632.2009.05421.x

coupled with redundancy, the dispersed arrangement of these systems may account, at least in part, for the observation that locomotion recovers in chronic partially spinalized preparations regardless of the specific funiculi selected for disruption.

It has been suggested that a polysynaptic neuronal relay in the dorsolateral region of the cat spinal cord, continuous with the pontomedullary locomotor region, may activate the spinal locomotor network.[18,19] However, acute lesions of the dorsolateral fasciculus (at the C2–3 level) do not interfere with hindlimb stepping induced by electrical stimulation of the pontomedullary or mesencephalic locomotor region.[7] Therefore, if the dorsal relay system is involved in the descending activation of locomotion, it is not essential.

Previous investigations have also shown that propriospinal neurons mediate forelimb–hindlimb coordination in quadrupeds, which includes descending cervicolumbar and ascending lumbocervical connections.[20–24] Propriospinal neurons are involved in organizing intersegmental phase relationships in lamprey,[25–28] selecting appropriate motor rhythms in the turtle,[29] and coordinating arm-leg movements during walking.[30] The present discussion does not further address forelimb–hindlimb coupling or ascending propriospinal systems. The focus of this review is on the potential role of propriospinal neurons in transmitting *descending* activation of the locomotor network, using the *in vitro* neonatal rat brainstem-spinal cord model.[31–34]

Propriospinal neurons—early descriptions and definition

By the end of the 19th century neuroanatomists recognized that the spinal cord gives rise to cells with short or long axons that ascend or descend in the white matter, and terminate within the spinal cord. In his 1889 and 1904 classical publications on the histology of the nervous system Cajal classified these cells, which projected ipsilateral or contralateral to their origin, as "funicular" and "commissural" neurons, respectively.[35] Sherrington and Laslett referred to intraspinal projections as "association fibres."[36] Based on their study of certain spinal reflexes, such as the scratch reflex, they emphasized that association fibres were also capable of transmitting in a caudal direction, in contrast to Pfluger's Fourth Law which stated that spinal reflex activity was conveyed only in a rostral direction, an idea apparently widely accepted up to that time.[36]

Proprio derives from the Latin word *proprius* meaning *one's own*; the adjective *propriospinal* thus denotes: "situated wholly within the spinal cord."[37] Accordingly, *propriospinal* neurons originate, project, and terminate within the spinal cord. Although this definition may seem unambiguous, use of the term *propriospinal* sometimes requires further qualification. One issue concerns the arbitrary distinction between propriospinal neurons and spinal interneurons. That is, how far rostrally or caudally must a spinal neuron axon travel before it is considered a propriospinal unit? Some propriospinal neurons are very long, for instance extending from C1 segment to the sacral spinal cord.[38] On the other hand the minimal distance is somewhat loosely defined as "more than a spinal segment,"[39] at least "a number of segments,"[40] or minimally "several segments."[41] Jankowska has highlighted the overlapping functional and anatomical features of propriospinal neurons, interneurons, and ascending tract cells.[41] For instance, an ascending tract cell may give off collaterals to a number of spinal cord segments before terminating in its supraspinal target, in which case the tract cell is also endowed with the propriospinal property of conveying information from one segment to another. An interneuron, classified as such, because it targets another cell in the same or neighboring segment of gray matter, may also project to neurons dispersed over multiple segments. Some investigators have defined propriospinal cells for the purpose of their own work as spinal neurons originating outside of the limb segments and projecting into them, while neurons originating and projecting within the limb enlargement (including funicular projections over several segments) were considered interneurons.[42]

Lloyd proposed a "bulbospinal correlation system" wherein brainstem impulses travel through long-projecting reticulospinal and long propriospinal fibres before transmission to motoneurons via a short propriospinal system that is distributed throughout the cord.[43] He suggested that the propriospinal system be viewed as an extension of brainstem reticular nuclei receiving vestibulospinal, corticospinal, and primary afferent input, and setting the state of the animal appropriate for initiation of voluntary movement. An organization analogous to Lloyd's concept of a bulbospinal cor- relation system might be well-suited for descending and peripheral afferent integration in spinal loco- motor networks. Bulbospinal projections can tar- get the propriospinal system throughout the length of the spinal cord; for instance, even single retic- ulospinal neurons can send collateral branches to both the cervical and lumbar enlargements.[44,45] If such an organization exists, a critical question with respect to functional recovery after spinal cord in- jury is whether re-establishing propriospinal trans- mission alone, in the absence of regeneration of the parallel long bulbospinal projection system, is suf- ficient for voluntary recruitment of locomotor net- work activity.

Activation of spinal locomotor networks in the *in vitro* neonatal rat using brainstem stimulation

In order to take advantage of the *in vitro* neona- tal rat brainstem-spinal cord model for the investi- gation of locomotor-related bulbospinal pathways, a reliable method of evoking locomotion in re- sponse to supraspinal stimulation had to be devel- oped. Neurochemical stimulation of the brainstem was reported in two early studies using this prepa- ration,[46,47] and we therefore incorporated neuro- chemical activation in our initial experiments on descending propriospinal systems.[31] However, com- pared to electrical stimulation (see below), where step cycle period displays a coefficient of variation (CV) of 12%, chemical stimulation of the brainstem is associated with less stable locomotor activity (CV 31%), and does not allow for rapid initiation or termination of locomotor rhythms.[31]

Induction of locomotion in the *in vitro* neona- tal rat preparation using electrical stimulation of the brainstem was first described by Atsuta and colleagues who applied micro-stimuli (40–280 μA) to the medioventral medulla.[48] In our attempts to duplicate their method technical difficulties were encountered, which we have detailed elsewhere.[32] Thus, through trial and error, our preference has been to use relatively long duration (4–20 ms), high amplitude (1–10 mA), low frequency (0.8–2.0 Hz) stimulus pulses applied to the medioventral surface of the brainstem via a large tip (200–300 μm) metal- in-glass electrode.[32] This method elicits locomotor- like activity for up to 45 min during continuous

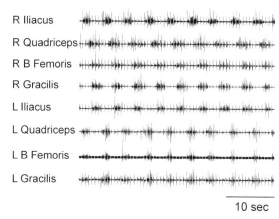

R Iliacus

R Quadriceps

R B Femoris

R Gracilis

L Iliacus

L Quadriceps

L B Femoris

L Gracilis

10 sec

Figure 1. Multichannel hindlimb electromyogram recordings of rhythmic discharge during electrical stim- ulation of the brainstem. Hip flexor (iliacus) activity al- ternates with hip extensor (biceps (B) femoris and gra- cilis) and knee extensor (quadriceps) activity. Stimula- tion artefact was partially suppressed using special pur- pose software. (Used with permission from Zaporozhets *et al.* 2004.)

stimulation in some preparations; but, more im- portantly, using shorter stimulation protocols (e.g., 60 sec) locomotor-like activity can be reliably and repeatedly evoked over the course of several hours (Fig. 1). Subsequently, Liu and Jordan reported a method involving micro-stimulation of the para- pyramidal region of the brainstem which appears to selectively target a population of serotonergic neu- rons.[49] Compared to the micro-stimulation meth- ods used by Atsuta *et al.*[48] and Liu and Jordan,[49] our macro-stimulation method is relatively indiscrimi- nate with respect to the neural elements activated in the brainstem; therefore, our method is also non- selective with respect to neurotransmitter systems released in the spinal cord. Nevertheless, because of its robustness we have found the macro-stimulation method valuable for the investigation of locomotor- related descending motor pathways.

Evidence that propriospinal pathways contribute to bulbospinal propagation of the locomotor command signal

To test whether propriospinal neurons have a role in the descending propagation of the locomo- tor command signal, we examined the effect of blocking synaptic transmission in selected cervi- cal and rostral thoracic spinal cord segments, using

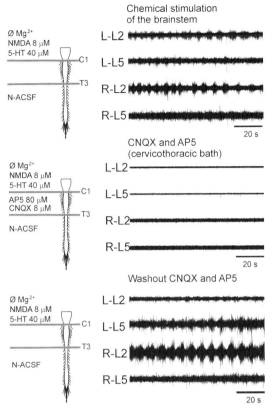

Figure 2. Suppression of synaptic transmission using glutamatergic receptor antagonists abolished locomotor-like activity evoked by chemical activation of the brainstem. The bath was partitioned at C1 and T3. Chemical stimulation of the brainstem induced lumbar locomotor-like activity (*left panel*). Application of AP5 and CNQX to the cervicothoracic region abolished rhythmic activity (*middle panel*). The effect was reversible (*right panel*). (Adapted with permission from Zaporozhets *et al.* 2006.)

double bath partitions.[31] Transmission along axons of passage, such as long direct bulbospinal projections, is unaffected using this protocol. Synaptic blockade using Ca^{2+}-free bath solutions, elevated Mg^{2+} ion concentration, or excitatory amino acid receptor antagonists (AP5 and CNQX) abolished locomotor-like discharge on lumbar ventral roots induced by either neurochemical or threshold electrical stimulation of the brainstem (Fig. 2).[31] The success of these manipulations in blocking locomotor output was related to the number of segments included. Thus, when synaptic transmission was suppressed in less than five cervicothoracic segments, brainstem-evoked locomotor-like discharge

was abolished (partially) in only 25% of preparations. Synaptic inhibition of five or more cervicothoracic segments completely abolished locomotor-like output in the lumbar region in 69% of preparations and partially blocked locomotor output in an additional 24%.

If the brainstem stimulus intensity was raised to 1.25–5 times the threshold level used to elicit locomotion in normal bath solution, exposure of the cervicothoracic segments to Ca^{2+}-free bath solution alone was usually insufficient to abolish lumbar locomotor-like activity. This was not due to electrotonic spread of the brainstem impulse through the Ca^{2+}-free compartment.[32] Complete blockade of rhythmic activity could be achieved, however, if synaptic transmission in the Ca^{2+}-free compartment was further suppressed by adding a Ca^{2+} chelating agent (ethylene glycol tetra-acetic acid, EGTA; Fig. 3) or increasing the Mg^{2+} ion concentration (to 15 mM). This observation is compatible with the fact that perfusion with Ca^{2+}-free solution alone may not guarantee the extracellular Ca^{2+} concentration is sufficiently low to block synaptic transmission.[31,50,51]

Figure 3 (*third panel*) illustrates that residual tonic discharge can persist on lumbar ventral roots after synaptic blockade of the cervicothoracic region. Tonic activity was not evident on cervical roots; this is not surprising given that last order synaptic input to cervical motoneurons, but not lumbar motoneurons, was suppressed in these experiments. Despite the absence of activity on cervical roots in the presence of Ca^{2+}-free solution shown in Figure 3, some degree of propriospinal relay activity must have persisted in the cervicothoracic region given that subsequent addition of EGTA was required to abolish rhythmic activity in the lumbar region. Persistent tonic discharge on lumbar roots, despite Ca^{2+}-free solution combined with EGTA, was likely related to transmission in long direct bulbospinal projections traversing the cervicothoracic region without synaptic relay. It appears however, that transmission in these long direct pathways alone was insufficient under these conditions for the activation of lumbar locomotor circuitry.

Glutamatergic receptor blockade using the *N*-methyl-D-aspartate (NMDA) receptor antagonist D-2-amino-5-phosphonovaleric acid (AP5) and/or the kainite/quisqualate receptor antagonist 6-cyano-7-nitorquinoxaline-2,3-dione (CNQX)

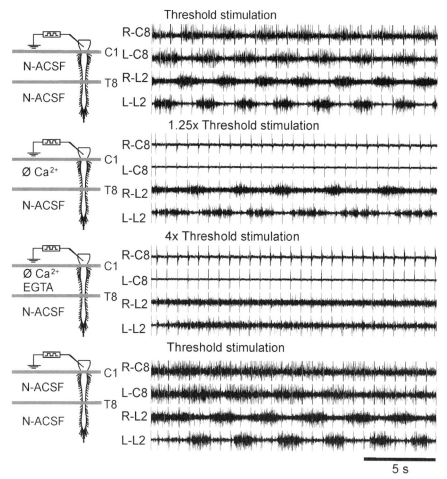

Figure 3. Ca^{2+}-free artificial cerebrospinal fluid (ACSF) abolished locomotor-like activity induced by electrical stimulation of the brainstem when combined with a Ca^{2+} ion chelator (EGTA). The bath was partitioned at C1 and T8. Cervical (C8) and lumbar (L2) ventral roots were monitored. Locomotor-like activity was elicited using threshold stimulation (*first panel*). Cervical root activity was abolished after removal of Ca^{2+} from the cervicothoracic region, although lumbar rhythmic activity persisted (*second panel*). Lumbar ventral root rhythm was also abolished, despite high intensity electrical stimulation (4T) of the brainstem, when EGTA (4 mM) was included in the bath (*third panel*). The effect was reversible (*fourth panel*). (Adapted with permission from Zaporozhets *et al.* 2006.)

blocked locomotor-like activity when threshold levels of brainstem stimulation were used, but failed to do so when higher intensity stimuli were applied. Therefore, although glutamatergic transmission appears to contribute to the activation of locomotor-related propriospinal neurons other transmitters must also participate. If a cholinergic propriospinal mechanism is involved, as previously postulated,[52] that role appears unessential in view of the observation that high concentrations of atropine (80 μM) failed to suppress lumbar locomotor-like activity.

Evidence that propriospinal neurons are sufficient for bulbospinal transmission of the locomotor command signal in the neonatal rat spinal cord

The data presented thus far, derived from the *in vitro* neonatal rat preparation, support a role for propriospinal relays, in addition to long direct bulbospinal pathways, in transmitting the locomotor command signal. In fact, the results suggest that the propriospinal contribution is *essential*. We then asked whether propriospinal pathways alone, in the

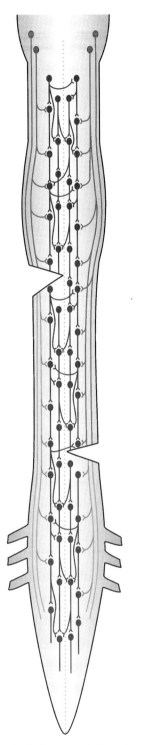

absence of long direct transmission, could be *sufficient*. This is an important issue, relevant to functional recovery, as successful regeneration of relatively short propriospinal links across the site of spinal cord injury is likely more feasible than regrowth of long direct bulbospinal projections over long distances.

To address this question we performed a series of experiments using *in vitro* neonatal rat brainstem spinal cord preparations with staggered bilateral spinal cord lesions.[33] The rostral hemisection was located between C1 and T3 and the contralateral caudal hemisection was made between T5 and mid-L1. These lesions disrupt direct long descending projections from the brainstem to the lumbar cord (Fig. 4). Propriospinal pathways are also disrupted by these lesions, which further reduces the chance of eliciting lumbar locomotor-like activity in response to brainstem stimulation. Nevertheless, locomotor-like activity was induced under these conditions (Fig. 5A). The rate of success (27%) was not related to the number of segments between the rostral and caudal hemisections (range 2–19). Success at inducing locomotor-like activity was also independent of whether the rostral hemisection was made above, below, or within the cervical enlargement.

This observation is compatible with propagation of the descending signal via a propriospinal system that includes a commissural component in the inter-lesion zone. The possibility that long direct bulbospinal projections can also cross the midline in the inter-lesion zone and then continue without an intervening synapse to the lumbar region is not absolutely excluded. However, we previously detailed evidence for and against the existence of such long commissural pathways and have discussed reasons why propriospinal commissural projections are more likely the substrate of rostrocaudal locomotor signal propagation in the presence of staggered contralateral hemisections.[33]

Lumbar locomotor-like activity was also successfully elicited by selectively stimulating

Figure 4. Hypothetical representation of propriospinal and direct bulbospinal systems involved in descending transmission of the locomotor command signal. Staggered contralateral hemisections shown are designed to disrupt all long direct descending bulbospinal projections to the lumbosacral segments. (Adapted with permission from Cowley *et al.* 2008.)

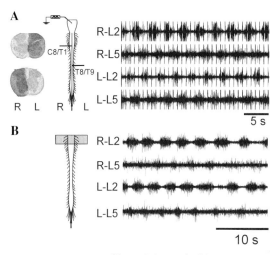

Figure 5. Locomotor-like activity evoked in response to electrical stimulation of the brainstem in the presence of staggered hemisections (A) and in response to chemical activation of the rostral spinal cord in an intact preparation (B). (A) Locomotor-like activity in this preparation was well developed (CV = 13%) despite hemisections located below the cervical enlargement (right C8/T1) and at left T8/9. Note, the dark region of the axial tissue sections indicates the extent of residual *intact* spinal cord at the lesion site, superimposed on the nearest section of nonlesioned bilaterally intact spinal cord. (B) Locomotor-like activity (CV = 19%) was evoked in the lumbar region by chemical stimulation of propriospinal neurons in the rostral cervical region. Bath application of 5-HT (50 μM) and NMDA (15 μM) to spinal cord segments C1–C4 produced rhythmic alternating activity of left and right sides as well as ipsilateral L2 and L5 alternation. (Adapted with permission from Cowley *et al.* 2008.)

(neurochemically) spinal neuronal cell bodies in the rostral cervical cord (Fig. 5B).[33] Because axons of passage, such as long bulbospinal projections, are not activated by this method, the finding further supports the concept of propriospinal relays alone having the capacity to transmit the descending locomotor activating signal.

Commissural projections support bulbospinal activation of locomotion

Given the aforementioned observation that commissural projections in the cervicothoracic region transfer descending locomotor command information from one side of the cord to the other, we examined the effect of midsagittal lesions made at various

rostrocaudal locations.[34] In some preparations midsagittal lesions throughout the entire spinal cord had no effect on the capacity to evoke locomotor-like activity in response to electrical stimulation of the brainstem, *provided at least two or three contiguous segments remained bilaterally intact*. More specifically, neither the potential for rhythm generation nor left–right coordination was affected by these extensive lesions of the commissural system. However, the remaining intact bridges had to include the T13 or L1 segments. Locomotor-like activity was also induced neurochemically in some preparations by applying 5-hydroxytryptamine and NMDA to the whole cord.[34] Appropriately coordinated left–right locomotor-like alternation was elicited even when only one segment remained bilaterally intact (Fig. 6A). However, single bridges located in the thoracolumbar junction region were most effective (Fig. 6B). Thus, the results of lesion experiments using brainstem stimulation and direct neurochemical activation of the spinal cord both suggest that preservation of commissural projections in the thoracolumbar junction region is critical for eliciting coordinated left–right alternating locomotor-like activity.

However, in other preparations, midsagittal separation from C1 to mid-L1, or from the conus medullaris to the T12/13 junction, had no effect on lumbar locomotor-like activity, despite these lesions interrupting commissural connections in the T13 and L1 segments. In addition, preparations bilaterally intact with the exception of midsagittal lesions restricted to the thoracolumbar junction region (from T12 to L2 inclusive) were also capable of developing coordinated left–right alternating locomotor-like activity in response to brainstem stimulation (Fig. 7). Thus, the combined midsagittal lesion data indicate that no specific rostrocaudal level of the spinal cord contains essential locomotor-related commissural projections. However, in the presence of extensive midsagittal separation of the left and right halves of the spinal cord, preservation of cross projections through the thoracolumbar junction (T13 or L1) appears to be particularly important for eliciting locomotor-like activity. These data also suggest that the left–right coordinating mechanism for locomotion is robust and redundantly distributed.

There is no doubt that commissural projections in the lumbar region have a role in inter-limb

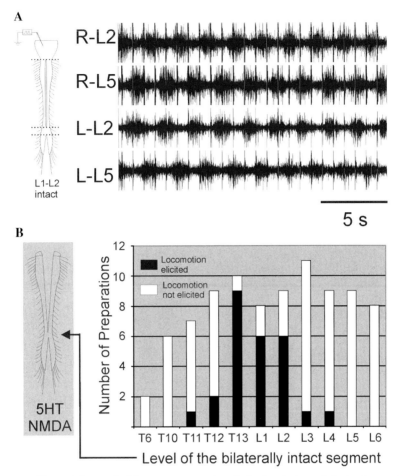

Figure 6. Locomotor-like activity evoked in response to electrical stimulation of the brainstem in preparations with only two or three segments bilaterally intact (**A**) whereas chemical stimulation evoked locomotor activity in preparations with only one segment bilaterally intact (**B**). (**B**) Summary of the induction of coordinated locomotor-like activity following application of 5HT and NMDA to preparations with a single bilaterally intact segment, as indicated on the *x*-axis. (Used with permission from Cowley *et al.* 2009.)

control during locomotion, as only they can maintain side-to-side coordination in isolated (bilaterally intact) lumbar or lumbosacral spinal cord preparations.[53–55] However, we observed that commissural connections in lumbar segments are not *essential* for left–right coordination during locomotion, as this function can be served by more rostrally located segments.[34,56] This finding is compatible with previous work using this preparation[57] as well as results from cat,[58] turtle,[59] and lamprey.[60]

One difference between whole-cord neurochemically induced activity and activity elicited by brainstem stimulation was that commissural connections had to be preserved in at least two or three contiguous segments in order for brainstem stimulation to induce rhythmic activity.[34] Similarly, complete disruption of the commissural system in larval lamprey abolishes locomotion in response to descending supraspinal inputs.[60] In contrast, direct neurochemical application can induce rhythmic activity in the completely isolated hemi-spinal cord of rodents[34,55–57,61] as well as the mudpuppy[62] and embryonic chick.[63] Thus, in the intact animal, in addition to mediating inter-limb coordination, commissural propriospinal neurons may target the locomotor rhythm-generating circuitry. This is compatible with the two level model of the central pattern generator proposed by McCrea and Rybak,

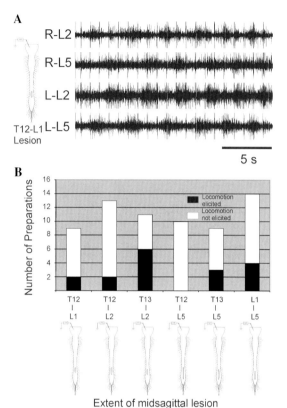

Figure 7. Midsagittal lesions restricted to the lower thoracic-upper lumbar region did not abolish locomotor-like activity. (**A**) Electrical stimulation of the brainstem evoked locomotor-like activity in this preparation with a midsagittal lesion from the T12 to L1 segments, inclusive. (**B**) Summary chart showing the number of preparations that developed locomotor-like activity in response to brainstem electrical stimulation after midsagittal lesions through the indicated segmental levels (inclusive). (Used with permission from Cowley *et al.* 2009.)

which suggests strong propriospinal connections are an important feature of a single widely distributed rhythm generator, which controls pattern formation circuitry.[64]

Discussion

Several studies have reported that staggered contralateral hemisections of the *in vivo* spinal cord of monkeys,[65] humans,[66] cats[8] and weanling and adult rats[13,67] is associated with permanent paralysis. Stelzner and Cullen demonstrated that newborn rats with staggered hemisections can recover stepping movements by 30 days of age; however, recov-

ery was attributed to intrinsic spinal cord mechanisms (subsequent complete transection, rostral to the level of initial hemisections, failed to abolish recovered locomotor activity[13]). Kato *et al.* came to a similar conclusion after observing hindlimb stepping in cats with chronic staggered contralateral hemisections.[68] In particular, they noted that hindlimb and forelimb rhythms were not phase-related. Therefore, they suggested that rather than propriospinal mechanisms the hindlimb stepping generators in their preparations were activated by hindlimb afferent input. In contrast, Courtine and colleagues recently concluded that propriospinal transmission, rather than autonomous spinal cord circuitry, accounted for recovery of locomotion in mice with chronic staggered bilateral spinal cord hemisections.[69] Mice receiving a T12 hemisection and then a contralateral T7 hemisection (10 weeks later) at a time when stepping had returned on the side of the initial lesion, recovered bilateral hindlimb locomotor ability over the course of four weeks. Retrograde labeling techniques showed an increasing number of propriospinal neurons, in the inter-lesion zone, during the recovery period.[69] Interestingly, and in contrast to our result using an *in vitro* preparation, when the staggered hemisections were made simultaneously at the time of the first operation mice failed to recover locomotor function during a four week observation period.

Extrapolation of our findings using an immature *in vitro* preparation to the adult intact animal is not without some obvious limitations. However, one advantage of the isolated brainstem-spinal cord model is that it provides unequivocal evidence that any observed lumbar locomotor-like activity is due to descending supraspinal activation (i.e., brainstem electrical stimulation). The fact that the hindlimbs are removed and the preparation is stationary further argues against the possibility that autonomous locomotor circuitry in the spinal cord was activated in response to hindlimb afferent input.

The results of the adult *in vivo* rodent preparation[69] combined with observations from the *in vitro* neonatal rat model strongly favor a role for the propriospinal system in the descending propagation of the locomotor command signal. Both the *in vitro* and *in vivo* results also suggest that propriospinal pathways are sufficient in this role during acute (*in vitro*) and chronic (*in vivo*) recovery from injury. The findings also expand the significance of earlier observations derived from the lamprey[70,71] and chick embryo[72] which demonstrated the recruitment of propriospinal circuitry during recovery of locomotion after spinal cord injury.

In conclusion, the mammalian propriospinal system is a logical target for interventions aimed at restoring function after spinal cord injury. Indeed it has already been shown, in the adult rat, that sprouts of transected corticospinal tract axons can project to propriospinal neurons as a means of rerouting cortical influence onto lumbar neurons.[73,74] Nonspecific intraspinal microstimulation of thoracic propriospinal neurons in the rat has a small but significant beneficial effect on hindlimb stepping.[75] Ultimately, a combination of electrical excitation, pharmacological stimulation, and regeneration strategies will likely be required to optimize functional recovery after spinal cord injury.

Acknowledgments

This work was supported by the Canadian Institutes of Health Research and a Will-to-Win scholarship awarded to KCC.

References

1. Graham Brown, T. 1911. The intrinsic factors in the act of progression in the mammal. *Proc. R. Soc. B.* **84:** 308–319.

2. Graham Brown, T. 1914. On the nature of the fundamental activity of the nervous centres; together with an analysis of the conditioning of rhythmic activity in progression, and a theory of the evolution of function in the nervous system. *J. Physiol.* **48:** 18–46.

3. Bussel, B., A. Roby-Brami, P. Azouvi, *et al.* 1988. Myoclonus in a patient with spinal cord transection. Possible involvement of the spinal stepping generator. *Brain* **111**(Pt 5): 1235–1245.

4. Calancie, B., B. Needham-Shropshire, P. Jacobs, *et al.* 1994. Involuntary stepping after chronic spinal cord injury. Evidence for a central rhythm generator for locomotion in man. *Brain* **117**(Pt 5): 1143–1159.

5. Dietz, V., G. Colombo & L. Jensen. 1994. Locomotor activity in spinal man. *Lancet* **344:** 1260–1263.

6. Hultborn, H. & J. B. Nielsen. 2007. Spinal control of locomotion—from cat to man. *Acta Physiol. (Oxf)* **189:** 111–121.

7. Noga, B.R., D.J. Kriellaars & L.M. Jordan. 1991. The effect of selective brainstem or spinal cord lesions on treadmill locomotion evoked by stimulation of the mesencephalic or pontomedullary locomotor regions. *J. Neurosci.* **11**(6): 1691–1700.

8. Jane, J.A., J.P. Evans & L.E. Fisher. 1964. An investigation concerning the restitution of motor function following injury to the spinal cord. *J. Neurosurg.* **21:** 167–171.

9. Afelt, Z. 1974. Functional significance of ventral descending tracts of the spinal cord in the cat. *Acta Neurobiol. Exp.* **34:** 393–407.

10. Eidelberg, E., J.L. Story, J.G. Walden, *et al.* 1981. Anatomical correlates of return of locomotor function after partial spinal cord lesions in cats. *Exp. Brain Res.* **42:** 81–88.

11. Little, J.W., R.M. Harris & R.C. Sohlberg. 1988. Locomotor recovery following subtotal spinal cord lesions in a rat model. *Neurosci. Lett.* **87:** 189–194.

12. Schucht, P., O. Raineteau, M. E. Schwab, *et al.* 2002. Anatomical correlates of locomotor recovery following dorsal and ventral lesions of the rat spinal cord. *Exp. Neurol.* **176:** 143–153.

13. Stelzner, D. J. & J. M. Cullen. 1991. Do propriospinal projections contribute to hindlimb recovery when all long tracts are cut in neonatal or weanling rats? *Exp. Neurol.* **114:** 193–205.

14. You, S.W., B.Y. Chen, H.L. Liu, *et al.* 2003. Spontaneous recovery of locomotion induced by remaining fibers after spinal cord transection in adult rats. *Restor. Neurol. Neurosci.* 21: 39–45.

15. Brustein, E. & S. Rossignol. 1998. Recovery of locomotion after ventral and ventrolateral spinal lesions in the cat. I. Deficits and adaptive mechanisms. *J. Neurophysiol.* **80:** 1245–1267.

16. Bem, T., T. Gorska, H. Majczynski, *et al.* 1995. Different patterns of fore-hindlimb coordination during overground locomotion in cats with ventral and lateral spinal lesions. *Exp. Brain Res.* **104:** 70–80.

17. Rossignol, S., C. Chau, E. Brustein, *et al.* 1996. Locomotor capacities after complete and partial lesions of the spinal cord. *Acta Neurobiol. Exp.* **56:** 449–463.

18. Shik, M.L. 1983. Action of the brainstem locomotor region on spinal stepping generators via propriospinal pathways. In *Spinal Cord Reconstruction.* C. C. Kao, R. P. Bunge & P. J. Reier, Eds.: 421–434. Raven Press. New York.

19. Yamaguchi, T. 1986. Descending pathways eliciting forelimb stepping in the lateral funiculus: experimental studies with stimulation and lesion of the cervical cord in decerebrate cats. *Brain Res.* **379:** 125–136.

20. Miller, S., J. Van Der Burg & F.G.A. Van Der Meche. 1975. Coordination of movements of the hindlimbs and forelimbs in different forms of locomotion in normal and decerebrate cats. *Brain Res.* **91:** 217–237.

21. Ballion, B., D. Morin & D. Viala. 2001. Forelimb loco-motor generators and quadrupedal locomotion in the neonatal rat. **14:** 1727–1738.

22. Juvin, L., J. Simmers & D. Morin. 2005. Propriospinal circuitry underlying interlimb coordination in mammalian quadrupedal locomotion. *J. Neurosci.* **25:** 6025–6035.

23. Reed, W.R., A. Shum-Siu, S.M. Onifer, *et al.* 2006. Inter-enlargement pathways in the ventrolateral funiculus of the adult rat spinal cord. *Neuroscience* **142:** 1195–1207.

24. English, A.W., J. Tigges & P.R. Lennard. 1985. Anatomical organization of long ascending propriospinal neurons in the cat spinal cord. *J. Comp. Neurol.* **240:** 349–358.

25. Matsushima, T. & S. Grillner. 1990. Intersegmental co-ordination of undulatory movements—a "trailing oscil-lator" hypothesis. *NeuroReport* **1:** 97–100.

26. Cohen, A.H., G.B. Ermentrout, T. Kiemel, *et al.* 1992. Modelling of intersegmental coordination in the lam-prey central pattern generator for locomotion. *Trends Neurosci.* **15:** 434–438.

27. Miller, W.L. & K.A. Sigvardt. 2000. Extent and role of multisegmental coupling in the lamprey spinal locomo-tor pattern generator. *J. Neurophysiol.* **83:** 465–476.

28. Buchanan, J.T. 1992. Neural network simulations of cou-pled locomotor oscillators in the lamprey spinal cord. *Biol. Cybern.* **66:** 367–374.

29. Berkowitz, A. & P.S. Stein. 1994. Activity of descending propriospinal axons in the turtle hindlimb enlargement during two forms of fictive scratching: phase analyses. *J. Neurosci.* **14:** 5105–5119.

30. Dietz, V. 2002. Do human bipeds use quadrupedal coor-dination? *Trends Neurosci.* **25:** 462–467.

31. Zaporozhets, E., K.C. Cowley & B.J. Schmidt. 2006. Pro-priospinal neurons contribute to bulbospinal transmis-sion of the locomotor command signal in the neonatal rat spinal cord. *J. Physiol.* **572:** 443–458.

32. Zaporozhets, E., K.C. Cowley & B.J. Schmidt. 2004. A reliable technique for the induction of locomotor-like activity in the *in vitro* neonatal rat spinal cord using brainstem electrical stimulation. *J. Neurosci. Meth.* **139:** 33–41.

33. Cowley, K.C., E. Zaporozhets & B.J. Schmidt. 2008. Pro-priospinal neurons are sufficient for bulbospinal trans-mission of the locomotor command signal in the neona-tal rat spinal cord. *J. Physiol.* **586:** 1623–1635.

34. Cowley, K.C., E. Zaporozhets, R.A. Joundi, *et al.* 2009. Contribution of commissural projections to bulbospinal activation of locomotion in the *in vitro* neonatal rat spinal cord. *J. Neurophysiol.* **101:** 1171–1178.

35. Cajal, S.R.y. 1995. *Histology of the Nervous System (Vol 1):*

General Principles, Spinal Cord, Spinal Ganglia, Medulla & Pons. Translated by Swanson, N. & L. W. Swanson. Oxford University Press. Oxford.

36. Sherrington, C.S. & E.E. Laslett. 1903. Observations on some spinal reflexes and the interconnection of spinal segments. *J. Physiol.* **29:** 58–96.

37. 1993. Propriospinal. In *The New Shorter Oxford English Dictionary*, Vol. 2. Oxford University Press. Oxford.

38. Miller, K.E., V.D. Douglas, A.B. Richards, *et al.* 1998. Propriospinal neurons in the C1–C2 spinal segments project to the L5-S1 segments of the rat spinal cord. *Brain Res. Bull.* **47:** 43–47.

39. Kostyuk, P.G. & D.A. Vasilenko. 1979. Spinal interneu-rons. *Annu. Rev. Physiol.* **41:** 115–126.

40. Burke, D. 2001. Clinical relevance of the putative C-3–4 propriospinal system in humans. *Muscle Nerve.* **24:** 1437–1439.

41. Jankowska, E. 1992. Interneuronal relay in spinal path-ways from proprioceptors. *Prog. Neurobiol.* **38:** 335–378.

42. Illert, M., A. Lundberg & R. Tanaka. 1977. Integration in descending motor pathways controlling the forelimb in the cat. Part 3. Convergence on propriospinal neurones transmitting disynaptic excitation from the corticospinal tract and other descending tracts. *Exp. Brain Res.* **29:** 323–346.

43. Lloyd, D.P.C. 1941. Activity in neurons of the bulbospinal correlation system. *J. Neurophysiol.* **4:** 115–134.

44. Peterson, B.W., R.A. Maunz, N.G. Pitts, *et al.* 1975. Pat-terns of projection and braching of reticulospinal neu-rons. *Exp. Brain Res.* **23:** 333–351.

45. Martin, G.F., T. Cabana & A.O. Humbertson, Jr. 1981. Evidence for collateral innervation of the cervical and lumbar enlargements of the spinal cord by single reticular and raphe neurons. Studies using fluorescent markers in double-labeling experiments on the North American opossum. *Neurosci. Lett.* **24:** 1–6.

46. Atsuta, Y., P. Abraham, T. Iwahara, *et al.* 1991. Con-trol of locomotion *in vitro*: II. Chemical stimulation. *Somatosens. Mot. Res.* **8:** 55–63.

47. Smith, J.C., J.L. Feldman & B.J. Schmidt. 1988. Neural mechanisms generating locomotion studied in mam-malian brainstem-spinal cord *in vitro*. *FASEB J.* **2:** 2283–2288.

48. Atsuta, Y., E. Garcia-Rill & R.D. Skinner. 1988. Electri-cally induced locomotion in the *in vitro* brainstem-spinal cord preparation. *Brain Res. Dev. Brain Res.* **42:** 309–312.

49. Liu, J. & L.M. Jordan. 2005. Stimulation of the parapyra-midal region of the neonatal rat brain stem produces locomotor-like activity involving spinal 5-HT7 and 5-HT2A receptors. *J. Neurophysiol.* **94:** 1392–1404.

Ann. N.Y. Acad. Sci. 1198 (2010) 42–53 © 2010 New York Academy of Sciences.

50. Kuwana, S., Y. Okada & T. Natsui. 1998. Effects of extracellular calcium and magnesium on central respiratory control in the brainstem-spinal cord of neonatal rat. *Brain Res.* **786:** 194–204.

51. Piccolino, M., A. Pignatelli & L. A. Rakotobe. 1999. Calcium-independent release of neurotransmitter in the retina: a "copernican" viewpoint change. *Prog. Retin. Eye Res.* **18:** 1–38.

52. Jordan, L.M. & B.J. Schmidt. 2002. Propriospinal neurons involved in the control of locomotion: potential targets for repair strategies? *Prog. Brain Res.* **137:** 125–139.

53. Barbeau, H. & S. Rossignol. 1987. Recovery of locomotion after chronic spinalization in the adult cat. *Brain Res.* **412:** 84–95.

54. Forssberg, H., S. Grillner, J. Halbertsma, *et al.* 1980. The locomotion of the low spinal cat. II. Interlimb coordination. *Acta Physiol. Scand.* **108:** 283–295.

55. Kudo, N. & T. Yamada. 1987. N-methyl-D,L-aspartate-induced locomotor activity in a spinal cord-hindlimb muscles preparation of the newborn rat studied *in vitro*. *Neurosci. Lett.* **75:** 43–48.

56. Cowley, K.C. & B.J. Schmidt. 1997. Regional distribution of the locomotor pattern-generating network in the neonatal rat spinal cord. *J. Neurophysiol.* **77:** 247–259.

57. Kremer, E. & A. Lev-Tov. 1997. Localization of the spinal network associated with generation of hindlimb locomotion in the neonatal rat and organization of its transverse coupling system. *J. Neurophysiol.* **77:** 1155–1170.

58. Kato, M. 1988. Longitudinal myelotomy of lumbar spinal cord has little effect on coordinated locomotor activities of bilateral hindlimbs of the chronic cats. *Neurosci. Lett.* **93:** 259–263.

59. Samara, R.F. & S.N. Currie. 2007. Crossed commissural pathways in the spinal hindlimb enlargement are not necessary for right left hindlimb alternation during turtle swimming. *J. Neurophysiol.* **98:** 2223–2231.

60. Jackson, A.W., D.F. Horinek, M.R. Boyd, *et al.* 2005. Disruption of left–right reciprocal coupling in the spinal cord of larval lamprey abolishes brain-initiated locomotor activity. *J. Neurophysiol.* **94:** 2031–2044.

61. Bonnot, A. & D. Morin. 1998. Hemisegmental localisation of rhythmic networks in the lumbosacral spinal cord of neonate mouse. *Brain Res.* **793:** 136–148.

62. Cheng, J., R.B. Stein, K. Jovanovic, *et al.* 1998. Identification, localization, and modulation of neural networks for walking in the mudpuppy (Necturus Maculatus) spinal cord. *J. Neurosci.* **18:** 4295–4304.

63. Ho, S. & M.J. O'Donovan. 1993. Regionalization and intersegmental coordination of rhythm-generating networks in the spinal cord of the chick embryo. *J. Neurosci.* **13:** 1354–1371.

64. McCrea, D. A. & I. A. Rybak. 2008. Organization of mammalian locomotor rhythm and pattern generation. *Brain Res. Rev.* **57:** 134–146.

65. Lassek, A.M. & P.A. Anderson. 1961. Motor function after spaced contralateral hemisections in the spinal cord. *Neurology* **11**(Pt 1): 362–365.

66. Nathan, P.W. & M.C. Smith. 1973. Effects of two unilateral cordotomies on the motility of the lower limbs. *Brain* **96:** 471–494.

67. Harris, R.M., J.W. Little & B. Goldstein. 1994. Spared descending pathways mediate locomotor recovery after subtotal spinal cord injury. *Neurosci. Lett.* **180:** 37–40.

68. Kato, M., S. Murakami, K. Yasuda & H. Hirayama. 1984. Disruption of fore- and hindlimb coordination during overground locomotion in cats with bilateral serial hemisection of the spinal cord. *Neurosci. Res.* **2:** 27–47.

69. Courtine, G., B. Song, R.R. Roy, *et al.* 2008. Recovery of supraspinal control of stepping via indirect propriospinal relay connections after spinal cord injury. *Nat. Med.* **14:** 69–74.

70. McClellan, A.D. 1994. Time course of locomotor recovery and functional regeneration in spinal cord-transected lamprey: *in vitro* preparations. *J. Neurophysiol.* **72:** 847–860.

71. Rouse, D.T., Jr. & A.D. McClellan. 1997. Descending propriospinal neurons in normal and spinal cord-transected lamprey. *Exp. Neurol.* **146:** 113–124.

72. Sholomenko, G.N. & K.R. Delaney. 1998. Restitution of functional neural connections in chick embryos assessed *in vitro* after spinal cord transection in ovo. *Exp. Neurol.* **154:** 430–451.

73. Bareyre, F.M., M. Kerschensteiner, O. Raineteau, *et al.* 2004. The injured spinal cord spontaneously forms a new intraspinal circuit in adult rats. *Nat Neurosci.* **7:** 269–277.

74. Vavrek, R., J. Girgis, W. Tetzlaff, *et al.* 2006. BDNF promotes connections of corticospinal neurons onto spared descending interneurons in spinal cord injured rats. *Brain* **129:** 1534–1545.

75. Yakovenko, S., J. Kowalczewski & A. Prochazka. 2007. Intraspinal stimulation caudal to spinal cord transections in rats. Testing the propriospinal hypothesis. *J. Neurophysiol.* **97:** 2570–2574.

Ann. N.Y. Acad. Sci. ISSN 0077-8923

ANNALS OF THE NEW YORK ACADEMY OF SCIENCES

Issue: *Neurons and Networks in the Spinal Cord*

Sensory-induced activation of pattern generators in the absence of supraspinal control

A. Lev-Tov,[1] A. Etlin,[1] and D. Blivis[1,2]

[1]Department of Medical Neurobiology, IMRIC, The Hebrew University Medical School, Jerusalem, Israel. [2]Current address of D. Blivis: The section of Developmental Neurobiology, NINDS, NIH, Bethesda, Maryland

Address for correspondence: Aharon Lev-Tov, Ph.D., Department of Medical Neurobiology, The Hebrew University Medical School, Jerusalem 91010, Israel. Voice: 972-2-675-8445; fax: 972-2-675-7451. aharonl@ekmd.huji.ac.il

Sacrocaudal afferent (SCA) stimulation is used in this work to study neural pathways involved in sensory-activation of central pattern generators (CPGs) in the isolated spinal cord of the neonatal rat. Surgical manipulations of the white matter funiculi and confocal imaging of back-labeled funicular pathways suggest that the CPGs are activated during SCA stimulation by crossed and uncrossed multifunicular projections of sacral neurons and that activation of short projecting proprioneurons is sufficient for the generation of the rhythm by SCA stimulation. The versatile organization of the pathways involved in the SCA-induced rhythm makes it a potent and durable activator of the CPGs in the absence of descending control from the brain. The significance of our findings and their potential clinical use are discussed.

Keywords: sacrocaudal afferents; propriospinal; ascending pathways; spinal motoneurons; locomotor

Introduction

The ability of sensory input to activate the spinal pattern generating circuitry and control the timing of stepping has long been reported for spinalized cats (reviewed in refs. 1 and 2) and rats[3] (reviewed in ref. 4). Recently, several clinical studies emphasized the importance of sensory activation of locomotor rhythms by showing that input from load and joint receptors can re-activate the locomotor central pattern generators (CPGs) and improve the mobility of patients with incomplete thoracic injury of the spinal cord.[5–8] Our studies of the isolated mammalian spinal cord preparation have revealed that stimulation of sacrocaudal afferents (SCAs) is a potent activator of motor rhythms in the sacral and thoracolumbar[9–12] spinal segments (Fig. 1), and that the thoracolumbar rhythm produced by SCA stimulation exhibits a typical locomotor-like pattern.[11,13] Thus, the SCA induced rhythm in the isolated rodent spinal cord preparation can be used to study the pathways and mechanisms involved in sensory activation of locomotor activity in the absence of the descending control from the brain. In the present work, we briefly review our recent findings concern-ing the neural pathways interposed between SCA and the thoracolumbar CPGs with special attention to the various factors that contribute to the unique potency of SCA stimulation to produce coordinated motor rhythms.

Different types of afferents can induce the rhythm

Figures 1A–C show ventral root recordings from three different spinal cord preparations of 3-day-old rats. The rhythmic activity in these preparations was induced by a transient mechanical stimulation of a sacrocaudal dermatome at the base of the tail in a hindlimb spinal cord preparation (Fig. 1A; e.g., see refs. 9 and 14), and by electrical stimulation of dorsal root afferents entering the first coccygeal dorsal root (Co1, Figs. 1B and C). The rhythm shown in Figure 1C was recorded from the left and right ventral roots of the flexor dominated L2, and the extensor dominated L5 segment. It is characterized by an alternating left–right and an alternating flexor extensor pattern. Thus, the rhythm can be generated by mechanical stimulation of dermatomes and by low- and

doi: 10.1111/j.1749-6632.2009.05424.x

 Ann. N.Y. Acad. Sci. 1198 (2010) 54–62 © 2010 New York Academy of Sciences.

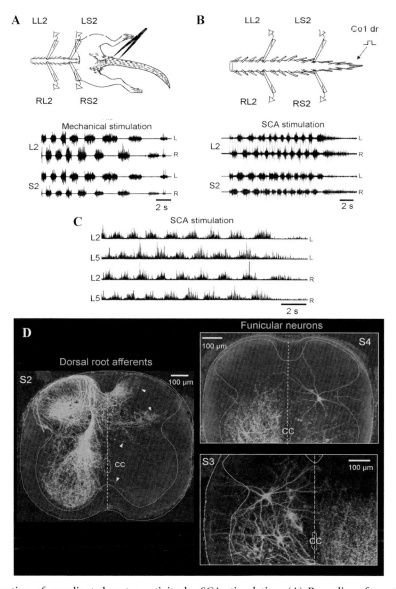

Figure 1. Generation of coordinated motor activity by SCA stimulation. (A) Recordings from the left (L) and right (R) ventral roots of the 2nd lumbar and sacral segments of the spinal cord (L2 and S2, respectively) show alternating left–right rhythmic bursts produced following a brief mechanical stimulation of sacrocaudal dermatomes in a hindlimb-tail-spinal cord preparation. (B) Recordings of an alternating left–right rhythm from the left and right L2 and S2 ventral roots during a 30-pulse 2.5 Hz stimulus train applied to the left Co1 dorsal root at 1.6× threshold (T). (C) The rhythm recorded from the left and right L2 and L5 ventral roots shows left–right alternation and alternating flexor-extensor bursts on a given side of the spinal cord. Data were high-pass filtered at 40 Hz and rectified. The 40 pulse, 3 Hz stimulus train to Co1 was applied at 1.8 T. (D) The branching pattern of sacrocaudal afferents and of the dendrites of funicular neurons. Confocal projected image of the caudal S2 segment following anterograde labeling of SCAs entering the right S3 dorsal root with fluorescein dextran (*left*). Afferents branching to the contralateral superficial and deep dorsal horn and to the intermediate and ventral laminae of the gray matter are pointed to by arrowheads. The dendrites of sacral neurons back-filled with fluorescein dextran through the VF at the S2 level, exhibit clear projections to the contralateral side in the confocal micrographs of the S3 and S4 segments in different preparations (*right*). CC = central canal; dashed line = midline.

high-intensity stimulation of afferents.[9,10,15] Moreover, we have shown that the rhythm could also be generated by radiant heat stimulation of sacrocaudal dermatomes[15] (see ref. 16 for cat studies) and that the rhythm produced by mechanical, radiant heat, and electrical stimulation is blocked by application of mu-opioids to the sacral but not the thoracolumbar segments of the spinal cord.[15] Further support to the involvement of pain-delivering pathways in the generation of the locomotor rhythm has been recently provided for the neonatal mouse spinal cord where application of transient receptor potential (TRP) channel agonists was found to be a potent modulator of the locomotor rhythm.[17] The ability of SCA stimulation to activate the CPGs has also been reported in spinal cats where perineal stimulation is routinely used to initiate stepping.[18] In summary, the rhythm can be produced by activation of different sensory modalities, and the nociceptive and nonnociceptive afferent pathways associated with them.[15]

The branching patterns of sacral afferents and the dendrites of the recipient neurons

The ability of afferent-stimulation to produce locomotor-like activity is not unique to the sacrocaudal region. Stimulation of hindlimb flexor reflex afferents (FRAs) has long been shown to produce a stepping-like pattern in spinal cats following systemic administration of L-Dopa and Nialamide[19–22] (for review see refs. 23 and 24), and stimulation of lumbar dorsal roots has been reported to induce locomotor-like activity in the isolated spinal cord preparation of the neonatal rat[14,25] and mouse.[13] However, it seems that stimulation of SCA has higher capacity to generate a robust and regular thoracolumbar and sacral rhythmic activity than stimulation of the pathways mentioned above. One of the factors that may contribute to this capacity is the branching pattern of the SCA and that of the dendrites of the recipient sacral neurons. Our recent studies revealed that the stimulated sacral afferents have a bilateral branching pattern and they can directly innervate sacral relay neurons located ipsi- and contralaterally to the stimulated dorsal root (Blivis, Mentis, O'Donovan & Lev-Tov, unpublished). Figure 1D (*left*) shows a confocal micrograph of a cross-section of the S2 segment following anterograde loading of SCAs entering the right S3

dorsal root with fluorescein dextran. The afferents ramify to innervate the left and right gray matter. The crossed afferent projections terminate in the superficial and deep dorsal horn laminae and in laminae IX and VII (yellow arrowheads). Some of these branches terminated close to the lateral most aspect of the contralateral gray matter. These findings resemble the crossed branching pattern described for various types of afferents in the sacrocaudal segments of the cat spinal cord.[26] Another finding that may assist the bilateral activation of sacral neurons by SCA stimulation is the branching pattern of the sacral relay neurons. Backfilling of cut funicular axons with fluorescent dextrans, showed that many of the labeled funicular neurons extended their dendrites across the midline. Examples of sacral neurons with crossed dendrites are shown in the projected confocal images in Figure 1D (*right*). A similar branching pattern of sacral neurons has been reported for HRP filled cells in the dorsal horn of the cat spinal cord.[27] Thus, the crossed and uncrossed afferent projections to the gray matter and their direct synaptic contacts with crossed and uncrossed dendritic projections of sacral neurons whose axons ascend rostrally to the lumbar cord (Blivis, Mentis, O'Donovan & Lev-Tov, unpublished) should provide a potent means for bilateral activation of these neurons during unilateral SCA stimulation.

Heterogeneous populations of sacral neurons with multifunicular projections are activated by sacrocaudal afferent stimulation to produce the rhythm

Our previous studies revealed that there are no direct contacts between SCA and CPGs circuitry in the thoracolumbar cord, and that the generation of the rhythm is made possible by synaptic activation of sacral relay neurons whose axons project rostrally through the white matter funiculi.[11,15,28,29] These studies also suggested that the axonal projections of these neurons through the ventral funiculi (VF) had a prominent contribution to the generation of the rhythm by SCA stimulation. More recent studies[30] revealed that bilateral interruption of any of the known divisions of the white matter funiculi did not block the rhythm produced by SCA stimulation. Moreover the sacral neurons projecting through the VF, ventrolateral and lateral funiculi (VLF/LF), and dorsolateral funiculi (DLF) but not those traveling through the dorsal funiculi (DF), were sufficient to ensure the generation of the rhythm by SCA stimulation when the rest of the funiculi were cut. The contribution of the VF projections in these latter studies was also found to be prominent. Figure 2B demonstrates that a bilateral lesion of the VF at the lumbosacral junction perturbed the rhythm produced by SCA stimulation but did not block it. The initial response to the stimulus train was characterized by a mixture of tonic and rhythmic discharge that developed at later stages of the train to a robust and regular rhythm with an alternating left–right pattern. Figure 2C, shows that the rhythm could be readily produced in the thoracolumbar segments by SCA stimulation following a multiple funicular lesion that spared the VF as the only intact funiculus. This rhythm was robust and regular.

The pathways projecting from the sacral to the thoracolumbar segments through the VF, VLF/LF, and DLF were studied using retrograde labeling of cut funicular axons with fluorescent dextrans at the lumbosacral junction, and visualized either from whole mount preparations that have been rendered transparent, or from serial sections of the labeled spinal cords using confocal microscopy imaging (Figs. 2D and 3A). Generally speaking, the pathways projecting through the VF at the lumbosacral junction were mainly crossed and those projecting via the VLF (not shown) were mainly uncrossed.[30] Moreover, most of the neurons labeled through the cut DLF were found ipsilateral to the fill (not shown, see ref. 30). Demonstration of the heterogeneity of the populations of neurons activated by SCA stimulation, and the assembly of their axonal projections through the VF is shown in Figures 2 and 3. The confocal projected image shown in Figure 2D, is a ventral view of a transparent whole mount-preparation labeled through the cut VF at the lumbosacral junction. Labeled sacral neurons were found mostly contralateral to the site of the fill. The number of the labeled neurons decreased in the caudal direction, and the axons of the contralaterally labeled neurons crossed the sacral cord through the ventral commissure and ascended rostrally (Fig. 2D). A confocal micrograph of a crossed section through the S2 segment in another VF labeled preparation is shown in Figure 3A. A dense ipsilateral neuropil of labeled VF fibers is shown on the lower left with retrogradely labeled propriospinal and tract neurons that are localized mainly to the ventral, intermediate, and deep dorsal horn laminae of the gray matter, contralateral to the fill. Three-dimensional (3-D) reconstructions of the sacral segments (S1–S4) of the spinal cord following back-loading of the left VF at the lumbosacral junction is shown in Figures 3B–D. A total of 2535 sacral neurons were labeled in this experiment. Seventy-five percent of them were found contralateral to the injection site and their spatial distribution is shown in Figure 3B. Twenty-five percent of the labeled neurons were localized ipsilateral to the fill as shown in Figure 3C. A rostral view of the reconstructed sacral segments with all the labeled neurons is shown in Figure 3D. The neurons in Figures 3B–D are color coded according to their laminar localization (for details see legend). The segmental and laminar distributions of the VF neurons in this preparation are summarized in a 3-D histogram in Figure 3E. This histogram shows that most of the neurons were found in the ventral (VIII, and IX) and intermediate (lamina VII) laminae of the gray matter, that a substantial number of neurons are localized to the deep dorsal horn laminae (mainly laminae V) and that fewer neurons are spread around the central canal (CC) within lamina X. This histogram also shows the rostrocaudal decrease in number of labeled neurons and the predominance of neurons associated with the crossed pathways. In summary, the generation of the thoracolumbar rhythm by SCA stimulation, cannot be attributed to a specific pathway. It involved activation of heterogeneous populations of sacral relay neurons. These neurons are distributed in different regions of the gray matter (e.g., Fig. 3). The neurons projecting through the VF, VLF, and LF reside in the deep-dorsal, intermediate, and ventral laminae of the gray matter, while those projecting via the DLF are localized to the dorsal laminae of the gray matter and the dorsolateral white matter (not shown). Moreover, the axonal projections of these pathways are crossed and uncrossed, and can be activated separately[11,12] or concurrently to produce the rhythm by SCA stimulation.

Chain activation of proprioneurons with short ascending projections is sufficient to produce the rhythm

Another factor that adds versatility to the SCA activating system and increases its resistance to neural damage concerns the mode of activation of the

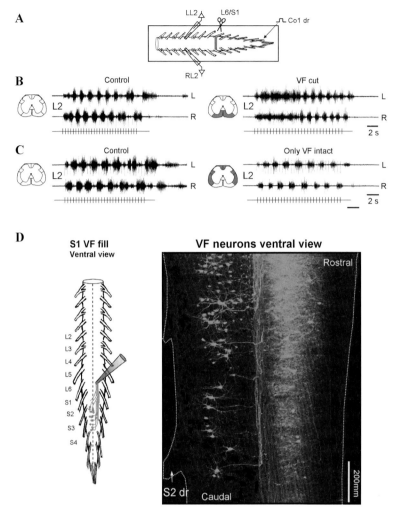

Figure 2. Sacral neurons projecting rostrally through the ventral funiculus have a prominent role in delivering the drive required to activate the lumbar CPGs by SCA stimulation. (**A**) Schematic ventral view of the spinal cord showing the stimulated Co1 dorsal root, the ventral root recordings from L2, and the location of the lumbosacral junction (*red line*), where the surgical lesions of the funiculi are inflicted. (**B**) Recordings from the left and right L2 ventral roots before (control) and after a bilateral interruption of the VF (VF cut) at the lumbosacral junction. Twenty pulse 1.25 Hz stimulus train was applied to the right Co1 dorsal root at 1.22 T to produce the rhythm. (**C**) Recordings from the left and right L2 ventral roots before (control) and after a bilateral interruption of the VLF/LF, DLF and DF (VF was left intact) at the lumbosacral junction. Thirty pulse 2 Hz stimulus train was applied to the left Co1 dorsal root at 1.88 T. (**D**) Rostrally projecting VF neurons. Schematic ventral view of backfilling of cut VF axon bundles with fluorescein dextran at the left lumbosacral junction (*left*) is superimposed with a projected confocal image of the labeled neurons in a whole mount transparent preparation of the spinal cord. Note the predominance of contralaterally filled neurons, the decrease in the number of cells in the caudal direction and, the course of the crossing axons onto the ascending VF. The projected image is composed of 20 optical slices, 8 μm each, scanned from the ventral aspect of the whole mount preparation (part of 70 consecutive optical slices).

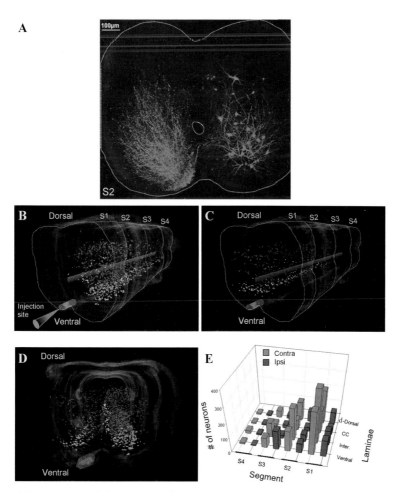

Figure 3. The spatial and segmental distribution of VF neurons in the sacral segments of the spinal cord. Projected confocal microscope image of a 70 μm cross section at the caudal S2 segment in the neonatal rat spinal cord following back loading of the right ventral funiculus with fluorescein dextran at the lumbosacral junction. Note the dense neuropil ipsilateral to the fill, the laminar distribution of the contralateral labeled cells, and the axonal projections of the labeled cells crossing through the ventral white commissure (**A**). Three-dimensional reconstruction of the sacral cord from a sample of cross sections shows labeled VF neurons contralateral to the fill (**B**), ipsilateral to the fill (**C**), and a frontal view of all the labeled neurons (**D**). Color coding: green = ventral laminae; red = lamina VII; blue = deep dorsal laminae; white = lamina X neurons (around the central canal). The brown cylinder denotes the CC in the spinal cord model. The 3D model was built using the 3D-doctor software package. Three-dimensional histogram describing the segmental and laminar distribution of the labeled neurons in this experiment is shown in (**E**). *Red =* ipsilateral, *green =* contralateral to the fill.

CPGs by the sacral neurons. Theoretically, the sacral neurons activated by SCA stimulation can activate the CPGs either directly or indirectly, by recruiting additional groups of propriospinal neurons that are interposed between the second-order relay neurons and the CPGs. Indeed in accord with this idea, our recent work has shown that the lumbar rhythm was maintained when the continuity of long ascending projections of propriospinal and tract neurons was interrupted at different loci along the sacral cord.[30] One such experiment is illustrated in Figure 4. The rhythm in this experiment was produced by stimulation of SCAs entering the spinal cord through the Co1 **dorsal root** (**control. A**). The rhythm persisted following a bilateral cut of the DF, DLF, VLF/LF at the S3/S4 **junction** (**B**). Thus, the drive required to

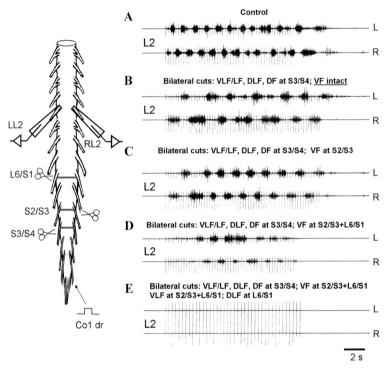

Figure 4. Direct contacts made by long-ascending axons from the sacral neurons to the thoracolumbar circuits are not essential for activation of the CPGs by SCA stimulation. Recordings from the left and right L2 ventral roots are shown during stimulus train applied to the left Co1 dorsal root, before (A) and after bilateral interruption of the VLF/LF, DLF, and DF at the S3/S4 junction with the VF as the only intact funiculi (B). The rhythm persists after bilateral interruptions of the VF first at the S2/S3 junction (C) and then the L6/S1 junction (D). The rhythm is blocked under these conditions when the VLF/LF was bilaterally cut at the S2/S3 junction and the DLF was bilaterally lesioned at the L6/S1 junction (E). Stimulus trains: 50-pulse 4 Hz at 1.75 T (A–D), 40 pulse, 3 Hz at 2.5 T (E).

activate the CPGs was delivered in this case only by sacral neurons projecting rostrally through the VF. The VF was then bilaterally lesioned first at the S2/S3 junction (C), and then the L6/S1 junction (D) and in each case the lumbar rhythm persisted. The rhythm was completely blocked only after extension of the S2/S3 lesion to the VLF and the L6/S1 lesion to the DLF (E), see ref. 30. These results suggest that chain activation of propriospinal neurons with short-range multifunicular projections is sufficient to excite the lumbar CPGs by SCA stimulation. Another series of experiments revealed that although activation of direct contacts between the sacral and lumbar cord can produce the rhythm, its efficacy was less compared to the serial activation mode.[30] Thus, direct synaptic contacts made by long ascending axons from the sacral cord to the thoracolumbar locomotor circuits are not necessarily required to attain activation of the CPGs by SCA stimulation. The

involvement of short ascending proprioneurons in the ascending control of the CPGs and in caudo-rostral communication in the spinal cord can be added to a growing body of evidence concerning the role of propriospinal neurons in descending control of the pattern-generating circuitry,[31] their function as alternative communication pathways following traumatic spinal cord injuries,[32,33] and their potential use in functional recovery from spinal cord injuries.[34,35]

In summary, the pathways involved in the SCA-induced rhythm described in this study exhibit high potency, substantial versatility, and a high level of redundancy that determines the extreme resistance of this system to neural damage of the spinal cord. It is suggested that the sacrocaudal sensory activating system may provide a possible basis of alternative therapeutic approaches following spinal cord injuries.

Acknowledgments

Supported by The Israel Science Foundation (ISF) grants no. 129/04, 1591/08, 1930/08 and by The United States-Israel Binational Science Foundation (BSF) grants no: 2001010 and 2005020, to ALT. We thank Dr. G.Z. Mentis for his advice and expertise in performance of the retrograde labeling experiments and Dr. M.J. O'Donovan for helpful comments on the manuscript.

Conflicts of interest

The authors declare no conflicts of interest.

References

1. Pearson, K.G. 2004. Generating the walking gait: role of sensory feedback. *Prog. Brain Res.* **143:** 123–129.
2. Rossignol, S., R. Dubuc & J.-P. Gossard. 2006. Dynamic sensorimotor interactions in locomotion. *Physiol. Rev.* **86:** 89–154.
3. Lavrov, I. *et al.* 2008. Facilitation of stepping with epidural stimulation in spinal rats: role of sensory input. *J. Neurosci.* **28:** 7774–7780.
4. Edgerton, V.R. *et al.* 2008. Training locomotor networks. *Brain Res. Rev.* **57:** 241–254.
5. Colombo, G., M. Wirz & V. Dietz. 2001. Driven gait orthosis for improvement of locomotor training in paraplegic patients. *Spinal Cord* **39:** 693–700.
6. Dietz, V., R. Müller & G. Colombo. 2002. Locomotor activity in spinal man: significance of afferent input from joint and load receptors. *Brain* **125:** 2626–2634.
7. Dietz, V. & S.J. Harkema. 2004. Locomotor activity in spinal cord-injured persons. *J. Appl. Physiol.* **92:** 1954–1960.
8. Dietz, V. 2009. Body weight supported gait training: from laboratory to clinical setting. *Brain Res. Bull.* **78:** I-VI.
9. Lev-Tov, A., I. Delvolve & E. Kremer. 2000. Sacrocaudal afferents induce rhythmic efferent bursting in isolated spinal cords of neonatal rats. *J. Neurophysiol.* **83:** 888–894.
10. Delvolve, I., H. Gabbay & A. Lev-Tov. 2001. The motor output and behavior produced by rhythmogenic sacrocaudal networks in spinal cords of neonatal rats. *J. Neurophysiol.* **85:** 2100–2110.
11. Strauss, I. & A. Lev-Tov. 2003. Neural pathways between sacrocaudal afferents and lumbar pattern generators in neonatal rats. *J. Neurophysiol.* **89:** 773–784.
12. Gabbay, H. & A. Lev-Tov. 2004. Alpha-1 adrenoceptor agonists generate a "fast" NMDA receptor-independent motor rhythm in the neonatal rat spinal cord. *J. Neurophysiol.* **92:** 997–1010.
13. Whelan, P., A. Bonnot & M.J. O'Donovan. 2000. Properties of rhythmic activity generated by the isolated spinal cord of the neonatal mouse. *J. Neurophysiol.* **84:** 2821–2833.
14. Smith, J. C., J.L. Feldman & B.J. Schmidt. 1988. Neural mechanisms generating locomotion studied in mammalian brain stem-spinal cord *in vitro. FASEB J.* **2:** 2283–2288.
15. Blivis, D., G.Z. Mentis, M.J. O'Donovan & A. Lev-Tov. 2007. Differential effects of opioids on sacrocaudal afferent pathways and central pattern generators in the neonatal rat spinal cord. *J. Neurophysiol.* **97:** 2875–2886.
16. Schomburg, E.D., H. Steffens & N. Wada. 2001. Parallel nociceptive reflex pathways with negative and positive feedback functions to foot extensors in the cat. *J. Physiol.* **536:** 605–613.
17. Mandadi, S. *et al.* 2009. Locomotor networks are targets of modulation by sensory transient receptor potential vanilloid 1 and transient receptor potential melastatin 8 channels. *Neuroscience* **162:** 1377–1397.
18. Pearson, K.G. & S. Rossignol, 1991. Fictive motor patterns in chronic spinal cats. *J. Neurophysiol.* **66:** 1874–1887.
19. Jankowska, E. *et al.* 1967. The effect of DOPA on the spinal cord. 6. Half-centre organization of interneurones transmitting effects from the flexor reflex afferents. *Acta Physiol. Scand.* **70:** 389–402.
20. Jankowska, E. *et al.* 1967. The effect of DOPA on the spinal cord. 5. Reciprocal organization of pathways transmitting excitatory action to alpha motoneurones of flexors and extensors. *Acta Physiol. Scand.* **70:** 369–388.
21. Lundberg, A. 1979. Multisensory control of spinal reflex pathways. *Prog. Brain Res.* **50:** 11–28.
22. Schomburg, E.D. *et al.* 1998. Flexor reflex afferents reset the step cycle during fictive locomotion in the cat. *Exp. Brain Res.* **122:** 339–350.
23. Burke, R.E. 1999. The use of state-dependent modulation of spinal reflexes as a tool to investigate the organization of spinal interneurons. *Exp. Brain Res.* **128:** 263–277.
24. Hultborn, H. *et al.* 1998. How do we approach the locomotor network in the mammalian spinal cord? *Ann. N.Y. Acad. Sci.* **860:** 70–82.
25. Marchetti, C., M. Beato & A. Nistri. 2001. Alternating rhythmic activity induced by dorsal root stimulation in the neonatal rat spinal cord. *J. Physiol.* **530:** 105–112.
26. Ritz, L.A., P.B. Brown & S.M. Bailey. 1989. Crossed and uncrossed projections to cat sacrocaudal spinal cord: I.

Axons from cutaneous receptors. *J. Comp. Neurol.* **289:** 284–293.

27. Gladfelter, W.E. *et al.* 1993. Crossed receptive field components and crossed dendrites in cat sacrocaudal dorsal horn. *J. Comp. Neurol.* **336:** 96–105.

28. Blivis, D., G.Z. Mentis, M.J. O'Donovan & A. Lev-Tov. Studies of sacral neurons involved in activation of the lumbar central pattern generator for locomotion in the neonatal rodent spinal cord. Program No. 564.7/DD59. 2009, Neuroscience Meeting Planner. Chicago, IL: Society for Neuroscience, 2009. Online.

29. Lev-Tov, A. & M.J. O'Donovan. 2009. Spinal cord: neonatal circuits. In *Encyclopedia of Neuroscience*. Larry R. Squire, Ed.: Academic Press. Oxford.

30. Etlin, A., D. Blivis, M. Ben Zwi & A. Lev-Tov. Proprioneurons with multifunicular projections are activated by sacrocaudal afferents to turn on the pattern generating circuitry in the absence of supraspinal control. Program No. 564.7/DD58. 2009, Neuroscience Meeting Planner. Chicago, IL: Society for Neuroscience, 2009. Online.

31. Cowley, K.C., E. Zaporozhets & B.J. Schmidt. 2006. Propriospinal neurons are sufficient for bulbospinal transmission of the locomotor command signal in the neonatal rat spinal cord. *J Physiol.* **572:** 443–458.

32. Courtine, G. *et al.* 2008. Recovery of supraspinal control of stepping via indirect propriospinal relay connections after spinal cord injury. *Nat. Med.* **14:** 69–74.

33. Guevremont, L. *et al.* 2006. Locomotor-related networks in the lumbosacral enlargement of the adult spinal cat: activation through intraspinal microstimulation. *IEEE Trans. Neural Syst. Rehabil. Eng.* **14:** 266–272.

34. Edgerton, V.R. & R.R. Roy. 2009. Robotic training and spinal cord plasticity. *Brain Res. Bull.* **78:** 4–12.

35. Yakovenko, S., J. Kowalczewski & A. Prochazka. 2007. Intraspinal stimulation caudal to spinal cord transections in rats. Testing the propriospinal hypothesis. *J. Neurophysiol.* **97:** 2570–2574.

Ann. N.Y. Acad. Sci. ISSN 0077-8923

ANNALS OF THE NEW YORK ACADEMY OF SCIENCES

Issue: *Neurons and Networks in the Spinal Cord*

Mechanisms of excitation of spinal networks by stimulation of the ventral roots

Michael J. O'Donovan,[1] Agnes Bonnot,[2] George Z. Mentis,[1] Nikolai Chub,[1] Avinash Pujala,[1] and Francisco J. Alvarez[3]

[1]Developmental Neurobiology Section, NINDS, NIH, Bethesda, Maryland. [2]RCCN, Neurobiologie des Processus Adaptatifs, Université PM Curie, Paris, France. [3]Department of Neurosciences, Cell Biology, and Physiology, Wright State University, Dayton, Ohio

Address for correspondence: Michael J. O'Donovan, Building 35, Room 3C-1014, 35 Convent Drive, Bethesda, MD 20892. odonovm@ninds.nih.gov

It has recently been demonstrated that motoneurons in neonatal rodents release an excitatory amino acid, in addition to acetylcholine, from their central terminals onto Renshaw cells. Although the function of this amino acid release is not understood, it may mediate the excitatory actions of motor axon stimulation on spinal motor networks. Stimulation of motor axons in the ventral roots or muscle nerves can activate the locomotor central pattern generator or entrain bursting in the disinhibited cord. Both of these effects persist in the presence of cholinergic antagonists and are abolished or diminished by ionotropic and metabotropic glutamate antagonists. Calcium imaging in the disinhibited cord shows that a ventral root stimulus evokes ventrolateral activity initially, which subsequently propagates to the rest of the cord. This finding suggests that excitatory interneurons excited by motoneuron recurrent collaterals are located in this region. However, motoneurons do not exhibit short latency excitatory potentials in response to ventral root stimulation indicating that the excitatory effects are mediated polysynaptically. We discuss the significance of these findings.

Keywords: calcium imaging; motoneuron; recurrent excitation; spinal cord

Introduction

The mammalian spinal cord contains the circuitry for several rhythmic motor behaviors. It is generally assumed that such behaviors are produced by networks of spinal interneurons and that motoneurons do not contribute causally to their generation.[1] However, recent work in the developing spinal cord suggests that motoneurons might play a more important role in rhythmogenesis than had been previously thought. In the *Xenopus* tadpole, for example, motoneurons are coupled to each other through cholinergic and electrical synapses and also to some of the interneurons involved in the generation of swimming.[2] Moreover, in the developing spinal cord of the chick[3,4] and mouse embryo[5] stimulation of motor axons can trigger bursting of spinal motor

circuits. In the early embryonic spinal cord, network excitation by motoneuron stimulation has been related to the depolarizing actions of GABA and glycine. However, the reversal potential of inhibitory synapses becomes more hyperpolarized in late embryonic and neonatal motoneurons[6] precluding the possibility that the excitatory effects of motoneuron stimulation are mediated through the depolarizing effects of GABA and glycine. Nevertheless, ventral root stimulation can synaptically excite motoneurons in the spinal cords of neonatal rats and mice,[7,8] and has been reported to evoke glutamatergic EPSPs in neonatal rat motoneurons.[9] In this review, we discuss our recent work on the excitatory actions of motoneurons in the neonatal spinal cord of the mouse and consider the possible role of motoneurons in locomotor rhythmogenesis.

doi: 10.1111/j.1749-6632.2010.05535.x

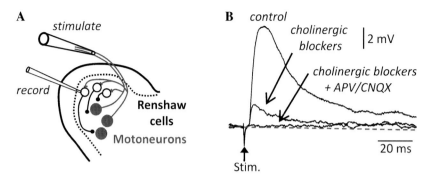

Figure 1. Motoneurons release an excitatory amino acid from their terminals onto Renshaw cells in addition to acetylcholine. (**A**) Schematic showing a whole cell recording from an identified Renshaw cell (*blue filled circles*) and a suction electrode on the ventral root to antidromically stimulate motoneurons (*gray filled circles*) in the isolated spinal cord *in vitro*. (**B**) Synaptic responses in response to a single antidromic stimulus applied to the ipsilateral ventral root. Addition of cholinergic blockers reduced but did not abolish the response. The response was abolished by the addition of the glutamatergic antagonists APV and CNQX. The data in B were modified from Ref. 10.

Motoneurons release an excitatory amino acid at their central terminals onto Renshaw cells

A single stimulus applied to a ventral root evokes a monosynaptic excitatory potential in Renshaw cells in the neonatal mouse spinal cord.[7,10] This potential can be reduced in amplitude, but not abolished, by a combination of bath applied antagonists to acetylcholine (Fig. 1B). The remaining noncholinergic components of the potential are abolished by a combination of the NMDA receptor antagonist APV and the non-NMDA antagonists CNQX[7,10] or NBQX.[11]

It has not been possible to identify the released excitatory amino acid as glutamate because motoneuron synaptic terminals on Renshaw cells do not contain immunocytochemically detectable levels any of any of the known vesicular glutamate transporters.[10,12] While this result may mean that a different, as yet unknown, vesicular glutamate transporter (VGLUT) is present on motoneuron terminals it is also possible that the motoneurons release significant amounts of aspartate rather than glutamate. Given that NMDA receptors are gated by both aspartate and glutamate, while AMPA receptors preferentially bind glutamate,[13] the presence of significant aspartate release together with the lack of an efficient synaptic vesicle packaging mechanism for glutamate could partly explain why NMDA components at this synapse are frequently larger and

less variable than AMPA components.[11] VGLUTs do not transport aspartate[14–17] therefore aspartate synaptic release must be VGLUT-independent. A recent report suggested that sialin (SLC17A5) packages aspartate and glutamate into hippocampal synaptic vesicles,[18] but results from our laboratories indicate that this transporter is not located at the intraspinal terminals of motor axon collaterals. Therefore, the release of an excitatory amino acid from motoneuron terminals must operate through a vesicular transport mechanism that is distinct from the currently known VGLUTs or sialin. Unfortunately, it is not possible to reliably distinguish between aspartate and glutamate release pharmacologically and for this reason electron microscopy studies are under way to analyze the relative enrichments of aspartate and glutamate inside motor axon synapses on Renshaw cells. Whatever the exact mechanism of release, or the particular excitatory amino acid being released, it is now well established that the intraspinal recurrent collaterals of motor axons can activate NMDA and AMPA receptors postsynaptically.

Ventral root stimulation can activate locomotor-like activity and entrain disinhibited bursting

Stimulation of motor axons in the ventral root or the sciatic nerve can trigger episodes of locomotor-like activity in the isolated neonatal mouse spinal cord[10] or can entrain the spontaneous bursting that occurs in the presence of bicuculline and strychnine.[8,19] Surprisingly neither of these excitatory effects is blocked by bath application of a cocktail of muscarinic and nicotinic cholinergic antagonists[10,19] (Fig. 2). Rather we found that the excitatory effects of ventral root stimulation could be reversibly abolished by ionotropic glutamatergic antagonists (Figs. 2C and 2D).

One unusual feature of the excitatory effects of ventral root stimulation was their lability and rostrocaudal variation in efficacy.[19] This is shown in Figure 2E, which displays the percentage of experiments in which a particular ventral root was effective at evoking locomotor-like activity or entraining disinhibited bursting. We found that even the most effective roots were capable of evoking excitatory actions in only ∼60–70% of experiments, while the efficacy of the least effective roots was substantially lower (∼30% of experiments). We do not know the reason for this lability. It suggests that some aspect of spinal cord function varies from animal to animal and from segment to segment in the isolated spinal cord preparation. These rostrocaudal variations do not appear to correlate with spinal segment size or the number of myelinated and unmyelinated axons in the roots. We found that L5 was more effective than L2 at evoking excitatory effects even though it is larger. Thus, we can eliminate the possibility that the lability is associated with the extent of tissue oxygenation, which is presumably poorer in the largest segments. Similarly, there was no correlation between the efficacy of a particular root and the number of myelinated or unmyelinated axons it contains in the adult mouse.[19,20] For example, the thinner L6 ventral root elicited excitatory effects as effectively as the much larger L4 and L5 ventral roots.

Ventral root evoked locomotor-like activity and the entrainment of disinhibited bursting exhibited similar pharmacological properties and rostrocaudal variations in efficacy, suggesting that the mechanisms underlying these excitatory effects are similar.[21] As a result, the disinhibited cord can be used as a model for investigating the excitatory effects of ventral root stimulation. This is advantageous experimentally because the synaptic output of Renshaw cells is blocked so that their activation cannot mediate the excitatory actions of ventral root stimulation. Although Renshaw cells are known to be inhibitory in the adult animal, during the neonatal period it is possible that some of their synaptic targets within the spinal cord might have an elevated chloride equilibrium potential rendering the synaptic actions of GABA and glycine excitatory.[22] In addition, the spontaneous bursting that occurs in the disinhibited cord is highly synchronized among spinal neurons, thereby facilitating calcium imaging of neuronal activity (see below).

Ventral root activation of spinal networks is reduced or abolished by bath application of the mGluR1 antagonist CPCCOEt

Locomotor-like activity evoked by ventral root stimulation usually appears after two to five stimuli (Fig. 3A). These initial stimuli, prior to the onset of locomotor bursting, evoke long latency responses that can be recorded from individual motoneurons or from the ventral roots (Fig. 3A, right hand panel). These long-latency ventral root potentials are abolished in the presence of bicuculline and strychnine.[19] However, it is unlikely that they are depolarizing inhibitory potentials because the chloride equilibrium potential in neonatal mouse motoneurons is at, or just below, the resting membrane potential.[6] Why these potentials should disappear in the presence of inhibitory antagonists is unclear unless their expression in motoneurons is somehow facilitated by the presence of depolarizing IPSPs in interneurons. The absence of short latency responses in motoneurons (Fig. 3A, right-hand panel) in response to ventral root stimulation indicates that motoneuron axon collaterals do not contact an excitatory interneuron that projects back onto motoneurons in a similar manner to Renshaw cells.

The bursts evoked by ventral root stimulation in the disinhibited cord were also characterized by their long-latency after the stimulus (Fig. 3B). Furthermore, the time from the stimulus train to the onset of the ventral root burst progressively lengthened with successive stimuli. As shown in Figure 3B, the first burst evoked by the ventral root stimulus exhibited a delay from the last stimulus in the train (5 pulses at 20 Hz) of ∼60 ms. This delay progressively lengthened with successive bursts so that by the fourth burst the delay was ∼700 ms.

These surprisingly long delays raised the possibility that the excitatory effects of ventral root stimulation might be mediated, at least in part, by

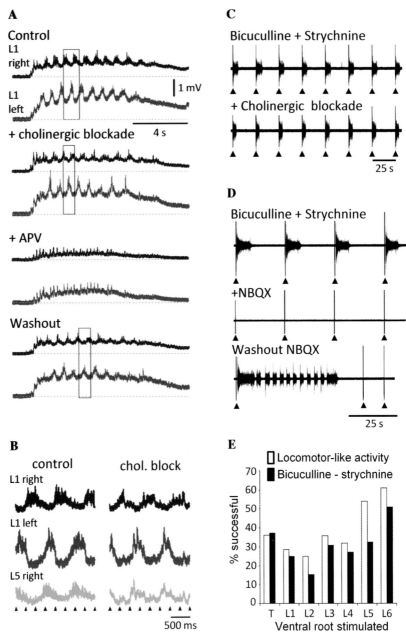

Figure 2. Locomotor-like activity and disinhibited bursting evoked by stimulation of motor axons exhibit similar properties in the neonatal spinal cord of the mouse. (A) Locomotor-like activity evoked by a train of stimuli applied to the sciatic nerve. To ensure exclusive stimulation of motor axons, the ipsilateral dorsal roots were cut. The records are direct coupled (DC) recordings of the electrical activity recorded from the *left* (*red* traces) and *right* (*blue* traces) lumbar 1 (L1) ventral roots. The rectangle in this and the subsequent panels highlights the alternation between the activity on the left and right sides. The top set of traces (control) show the activity induced by sciatic nerve stimulation in the absence of drugs. The next traces show that the locomotor-like activity persists in the presence of a cocktail of cholinergic antagonists (50 μM mecamylamine, 50 μM dihydro-β-erythroidine, and 5 μM atropine), although the discharge has been reduced. In the presence of the NMDA antagonist APV, the locomotor-like activity is abolished and it recovers when the drugs are washed out (Washout). (B) The phase relations between the activity

metabotropic glutamate receptor activation, which is known to be slow. Consistent with this idea, we found that the mGluR1 antagonist CPCCOEt reduced the ability of a ventral root stimulus to entrain disinhibited bursting and reversibly blocked the locomotor-like activity evoked by ventral root stimulation[19] (Fig. 3C). The sensitivity of locomotor-like activity and disinhibited bursting to mGluR1 antagonists is consistent with previous work showing that mGluR1 activation can accelerate the locomotor rhythm in the lamprey[23] and in the rat spinal cords.[24]

The most parsimonious explanation to account for the excitatory effects of ventral root stimulation is that an excitatory amino acid released from motoneuron terminals acts on metabotropic glutamate receptors on interneurons other than Renshaw cells (2 in Fig. 3D). Alternatively, a glutamatergic interneuron activated by motoneuron collaterals might be responsible for activating the metabotropic receptors within the burst generating network (3 in Fig. 3D). The location and identity of such cells is currently unknown, so we used calcium imaging in the disinhibited cord to identify the origin of the earliest optical activity following stimuli applied to the ventral roots.

Calcium imaging reveals the existence of a ventro laterally located network activated by ventral root stimulation

We used calcium imaging of either the lateral aspect of the spinal cord or the cut face (rostral L5) to identify the locus of the initial optical activity following a ventral root stimulus. As illustrated in Figure 4, the earliest optical activity appeared in the ventrolateral area from where it spread to encompass the rest of the cord. In ~40% of spontaneously occurring bursts a similar pattern of propagation was observed.[19] The fact that this pattern of prop-

agation can be observed in spontaneous bursts is significant, because it suggests the existence of a functionally discrete ventrolateral network that can be recruited either spontaneously or in response to ventral root stimulation.

However, as pointed out earlier, the maturation of chloride equilibrium potentials makes it highly unlikely that the Renshaw cell circuit is responsible for the propagation of ventral root antidromic activity into the spinal network of neonatal mice. Moreover, because the output of Renshaw cells is blocked in the disinhibited mouse spinal cord, the excitatory actions of ventral root stimulation are probably mediated through activation of excitatory interneurons by the ventral root stimulus. A hint to the mechanism of propagation can be inferred from the velocity of the ventro dorsal wave of excitation. This is approximately 10 μm/ms, which is much too slow to be accounted for by conduction delays. The most likely explanation is that it represents the sequential synaptic activation of groups of neurons coupled by short-range excitatory synaptic connections.

Concluding remarks

The existence of recurrent excitatory pathways from motoneurons into spinal cord networks may have gone undetected for so long because the pathways are labile, operate through a noncholinergic mechanism and are not easily activated in the neonatal spinal cord. This is consistent with the suggestion of Machacek and Hochman[8] that the excitatory circuit activated by motoneurons might be under noradrenergic or some other form of neuromodulatory control, which may vary from animal to animal. It is also possible that this pathway is only functional in the neonatal animal and is "deselected" as the animal matures. A precedent for such

---

recorded from the left and right L1 and the right L5 ventral roots under control conditions (control) are unchanged in the presence of cholinergic blockade (chol. block). (C) Spontaneous bursting in the presence of the inhibitory antagonists bicuculline and strychnine can be entrained by a brief train of five stimuli (20 Hz, *arrowheads*) applied to an adjacent ventral root. The effect is maintained in the presence of cholinergic blockade but abolished in the presence of the AMPA/kainate antagonist NBQX (panel D). (E) Histogram comparing the efficacy of ventral root stimulation at evoking locomotor-like activity (*open bars*) or the entrainment of disinhibited bursting (*filled bars*). The ordinate shows the percentage of experiments in which the ventral root stimulus produced locomotor-like activity or entrained disinhibited bursting. Modified from Refs. 10 (A and B) and 19 (C–E).

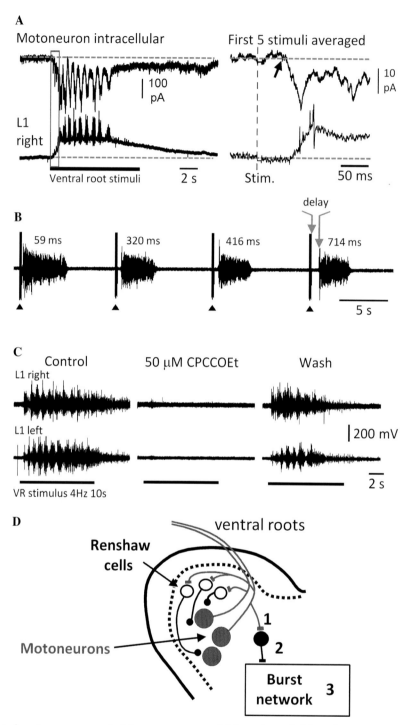

Figure 3. Ventral root responses evoked in motoneurons exhibit prolonged delays that may reflect metabotropic glutamate receptor activation. (A) Whole cell voltage clamp recording from an identified motoneuron together with the DC extracellular signal recorded from the right L1 ventral root during an episode of locomotor-like activity evoked by a train (4 Hz, 10 s) of ventral root stimuli. The responses evoked by the first five stimuli (delineated by the *gray rectangle*) were averaged and are displayed in the expanded traces on the right. The *arrow* marks the onset

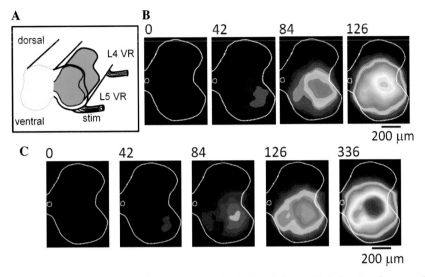

Figure 4. Calcium imaging of the cut face of the disinhibited spinal cord (rostral L5) showing the ventrolateral origin of optical activity following a ventral root stimulus or at the onset of some spontaneous bursts. (A) Schematic of the spinal cord preparation showing the cut face of the rostral L5 segment. One hemi-segment was injected with the calcium-sensitive dye fluo-3 (*green* region). (B) Series of images showing the ventrolateral origin of activity following a brief stimulus train (five stimuli, 20 Hz) applied to the ipsilateral L5 ventral root. Each image is a difference image obtained by subtracting a pre-stimulus control image from the active frame. The time of acquisition of the frame (ms) is indicated above the images. (C) A similar pattern of activation can be observed during ~40% of the spontaneously occurring bursts. Modified from Ref. 19.

deselection is observed in the gradual weakening of primary afferent input onto Renshaw cells in the mouse.[25]

The functional role of this pathway in locomotion is unclear. Mice do not begin weight bearing locomotion until the second week postnatally. It is possible that the interneuronal circuitry responsible for the locomotor drive to motoneurons is immature at this stage so that the recurrent excitation derived from motoneurons is necessary to maintain adequate motoneuronal drive to muscle. As the interneuronal circuitry matures the contribution of motoneurons to the excitatory drive would decrease. Alternatively, recurrent excitatory motoneuron circuits may persist into adulthood. Ultimately, these issues can only be resolved by identifying the

---

of the evoked inward current with a latency of 50 ms from the ventral root stimulus (*red dotted line*). (B) During disinhibited bursting entrained by a brief train of stimuli (five stimuli at 20 Hz) applied to an adjacent ventral root the delay between the last stimulus in the train and the onset of the evoked burst (*arrows* and delay on 4th burst) progressively increases. The delays are indicated over the individual bursts. (C) Locomotor-like activity evoked by a ventral root stimulus train is reversibly abolished in the presence of the mGluR1 receptor antagonist CPCCOEt. The bars below the records indicate the duration of the stimulus train. (D) Schematic of the ventral part of the cord showing the possible loci of action of CPCCOEt. It is assumed that motoneuron collaterals release glutamate at an excitatory interneuron that is distinct from Renshaw cells. This interneuron in turn projects to the burst generating network. CPCCOEt could act presynaptically on motoneuron synaptic terminals (1), pre- and/or postsynaptically on the excitatory interneuron (2) or within the burst network itself (3). Parts of (B) and (C) were modified from Ref. 19.

interneurons responsible for transmitting ventral root excitation into spinal networks.

Acknowledgment

This work was supported by the intramural program of NINDS.

Conflicts of interest

The authors declare no conflicts of interest.

References

1. Kiehn, O. 2006. Locomotor circuits in the mammalian spinal cord. *Annu. Rev. Neurosci.* **29:** 279–306.

2. Perrins, R. & A. Roberts. 1995. Cholinergic contribution to excitation in a spinal locomotor central pattern generator in Xenopus embryos. *J. Neurophysiol.* **73:** 1013–1019.

3. Wenner, P. & M.J. O'Donovan. 1999. Identification of an interneuronal population that mediates recurrent inhibition of motoneurons in the developing spinal cord. *J. Neurosci.* **19:** 7557–7567.

4. Wenner, P. & M.J. O'Donovan. 2001. Mechanisms that initiate spontaneous network activity in the developing chick spinal cord. *J. Neurophysiol.* **86:** 1481–1498.

5. Hanson, M.G. & L.T. Landmesser. 2003. Characterization of the circuits that generate spontaneous episodes of activity in the early embryonic mouse spinal cord. *J. Neurosci.* **23:** 587–600.

6. Delpy, A., A.E. Allain, P. Meyrand & P. Branchereau. 2008. NKCC1 cotransporter inactivation underlies embryonic development of chloride-mediated inhibition in mouse spinal motoneuron. *J. Physiol.* **586:** 1059–1075.

7. Nishimaru, H., C.E. Restrepo, J. Ryge, *et al.* 2005. Mammalian motor neurons corelease glutamate and acetylcholine at central synapses 2005. *Proc. Natl. Acad. Sci. USA* **102:** 5245–5249.

8. Machacek, D.W. & S. Hochman. 2006. Noradrenaline unmasks novel self-reinforcing motor circuits within the mammalian spinal cord. *J. Neurosci.* **26:** 5920–5928.

9. Jiang, Z.G., E. Shen, M.Y. Wang & N.J. Dun. 1991. Excitatory postsynaptic potentials evoked by ventral root stimulation in neonate rat motoneurons in vitro. *J. Neurophysiol.* **65:** 57–65.

10. Mentis, G.Z., F.J. Alvarez, A. Bonnot, *et al.* 2005. Noncholinergic excitatory actions of motoneurons in the neonatal mammalian spinal cord. *Proc. Natl. Acad. Sci. USA* **102:** 7344–7349.

11. Lamotte d'Incamps, B. & P. Ascher. 2008. Four excitatory postsynaptic ionotropic receptors coactivated at the motoneuron-Renshaw cell synapse. *J. Neurosci.* **28:** 14121–14131.

12. Liu, T.T., B.A. Bannatyne, E. Jankowska & D.J. Maxwell. 2009. Cholinergic terminals in the ventral horn of adult rat and cat: evidence that glutamate is a cotransmitter at putative interneuron synapses but not at central synapses of motoneurons. *Neuroscience* **161:** 111–122.

13. Curras, M.C. & R. Dingledine. 1992. Selectivity of amino acid transmitters acting at N-methyl-D-aspartate and amino-3-hydroxy-5-methyl-4-isoxazolepropionate receptors. *Mol. Pharmacol.* **41:** 520–526.

14. Bellocchio, E.E., R.J. Reimer, R.T. Fremeau, Jr. & R.H. Edwards. 2000. Uptake of glutamate into synaptic vesicles by an inorganic phosphate transporter. *Science* **289:** 957–960.

15. Herzog, E., G.C. Bellenchi, C. Gras, *et al.* 2001. The existence of a second vesicular glutamate transporter specifies subpopulations of glutamatergic neurons. *J. Neurosci.* **21:** RC181.

16. Fremeau, R.T., Jr., J. Burman, T. Qureshi, *et al.* 2002. The identification of vesicular glutamate transporter 3 suggests novel modes of signaling by glutamate. *Proc. Natl. Acad. Sci. USA* **99:** 14488–14493.

17. Varoqui, H., M.K. Schäfer, H. Zhu, *et al.* 2002. Identification of the differentiation-associated Na+/PI transporter as a novel vesicular glutamate transporter expressed in a distinct set of glutamatergic synapses. *J. Neurosci.* **22:** 142–155.

18. Miyaji, T., N. Echigo, M. Hiasa, *et al.* 2008. Identification of a vesicular aspartate transporter. *Proc. Natl. Acad. Sci. USA* **105:** 11720–11724.

19. Bonnot, A., N. Chub, A. Pujala & M.J. O'Donovan. 2009. Excitatory actions of ventral root stimulation during network activity generated by the disinhibited neonatal mouse spinal cord. *J. Neurophysiol.* **101:** 2995–3011.

20. Biscoe, T.J., S.M. Nickels & C.A. Stirling. 1982. Numbers and sizes of nerve fibres in mouse spinal roots. *Q. J. Exp. Physiol.* **67:** 473–494.

21. Beato, M. & A. Nistri. 1999. Interaction between disinhibited bursting and fictive locomotor patterns in the rat isolated spinal cord. *J. Neurophysiol.* **82:** 2029–2038.

22. Chub, N. & M.J. O'Donovan. 2001. Post-episode depression of GABAergic transmission in spinal neurons of the chick embryo. *J. Neurophysiol.* **85:** 2166–2176.

23. Krieger, P., S. Grillner & A. El Manira. 1998. Endoge-
    nous activation of metabotropic glutamate receptors
    contributes to burst frequency regulation in the lamprey
    locomotor network. *Eur. J. Neurosci.* **10:** 3333–3342.

24. Taccola, G., C. Marchetti & A. Nistri. 2004. Modulation
    of rhythmic patterns and cumulative depolarization by

    group I metabotropic glutamate receptors in the neona-
    tal rat spinal cord in vitro. *Eur. J. Neurosci.* **19:** 533–
    541.

25. Mentis, G.Z., V.C. Siembab, R. Zerda, *et al.* 2006. Pri-
    mary afferent synapses on developing Renshaw cells. *J.
    Neurosci.* **26:** 13297–13310.

Ann. N.Y. Acad. Sci. ISSN 0077-8923

ANNALS OF THE NEW YORK ACADEMY OF SCIENCES
Issue: *Neurons and Networks in the Spinal Cord*

Synaptic integration of rhythmogenic neurons in the locomotor circuitry: the case of Hb9 interneurons

Lea Ziskind-Conhaim,[1] George Z. Mentis,[2] Eric P. Wiesner,[1] and David J. Titus[1]

[1]Department of Physiology and Center for Neuroscience, University of Wisconsin School of Medicine and Public Health, Madison, Wisconsin. [2]Section of Developmental Neurobiology, NINDS, NIH, Bethesda, Maryland

Address for correspondence: Lea Ziskind-Conhaim, Department of Physiology, 129 SMI, University of Wisconsin School of Medicine and Public Health, 1300 University Avenue, Madison, WI 53706. lconhaim@physiology.wisc.edu

Innovative molecular and genetic techniques have recently led to the identification of genetically defined populations of ipsilaterally projecting excitatory interneurons with probable functions in the rhythm-generating kernel of the central pattern generators (CPGs). The role of interneuronal populations in specific motor function is determined by their synaptic inputs, intrinsic properties, and target neurons. In this review we examine whether Hb9-expressing interneurons (Hb9 INs) fulfill a set of criteria that are the hallmarks of rhythm generators in the locomotor circuitry. Induced locomotor-like activity in this distinct population of ventral interneurons is in phase with bursts of motor activity, raising the possibility that they are part of the locomotor generator. To increase our understanding of the integrative function of Hb9 INs in the locomotor CPG, we investigated the cellular mechanisms underlying their rhythmic activity and examined the properties of synaptic inputs from low-threshold afferents and possible synaptic contacts with segmental motoneurons. Our findings suggest that the rhythmogenic Hb9 INs are integral components of the sensorimotor circuitry that regulate locomotor-like activity in the spinal cord.

Keywords: locomotor-like rhythms; rhythmogenic interneurons; Hb9 interneurons; rhythm-generating kernel; locomotor central pattern generator; Hb9::eGFP transgenic mouse

Introduction

In all walking vertebrates, alternating hindlimb movements on the two sides of the body are controlled by the locomotor central pattern generators (CPGs), spinal networks that can generate a coordinated pattern of motor rhythms independently of sensory inputs.[1–4] In the isolated spinal cord, in the absence of descending inputs, the autonomous CPG can be stimulated to produce coordinated locomotor-like rhythms by either exposure to various neurotransmitter agonists[5–11] or by excitation of sensory afferents.[12–15] The CPGs for flexor- or extensor-related activity comprise ipsilateral excitatory interneurons that form the rhythm-generating kernel and commissural interneurons that coordinate the left–right alternating patterns of rhythmic activity.[16] Ipsilaterally projecting inhibitory interneurons are responsible for the alternating rhythms between flexor- and extensor-related motoneurons. Classical electrophysiological approaches combined with pharmacological manipulations have identified interneuronal populations that are part of the sensorimotor networks in the cat spinal cord.[17–19] These studies provided important information about the complex interactions between sensory inputs and interneurons in the locomotor networks, but because of technical limitations manipulating interneurons with various functions, the organization of these interneurons in the locomotor circuitry remains largely unknown.

Experimental manipulations helped identify groups of interneurons that might play a role in rhythm-generation and pattern coordination of motor activity in the isolated rodent spinal cords. Electrophysiological and morphological studies have characterized several classes of inhibitory interneurons that have been identified as key components in rhythm-coordinating networks.[20–23]

doi: 10.1111/j.1749-6632.2010.05533.x

However, up until a few years ago little was known about the identity of rhythmogenic interneurons that provide excitatory drive to ipsilateral motoneurons in quadrupeds. The development of novel molecular and genetic techniques[24,25] facilitated the discovery of genetically defined excitatory neuronal populations that might play a fundamental role in controlling rhythmic excitation in corresponding motoneurons. These populations include interneurons that express the Hb9 transcription factor (Hb9 INs),[26,27] the EphA4-positive neurons,[28] V2a interneurons,[29,30] and V3 interneurons.[31] Ablation or silencing the latter three classes of interneurons significantly altered the coordinated patterns of rhythmic motor activity, leading to the conclusion that they are essential components of the locomotor CPGs. These exciting findings are the first step in the identification of interneuronal populations with possible role in rhythmogenesis. To gain insight into the specific function of these interneurons in the complex architecture of the locomotor circuitry future studies will have to: (1) determine the regulatory actions of peripheral sensory projections and descending inputs on their activity patterns, (2) classify their intrasegmental synaptic interactions with other groups of interneurons with known functions, and (3) identify their target neurons.

Our review focuses on Hb9 INs, a cluster of rhythmogenic interneurons that fulfill important criteria that define a specific group of neurons as part of the rhythm-generating kernel of the locomotor CPG.[32] We briefly summarize the properties that make Hb9 INs appealing candidates for ipsilateral CPGs and introduce new findings that support the concept that they are integrated in the sensorimotor circuitry that modulate rhythmic motor activity.

Properties of Hb9 INs: hallmarks of rhythm-generating neurons

The discovery of Hb9 INs is credited to the development of the Hb9::eFGP transgenic mouse line[33] in which a group of Hb9::GFP interneurons can be visually identified for repeated experimental procedures.[26,27] Hb9 INs are clustered in medial lamina VIII of the lower thoracic and upper lumbar segments of the cord (Fig. 1), which are considered "hot" rhythmogenic areas along the rostrocaudal and ventrodorsal axes of the cord.[34,35] The interneurons are also visible in medial lamina VIII of cervical but not sacral segments (unpublished data). Their location and morphological appearance facilitate their visual identification, but their identity is confirmed unambiguously by a set of established electrophysiological criteria.[27,36,37]

Hb9 INs drew significant attention in recent years because they were the first class of genetically identified locomotor-related interneurons with probable role in rhythmogenesis in the isolated spinal cord of neonatal mice. They possess several properties that substantiate their putative contribution to rhythm generation in predominantly flexor-related motoneurons in upper lumbar segments L1–L3.[38] The main characteristics are as follows: (1) Neurochemically induced locomotor-like voltage oscillations are in-phase with ipsilateral motor activity in flexor-related segments (L1–L3, Fig. 1A).[26,36,39] (2) The induced membrane oscillations persist in the absence of fast primary excitatory and inhibitory synaptic transmission (Fig. 1C).[27,36,37,39–41] (3) Electrical coupling between them (Fig. 1B)[40] and with adjacent interneurons[39] synchronizes their outputs to target cells and might contribute to the synchronization of network activity. Although these observations raise the intriguing possibility that Hb9 INs are important components of the rhythm-generating circuitry, their synaptic integration in the complex locomotor networks remains unknown. Examining their intrasegmental synaptic connections is a crucial step in shedding light into their functional hierarchy in the locomotor circuitry. However, it should be emphasized that even if Hb9 INs are part of the generator that dictates the timing of motoneurons excitation, it is unlikely that they are the sole timing controller for flexor-related activity. Hindlimb movements require coordinated excitation of many groups of flexor muscles that are probably controlled by numerous synaptically connected rhythm generators.

A recent study has demonstrated that during neurochemically induced rhythmic activity, the onset of action potential firing in the majority of Hb9 INs lags the start of ipsilateral ventral root burst.[42] Moreover, rhythms generated by stimulating the conus midualis of the cord are more variable in Hb9 INs than in corresponding motoneurons so that the phase correlation between them is not maintained. On the basis of these findings, it has been proposed that Hb9 INs cannot serve as the sole rhythm generator at the upper lumbar segments.

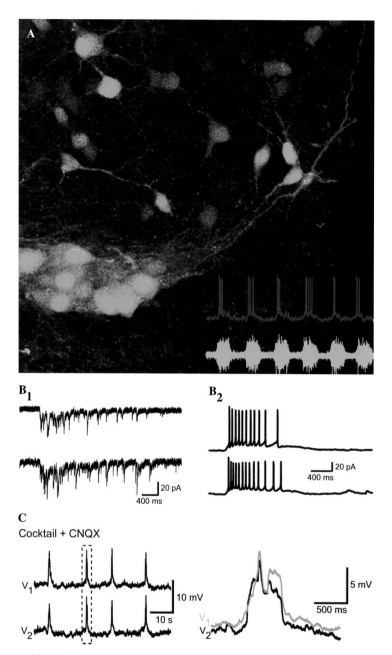

Figure 1. Locomotor-like rhythms in Hb9 INs. (A) Neurobiotin-filled Hb9 IN in medial lamina VIII, adjacent to 2–3 GFP+ putative Hb9 INs. Axon projection is visible in the proximity of motoneurons in the medial motor column. Subthreshold membrane oscillations and firing episodes in a Hb9 IN (*red*) are in-phase with ventral root bursts (*green*). (B) *Spontaneous,* synchronous burst of excitatory postsynaptic currents (B_1) and firing (B_2) recorded in two sets of electrically coupled Hb9 INs. (C) Synchronous, neurochemically induced subthreshold membrane oscillations in electrically coupled Hb9 INs. TEA (10 mM) and higher Ca^{2+} concentration (3 mM) were included in the extracellular solution. The similar wave form voltage oscillations were attributed to the homogeneous electrophysiological properties of Hb9 INs. Marked traces (*dotted box*) were expanded to show their similarities (*right-hand panel*). The rhythms persisted in the presence of CNQX (10 μM), indicating that they were independent of primary excitatory inputs mediated via non-NMDA receptors. Modified with permission from Hinckley *et al.*[26] and Hinckley and Ziskind-Conhaim.[40]

These interesting findings should be interpreted cautiously. Ventral root bursts in segments L1–L3 represent motoneuron activity in both the medial and lateral motor columns. Motoneurons in the two columns have different functions: the lateral motoneurons innervate the limb, while medial motoneurons innervate primarily axial musculature and some hip flexor muscles.[43] It is conceivable the two groups of motoneurons are active at a slightly different time and Hb9 INs regulate the burst onset of the slower motoneuron population. Moreover, sympathetic preganglionic motoneurons also project out of segment L1 and L2 and their activity, which may be synchronized with somatic motoneurons[44] could precede the rhythms generated by Hb9 INs and somatic motoneurons. The fact that stimulation of the caudal cord produces irregular rhythms in Hb9 INs can be explained if different CPGs are activated by descending and ascending projections. It is unknown whether stimulation of the conus midualis of the cord, which co-excites commissural and ipsilateral ascending/propriospinal pathways[45] activates the same CPGs that are controlled by descending/propriospinal networks.[46] Hb9 INs might receive their primary regulatory inputs from descending pathways.

Cellular mechanisms underlying rhythm generation in Hb9 INs

Intrinsic properties that contribute to voltage membrane oscillations

Our experiments were carried out using the hemisected mouse spinal cord with a longitudinal split that severed contralaterally projecting axons, thereby eliminating the contribution of commissural networks.[26] Unless otherwise stated, locomotor-like rhythms were generated by rhythmogenic cocktail containing: *N*-methyl-DL-aspartic acid (NMA, 5 μM), 5-hydroxytryptamine creatinine sulfate complex (5-HT, 10 μM) and dopamine (50 μM).

Spontaneous repetitive firing is not apparent in Hb9 INs, but endogenous episodes of membrane voltage oscillations similar to those induced by the rhythmogenic cocktail can be recorded periodically (Figs. 1B and 2A). Similarly, spontaneous oscillatory activity emerge in these neurons after removing extracellular calcium.[41] Bursts of spontaneous excitatory postsynaptic currents (EPSCs)

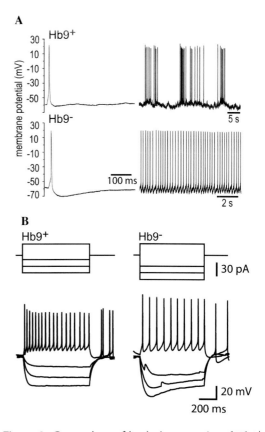

Figure 2. Comparison of intrinsic properties of Hb9+ and adjacent Hb9− negative interneurons. (**A**) Differences between action potential waveforms and spontaneous firing in Hb9+ and Hb9− INs in hemicords of newborn mice. Hb9+ INs generate smaller afterhyperpolarizations than Hb9− INs. Infrequent, small membrane oscillations (3–5 mV) and firing episodes develop spontaneously in Hb9+ INs, while firing at relatively constant frequency (5 Hz in this example) characterize adjacent Hb9− INs. (**B**) Current-clamp recordings from a different Hb9+ IN and a neighboring Hb9− IN. Resting membrane potentials were ∼ −60 mV in both interneurons. Spike-frequency adaptation is apparent Hb9+ IN. Linear I–V relationships at potentials more negative than resting membrane characterize Hb9+ INs. In most adjacent Hb9− INs, negative current injections produce hyperpolarization-dependent depolarization sags. *Panel B was used with permission from Hinckley and Ziskind-Conhaim.*[40]

(Fig. 1B$_1$) might initiate some of the endogenous firing episodes in the highly excitable Hb9 INs (input resistance ranging from approximately 1.0–1.5 GΩ). Typically, non-Hb9 interneurons in medial laminae VII–VIII fire at relatively constant frequency of 3–7 Hz (Fig. 2A). The constant firing might be attributed to the large (>10 mV) action potential afterhyperpolarization and the hyperpolarization-dependent depolarization sags that characterized these interneurons (Figs. 2A and 2B). Hb9 INs are characterized by a relatively small afterhyperpolarization and linear current-voltage relationship without the sag. Two of their cellular properties that are likely to contribute to the episodes of rhythmic firing include: (1) strong postinhibitory rebound and (2) spike frequency adaptation (Fig. 2B).

Voltage-dependent currents that underlie induced voltage oscillations

The ability of rhythmogenic neurons to produce subthreshold voltage oscillations relies on a dynamic interplay between voltage-dependent ionic currents and signal transduction pathways independently of fast synaptic transmission.[47] Fast and slow synaptic transmission regulates the onset and termination of rhythmic activity in unidentified spinal interneurons and commissural interneurons,[48,49] but not in Hb9 INs (Fig. 3). Blocking fast excitatory and inhibitory synaptic inputs does not alter the frequency of neurochemically induced voltage oscillations in Hb9 INs (Fig. 3A).[37] To elucidate the voltage-gated currents that mediate the slow membrane oscillations independently of synaptic transmission, experiments were performed in synaptically isolated hemisected spinal cords (in the presence of CNQX, picrotoxin and strychnine; antagonists of non-NMDA, GABA$_A$, and glycine receptors, respectively). The importance of persistent sodium current (I_{NaP}) to rhythm generation has been demonstrated in neuronal groups associated with rhythmic motor outputs controlling respiratory functions and mastication,[50–53] but see Ref. 54. Therefore, we examined whether it plays a role in mediating voltage oscillations in Hb9 INs. Exposure to rhythmogenic cocktail containing low concentrations of NMA (5 μM), 5-HT (10 μM) and dopamine (50 μM) triggered relatively small (<10 mV) and slow (∼0.1 Hz) locomotor-like voltage oscillations that were blocked by riluzole (10 μM), a blocker of I_{NaP} (Fig. 3B) and TTX (1 μM) that blocks both the fast- and slow-inactivating sodium channels. These data indicate that I_{NaP} is essential for generating the in-

duced membrane oscillations in Hb9 INs. I_{NaP} plays an important role in controlling rhythmic activity in Hb9 INs following the removal of extracellular calcium.[41] The current is activated at subthreshold potentials (average of −58 mV[37]), which might contribute to the synchronization of network activity as hypothesized in the respiratory circuitry.[55] Our finding that I_{NaP} regulates locomotor-like rhythmic activity in Hb9 INs independently of fast synaptic transmission provides additional support to the hypothesis that they function as integrated components in the rhythmogenic locomotor circuitry.

Recently it became apparent that increasing the concentration of N-methyl-D-aspartic acid (NMDA, 20 μM) in the rhythmogenic cocktail triggers different ionic mechanisms that generate larger (>10 mV) and faster (0.2–0.3 Hz) voltage oscillations than those produced during exposure to lower NMA concentration (5 μM).[37] TTX does not alter the frequency of the faster subthreshold oscillations but it reduces their amplitude, implying that currents stronger than I_{NaP} control their frequency.[27,36,37] NMDA receptor activation alone is sufficient to trigger voltage oscillations in motoneurons and interneurons near the central canal.[56,57] Similarly, exposure to high concentration of NMDA (10–20 μM) can produce rhythmic activity in Hb9 INs that are not regulated by I_{NaP} (not shown). It has been proposed that low-voltage activated (LVA) calcium current underlies the large amplitude membrane oscillations produced by rhythmogenic cocktail with high concentration of NMDA.[27] The conclusion is based primarily on the observation that nickel, a relatively specific blocker of LVA calcium current, suppresses the rhythmic activity. We have also documented that nickel (100 μM) blocks both the small and large membrane oscillations in synaptically isolated Hb9 INs (Fig. 4A). However, our preliminary data show that nickel-sensitive calcium current cannot be evoked by step depolarizations from a holding potential of −60 mV to −40 mV confirming the generally accepted assumption that LVA calcium current is partially inactivated at resting membrane potential. Small nickel-sensitive calcium currents can be generated by step depolarizations from a holding potential of −90 mV to −60 mV (not shown). The finding that LVA calcium current

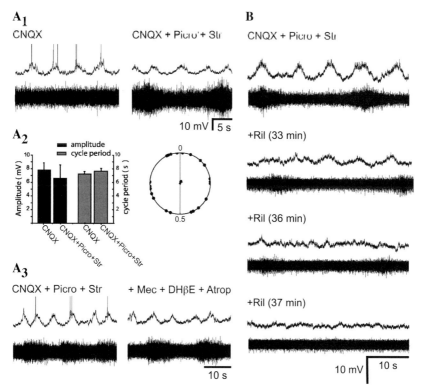

Figure 3. Cocktail-induced locomotor-like oscillations in synaptically isolated spinal cord are mediated by I_{NaP}. Simultaneous recording of neurochemically induced locomotor-like rhythms in Hb9 IN (*upper trace*) and electroneurograms of L1 or L2 ventral roots (*lower trace*). (A$_1$) The amplitude and frequency of induced CNQX-resistant voltage oscillations did not change after blocking glycinergic and GABAergic transmission (10 μM CNQX + 15 μM picrotoxin (Picro) + 0.5 μM strychnine (Str)). Ventral root bursts were suppressed in the presence of CNQX. Action potentials are truncated. (A$_2$) Histogram of the amplitude and cycle period (mean ± SE, $n = 6$) as a function of blocking non-NMDARs (CNQX) or inhibiting both fast excitatory and inhibitory transmission (CNQX + Picro + Str). Disinhibition did not significantly change the amplitude of CNQX-resistant membrane oscillations. Circular phase analysis demonstrates broadly distributed phase values, reflecting the lack of correlation between rhythmic activities in Hb9 INs and motoneurons in the synaptically isolated hemicord ($r = 0.12$). (A$_3$) In a different Hb9 IN, blocking nicotinic and muscarinic receptors did not significantly alter the properties of membrane voltage oscillations in Hb9 INs. Nicotinic transmission was blocked with mecamylamine (Mec, 10 μM) and dihydro-beta-erythroidine (DHβE, 50 μM), and muscarinic receptors were blocked with atropine (Atrop, 10 μM). Resting potentials varied between −52 and −56 mV. (B) Riluzole (Ril, 10 μM), a blocker of I_{NaP}, suppressed voltage oscillations in synaptically isolated Hb9 INs. Membrane potential was −50 mV. Modified with permission from Ziskind-Conhaim.[37]

cannot be produced at membrane potential of −60 mV requires an alternative explanation for the action of nickel on induced locomotor-like oscillations.

It is conceivable that nickel blocks NMDA receptor-mediated currents as reported in cultured neurons.[58] To test this possibility, we examined the effect of mibefradil, another relatively specific blocker of LVA calcium current[59,60] on voltage oscillations triggered by high NMDA concentration.

Mibefradil (10 μM) as well as nickel (100 μM) blocked the small (4–7 mV) rebound postinhibitory potentials (RIPs) generated in the presence of TTX in response to a break from hyperpolarizing current pulse to ∼ −100 mV ($n = 5$ Hb9 INs). The RIPs are thought to be mediated by LVA calcium current. In synaptically isolated Hb9 INs, the amplitude or frequency of membrane oscillations produced by NMDA (20 μM) did not significantly change during up to 40 min exposure to mibefradil

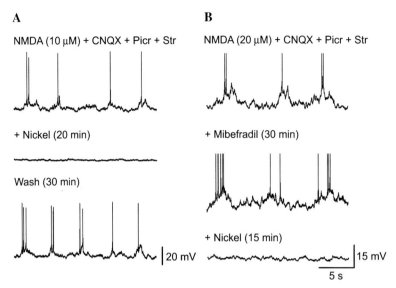

Figure 4. Nickel but not mibefradil suppressed cocktail-induced voltage oscillations triggered by high concentrations of NMDA. (**A**) NMDA alone triggered membrane oscillations that were blocked after 20 min exposure to nickel. The inhibition was reversible within 30 min of nickel removal. Membrane potentials: −55 to −60 mV. (**B**) In a different Hb9 IN, exposure to mibefradil did not block membrane voltage oscillations, but those were blocked by nickel. Membrane potentials: −53 to −57 mV. Action potentials are truncated.

(10 μM) (Fig. 4B). The mean amplitude and frequency of subthreshold oscillations were 8.0 mV ± 2.3 (SE, $n = 3$) and 0.35 Hz ± 0.04 Hz (7.2 ± 1.7 mV), respectively before mibefradil application and 7.2 ± 1.7 mV and 0.44 ± 0.11 Hz in its presence. Mibefradil had no effect on amplitude and frequency of lower frequency oscillation (0.07 Hz) induced by cocktail with low NMA concentration (5 μM, $n = 2$). Mibefradil-resistant membrane oscillations were blocked by nickel (Fig. 4B). Therefore, it is possible nickel suppresses induced locomotor-like membrane oscillations by blocking NMDA receptors rather than LVA calcium current.

It is reasonable to assume that the slow voltage oscillations that are generated by I_{NaP} (low NMA) are terminated by the slow inactivation of persistent sodium channels.[61,62] However, little was known about the current responsible for terminating the faster oscillations triggered by high NMDA. We hypothesized that if NMDA produces a large calcium influx, it might activate calcium-dependent potassium channels that play a role in burst termination in rhythmic neurons in the lamprey.[63] Exposure to charybdotoxin (100 nM), a blocker of high conductance calcium-dependent potassium channels (BKCa), did not suppress membrane oscilla-

tions triggered by low-NMA rhythmogenic cocktail (Fig. 5A), but the rhythms became less regular in its presence. An average amplitude of 7.2 ± 0.6 mV (S.E., $n = 3$) and frequency of 0.24 ± 0.04 Hz were recorded before charybdotoxin application, changing to 5.2 ± 1.9 mV and 0.4 ± 0.22 Hz in its presence. In contrast, the blocker eliminated voltage oscillations induced by high-NMDA cocktail (Fig. 5B), indicating that BKCa channels play an important role in voltage oscillations triggered by high NMDA. The contribution of calcium-dependent potassium currents to shortening the duration of oscillatory activity might explain the higher frequency membrane oscillations generated by a cocktail with higher NMDA concentration. Apamin (100 nM), a blocker of the small conductance calcium-dependent potassium channels, did not affect the properties of high NMDA-induced voltage oscillations (not shown).

Monosynaptic inputs from low-threshold afferents modulate locomotor-like rhythms in Hb9 INs

The activity pattern of motor circuits is influenced by peripheral sensory inputs that adjust locomotor activity to external stimuli. To increase our

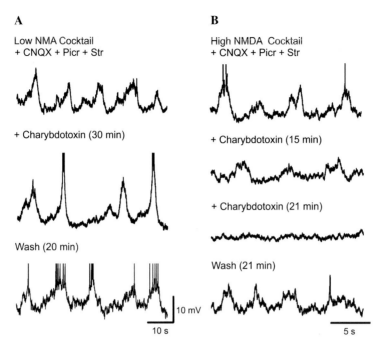

Figure 5. Blocking BKCa channels suppressed the membrane oscillations generated by high-NMDA rhythmogenic cocktail. (**A**) Exposure to cocktail with low NMA (5 μM) triggered voltage oscillations that became less regular but were not blocked in the presence of charybdotoxin. More regular pattern of voltage oscillations was apparent 20 min after removing charybdotoxin. Membrane potential: −52 to −55 mV. Action potentials are truncated. (**B**) In a different Hb9 IN, membrane oscillations triggered by high NMDA (20 μM) cocktail were blocked within 21 min exposure to charybdotoxin. The inhibitory action was reversible. Membrane potential: −50 to −54 mV.

understanding of the possible role of Hb9 INs in the locomotor circuitry, we examined whether their rhythmic activity is modulated by low-threshold afferents. In the hemisected spinal cord, stimulating low-threshold afferents (two time threshold) generated short-latency EPSCs in 62% of Hb9 INs (Fig. 6). These were monosynaptic EPSCs based on their stable latency during high-frequency stimulation and their resistance to mephenesin, a barbiturate that suppresses polysynaptic responses.[64]

Concomitant morphological analysis revealed that most boutons that expressed vesicular glutamate transporter-1 (VGluT-1) and parvalbumin, markers of primary afferents in neonatal rodents[65,66] were in close apposition to dendrites of neurobiotin-filled Hb9 INs (Fig. 6, $n = 4$). Quantitative analysis showed that most of the putative synaptic contacts were on distal dendrites. The number of boutons in close proximity to tertiary dendrites was two- to threefold higher than that on primary dendrites. The morphological data strongly support the electrophysiological findings that low-threshold afferents, presumably muscle afferents, provide direct sensory inputs to the majority of Hb9 INs.

If Hb9 INs are part of the locomotor networks, inputs from muscle afferents are likely to regulate their induced locomotor-like rhythms. In recent experiments we have shown that excitation of flexor-related, low-threshold afferents (L1–L3) during the flexor phase reset the rhythms in both Hb9 INs and segmental motoneurons while maintaining the phase relation between them.[67] These findings provide additional support to the hypothesis that Hb9 INs are part of the sensorimotor circuitry that contribute to locomotor rhythm generation.

Putative synaptic contacts between Hb9 INs and ipsilateral motoneurons

Identifying the target neurons of a given interneuronal population is fundamental for understanding their role in a network of known motor function. Several models have been proposed to describe the

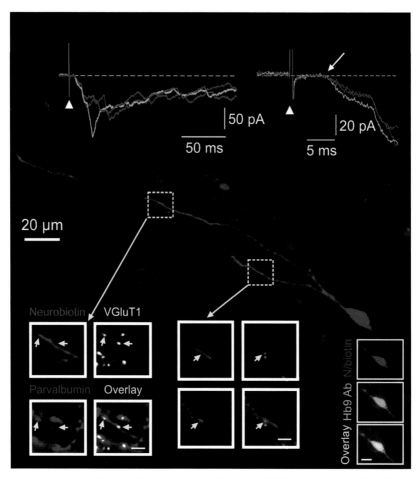

Figure 6. Putative glutamatergic boutons from primary afferents on Hb9 interneurons. Stimulation of dorsal root afferents at two times threshold evoked short-latency EPSCs in a Hb9 IN. Top left: superimposed are three successive traces recorded at 0.1 Hz. Top right: expanded time scale to show that the onset of the evoked response (*white arrow*) was time-locked to the stimulus artifact (*triangle*), suggesting that these were monosynaptic EPSCs. The Hb9 IN was filled with neurobiotin (*red*). Combined immunohistochemistry against VGluT1 (*white*), parvalbumin (*blue*), and the Hb9 protein (*green*) revealed that proximal and distal dendrites receive putative primary afferent synapses (VGluT1$^+$ and Parvalbumin$^+$; both sets of four images acquired at the single optical level). The Hb9 IN was reconstructed from individually acquired *z*-axis images and shown as a projection (main image; Hb9 shown in *red*). The soma of the neuron recorded from (neurobiotin) was positive for the Hb9 protein (set of three images at the bottom right), confirming its identity as a Hb9 IN.

interactions between excitatory neuronal components of the CPG and motoneurons. Based on the single-level CPG, the rhythm generators directly excite functionally related motoneurons, while in more complex architectures that consist of two- and three-level CPGs, motoneurons are driven by excitatory interneurons that are part of the pattern formation networks or last order interneurons.[68] Therefore, if the rhythmogenic Hb9 INs synapse onto segmental motoneurons they might function as the generator based on the single-level model but not according to the two-level network organization.

We have previously shown that axons of neurobiotin-filled Hb9 INs project toward ipsilateral motoneuron nuclei and their bouton-like varicosities are in close apposition to GFP-expressing proximal dendrites of large neurons in lamina IX.[26] The neurobiotin-filled boutons express VGluT2, a

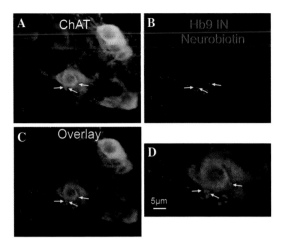

Figure 7. Putative contacts of Hb9 INs on motoneurons in the medial motor column. (**A**) Motoneurons were labeled with ChAT (*white*) to reveal the extent of somatic membrane. The image is a short *z*-stack projection from individual images. (**B**) The putative axon of a single-filled Hb9 interneuron. Neurobiotin was visualized with the ABC method and revealed with Rhodamine as the fluorochrome (*red*). (**C**) An overlay image from A and B. (**D**) Note the close apposition of three individual synaptic boutons from the Hb9 IN (*arrows*) to the soma of two medially located motoneurons.

marker of glutamatergic interneurons,[26,29,31] implying that Hb9 INs form synaptic contacts onto motoneurons in the medial and/or lateral motor columns. However, in that study we could not rule out the possibility that the VGluT2-expressing boutons are in close proximity to GFP positive dendrites of excitatory interneurons rather than motoneurons. Moreover, a different study has reported that contacts between GFP positive and VGluT2-expressing boutons and motoneurons are rare in spinal cords of juvenile mice, concluding that it is unlikely that Hb9 INs have a significant number of inputs onto motoneurons.[27]

We recently began a new set of experiments in which motoneurons were identified by the enzyme choline acetyltransferase (ChAT) and we investigated whether neurobiotin-filled axon terminals were in close proximity to ChAT-expressing motoneurons. Preliminary experiments have identified putative synaptic contacts between neurobiotin-filled boutons and ChAT-expressing motoneurons in the medial motor column (Fig. 7). The identity and properties of synaptic transmission be-

tween Hb9 INs and motoneurons will have to be carefully examined using paired whole-cell recordings.

Conclusions

Hb9 INs have been examined in great detail by several groups and accumulated data support the concept that they are part of the rhythm-generating kernel of the locomotor CPG.

However, one of the most conclusive tests, ablation or silencing Hb9 INs to determine the effects on locomotor activity has not been performed. The Hb9 gene that distinguishes Hb9 INs from most glutamatergic interneurons is also expressed in motoneurons, therefore genetic manipulations that alter their function will disrupt motoneuron activity. Testing the effect of silencing Hb9 INs on rhythmic motor activity is important for elucidating their probable role in the locomotor circuitry, but their functional hierarchy as rhythm generator, pattern formation neurons, or last order interneurons will be determined by: (1) the regulation of their activity by descending pathways, (2) their synaptic interactions with excitatory and inhibitory interneurons that are thought to be part of the rhythm-generating and rhythm-coordinating networks, and (3) the identification of their target neurons.

Acknowledgment

This work was supported by a NINDS/NIH grant NS-23808 to Lea Ziskind-Conhaim and NINDS intramural funds to George Z. Mentis.

Conflicts of interest

The authors declare no conflicts of interest.

References

1. Graham Brown, T. 1911. Intrinsic factors in the act of progression in the mammal. *Proc. R. Soc. Lond. Series B,* **84:** 308–319.
2. Grillner, S. & P. Wallen. 1985. Central pattern generators for locomotion, with special reference to vertebrates. *Ann. Rev. Neurosci.* **8:** 233–261.
3. Kiehn, O. & S.J. Butt. 2003. Physiological, anatomical and genetic identification of CPG neurons in the developing mammalian spinal cord. *Prog. Neurobiol.* **70:** 347–361.

4. Grillner, S. 2006. Biological pattern generation: the cellular and computational logic of networks in motion. *Neuron* **52:** 751–766.

5. Kudo, N. & T. Yamada. 1987. *N*-methyl-d,l-aspartate-induced locomotor activity in a spinal cord-hindlimb muscles preparation of the newborn rat studied *in vitro. Neurosci. Lett.* **75:** 43–48.

6. Smith, J.C. & J.L. Feldman. 1987. *In vitro* brainstem-spinal cord preparations for study of motor systems for mammalian respiration and locomotion. *J. Neurosci. Meth.* **21:** 321–333.

7. Cazalets, J.R., Y. Sqalli-Houssaini & F. Clarac. 1992. Activation of the central pattern generators for locomotion by serotonin and excitatory amino acids in neonatal rat. *J. Physiol.* **455:** 187–204.

8. Cowley, K.C. & B.J. Schmidt. 1997. Regional distribution of the locomotor pattern-generating network in the neonatal rat spinal cord. *J. Neurophysiol.* **77:** 247–259.

9. Kiehn, O. & O. Kjaerulff. 1998. Distribution of central pattern generators for rhythmic motor outputs in the spinal cord of limbed vertebrates. *Ann. N.Y Acad. Sci.* **860:** 110–129.

10. Whelan, P., A. Bonnot & M.J. O'Donovan. 2000. Properties of rhythmic activity generated by the isolated spinal cord of the neonatal mouse. *J. Neurophysiol.* **84:** 2821–2833.

11. Kiehn, O. 2006. Locomotor circuits in the mammalian spinal cord. *Ann. Rev. Neurosci.* **29:** 279–306.

12. Lev-Tov, A., I. Delvolve & E. Kremer. 2000. Sacrocaudal afferents induce rhythmic efferent bursting in isolated spinal cords of neonatal rats. *J. Neurophysiol.* **83:** 888–894.

13. Bonnot, A. *et al.* 2002. Locomotor-like activity generated by the neonatal mouse spinal cord. *Brain Res. Brain Res. Rev.* **40:** 141–151.

14. Gordon, I.T. & P.J. Whelan. 2006. Monoaminergic control of cauda equina evoked locomotion in the neonatal mouse spinal cord. *J. Neurophysiol.* **96:** 3122–3129.

15. Zhong, G., M.A. Masino & R.M. Harris-Warrick. 2007. Persistent sodium currents participate in fictive locomotion generation in neonatal mouse spinal cord. *J. Neurosci.* **27:** 4507–4518.

16. Goulding, M. 2009. Circuits controlling vertebrate locomotion: moving in a new direction. *Nat. Rev. Neurosci.* **10:** 507–518.

17. Lundberg, A. 1979. Multisensory control of spinal reflex pathways. *Prog. Brain Res.* **50:** 11–28.

18. Jankowska, E. & S. Edgley. 1993. Interactions between pathways controlling posture and gait at the level of spinal interneurones in the cat. *Prog. Brain Res.* **97:** 161–171.

19. Jankowska, E. 2008. Spinal interneuronal networks in the cat: elementary components. *Brain Res. Rev.* **1:** 46–55.

20. Butt, S.J. & O. Kiehn. 2003. Functional identification of interneurons responsible for left–right coordination of hindlimbs in mammals. *Neuron* **38:** 953–963.

21. Lanuza, G.M. *et al.* 2004. Genetic identification of spinal interneurons that coordinate left–right locomotor activity necessary for walking movements. *Neuron* **42:** 375–386.

22. Zhong, G., M. Diaz-Rios & R.M. Harris-Warrick. 2006. Intrinsic and functional differences among commissural interneurons during fictive locomotion and serotonergic modulation in the neonatal mouse. *J. Neurosci.* 26: 6509–6517.

23. Butt, S.J., J.M. Lebret & O. Kiehn. 2002. Organization of left–right coordination in the mammalian locomotor network. *Brain Res. Rev.* **40:** 107–117.

24. Jessell, T. M. 2000. Neuronal specification in the spinal cord: inductive signals and transcriptional codes. *Nat. Rev. Genet.* **1:** 20–29.

25. Goulding, M. & S.L. Pfaff. 2005. Development of circuits that generate simple rhythmic behaviors in vertebrates. *Curr. Opin. Neurobiol.* **15:** 14–20.

26. Hinckley, C.A. *et al.* 2005. Locomotor-like rhythms in a genetically distinct cluster of interneurons in the mammalian spinal cord. *J. Neurophysiol.* **93:** 1439–1449.

27. Wilson, J.M. *et al.* 2005. Conditional rhythmicity of ventral spinal interneurons defined by expression of the Hb9 homeodomain protein. *J. Neurosci.* **25:** 5710–5719.

28. Butt, S.J., L. Lundfald & O. Kiehn. 2005. EphA4 defines a class of excitatory locomotor-related interneurons. *Proc. Natl. Acad. Sci. USA* **102:** 14098–14103.

29. Crone, S. A. *et al.* 2008. Genetic ablation of V2a ipsilateral interneurons disrupts left-right locomotor coordination in mammalian spinal cord. *Neuron* **60:** 70–83.

30. Crone, S.A. *et al.* 2009. In mice lacking V2a interneurons, gait depends on speed of locomotion. *J. Neurosci.* **29:** 7098–7109.

31. Zhang, Y.S. *et al.* 2008. V3 spinal neurons establish a robust and balanced locomotor rhythm during walking. *Neuron* **60:** 84–96.

32. Brownstone R.M. & J.M. Wilson. 2008. Strategies for delineating spinal locomotor rhythm-generating networks and the possible role of Hb9 interneurones in rhythmogenesis. *Brain Res. Rev.* **57:** 64–76.

33. Wichterle, H. *et al.* 2002. Directed differentiation of embryonic stem cells into motor neurons. *Cell* **110:** 385–397.

34. Kjaerulff, O. & O. Kiehn. 1996. Distribution of networks generating and coordinating locomotor activity in the neonatal rat spinal cord *in vitro*: a lesion study. *J. Neurosci.* **16:** 5777–5794.

35. Kremer, E. & A. Lev-Tov. 1997. Localization of the spinal network associated with generation of hindlimb locomotion in the neonatal rat and organization of its transverse coupling system. *J. Neurophysiol.* **77:** 1155–1170.

36. Han, P. *et al.* 2007. Dopaminergic modulation of spinal neuronal excitability. *J. Neurosci.* **27:** 13192–13204.

37. Ziskind-Conhaim, L., L. Wu & E.P. Wiesner. 2008. Persistent sodium current contributes to induced voltage oscillations in locomotor-related Hb9 interneurons in the mouse spinal cord. *J. Neurophysiol.* **100:** 2254–2264.

38. Kiehn, O. & O. Kjaerulff. 1996. Spatiotemporal characteristics of 5-HT and dopamine-induced rhythmic hindlimb activity in the *in vitro* neonatal rat. *J. Neuorphysiol.* **75:** 1472–1482.

39. Wilson, J. M., A.I. Cowan & R.M. Brownstone. 2007. Heterogeneous electrotonic coupling and synchronization of rhythmic bursting activity in mouse hb9 interneurons. *J. Neurophysiol.* **98:** 2370–2381.

40. Hinckley, C.A. & L. Ziskind-Conhaim. 2006. Electrical coupling between locomotor-related excitatory interneurons in the mammalian spinal cord. *J. Neurosci.* **26:** 8477–8483.

41. Tazerart, S., L. Vinay & F. Brocard. 2008. The persistent sodium current generates pacemaker activities in the central pattern generator for locomotion and regulates the locomotor rhythm. *J. Neurosci.* **28:** 8577–8589.

42. Kwan, A.C. *et al.* 2009. Activity of Hb9 interneurons during fictive locomotion in mouse spinal cord. *J. Neurosci.* **29:** 11601–11612.

43. Vanderhorst, V.G. & G. Holstege. 1997. Organization of lumbosacral motoneuronal cell groups innervating hindlimb, pelvic floor, and axial muscles in the cat. *J. Comp. Neurol.* **382:** 46–76.

44. Schomburg, E.D., H. Steffens & K. Dembowsky. 2003. Rhythmic phrenic, intercostals and sympathetic activity in relation to limb and trunk motor activity in spinal cats. *Neurosci. Res.* **46:** 229–240.

45. Strauss, I. & A. Lev-Tov. 2003. Neural pathways between sacrocaudal afferents and lumbar pattern generators in neonatal rats. *J. Neurophysiol.* **89:** 773–784.

46. Cowley, K.C., E. Zaporozhets & B.J. Schmidt. 2008. Propriospinal neurons are sufficient for bulbospinal transmission of the locomotor command signal in the neonatal rat spinal cord. *J. Physiol.* **586:** 1623–1635.

47. Ramirez, J. M., A.K. Tryba & F. Pena. 2004. Pacemaker neurons and neuronal networks: an integrative view. *Curr. Opin. Neurobiol.* **14:** 665–674.

48. Raastad, M., B.R. Johnson & O. Kiehn. 1997. Analysis of EPSCs and IPSCs carrying rhythmic, locomotor-related information in the isolated spinal cord of the neonatal rat. *J. Neurophysiol.* **78:** 1851–1859.

49. Butt, S.J., R.M. Harris-Warrick & O. Kiehn. 2002. Firing properties of identified interneuron populations in the mammalian hindlimb central pattern generator. *J. Neurosci.* **22:** 9961–9971.

50. Del Negro, C.A. *et al.* 2002. Persistent sodium current, membrane properties and bursting behavior of pre-botzinger complex inspiratory neurons *in vitro*. *J. Neurophysiol.* **88:** 2242–2250.

51. Pena, F. *et al.* 2004. Differential contribution of pacemaker properties to the generation of respiratory rhythms during normoxia and hypoxia. *Neuron* **43:** 105–117.

52. Wu, N. *et al.* 2005. Persistent sodium currents in mesencephalic v neurons participate in burst generation and control of membrane excitability. *J. Neurophysiol.* **93:** 2710–2722.

53. Enomoto, A. *et al.* 2006. Participation of sodium currents in burst generation and control of membrane excitability in mesencephalic trigeminal neurons. *J. Neurosci.* **26:** 3412–3422.

54. Pace, R.W. *et al.* 2007. Inspiratory bursts in the pre-Botzinger complex depend on a calcium-activated nonspecific cation current linked to glutamate receptors in neonatal mice. *J. Physiol.* **582:** 113–125.

55. Koizumi, H. & J.C. Smith. 2008. Persistent Na+ and K+-dominated leak currents contribute to respiratory rhythm generation in the pre-Botzinger complex *in vitro*. *J. Neurosci.* **28:** 1773–1785.

56. Hochman, S., L.M. Jordan & J.F. MacDonald. 1994. *N*-methyl-D-aspartate receptor-mediated voltage oscillations in neurons surrounding the central canal in slices of rat spinal cord. *J. Neurophysiol.* **72:** 565–577.

57. Schmidt, B.J., S. Hochman & J.N. MacLean. 1998. NMDA receptor-mediated oscillatory properties: potential role in rhythm generation in the mammalian spinal cord. *Ann. N.Y. Acad. Sci.* **860:** 189–202.

58. Marchetti, C. & P. Gavazzo. 2003. Subunit-dependent effects of nickel on NMDA receptor channels. *Brain Res. Mol. Brain Res.* **117:** 139–144.

59. Bezprozvanny, I. & R.W. Tsien. 1995. Voltage-dependent blockade of diverse types of voltage-gated Ca^{2+} channels expressed in *Xenopus* oocytes by the Ca^{2+} channel antagonist mibefradil (Ro 40–5967). *Mol. Pharmacol.* **48:** 540–549.

60. McDonough, S. I. & B.P. Bean. 1998. Mibefradil inhibition of T-type calcium channels in cerebellar purkinje neurons. *Mol. Pharmacol.* **54:** 1080–1087.

61. Butera R.J., Jr., J. Rinzel & J.C. Smith. 1999. Models of respiratory rhythm generation in the pre-Botzinger complex. Part I. Bursting pacemaker neurons. *J. Neurophysiol.* **82:** 382–397.

62. Magistretti, J. & A. Alonso. 1999. Biophysical properties and slow voltage-dependent inactivation of a sustained sodium current in entorhinal cortex layer-II principal neurons: a whole-cell and single-channel study. *J. Gen. Physiol.* **114:** 491–509.

63. Manira, A., J. Tegner & S. Grillner. 1994. Calcium-dependent potassium channels play a critical role for burst termination in the locomotor network in lamprey. *J. Neurophysiol.* **72:** 1852–1861.

64. Ziskind-Conhaim, L. 1990. NMDA receptors mediate poly- and monosynaptic potentials in motoneurons of rat embryos. *J. Neurosci.* **10:** 125–135.

65. Oliveira, A.L. *et al.* 2003. Cellular localization of three vesicular glutamate transporter mRNAs and proteins in rat spinal cord and dorsal root ganglia. *Synapse* **50:** 117–129.

66. Alvarez, F. J. *et al.* 2004. Vesicular glutamate transporters in the spinal cord, with special reference to sensory primary afferent synapses. *J. Comp. Neurol.* **472:** 257–280.

67. Hinckley, C.A & L. Ziskind-Conhaim. 2005. Sensory Modulation of Locomotor-Like Rhythms in HB9-Expressing Interneurons. Program No. 516.12. 2005 Abstract Viewer/Itinerary Planner. Washington, DC: Society for Neuroscience. http://www.sfn.org/index.cfm?pagename=abstracts_archive&task=browse&action=results&start=2101.

68. McCrea, D. A. & I.A. Rybak. 2008. Organization of mammalian locomotor rhythm and pattern generation. *Brain Res. Rev.* **57:** 134–146.

Ann. N.Y. Acad. Sci. ISSN 0077-8923

ANNALS OF THE NEW YORK ACADEMY OF SCIENCES
Issue: *Neurons and Networks in the Spinal Cord*

Functional organization of V2a-related locomotor circuits in the rodent spinal cord

Kimberly J. Dougherty and Ole Kiehn

Mammalian Locomotor Laboratory, Department of Neuroscience, Karolinska Institutet, Stockholm, Sweden

Address for correspondence: Prof. Ole Kiehn, Mammalian Locomotor Laboratory, Department of Neuroscience, Karolinska Institutet, Stockholm S-171 77, Sweden. O.Kiehn@ki.se

Studies of mammalian locomotion have been greatly facilitated by the use of the isolated rodent spinal cord preparation that retains the locomotor circuits needed to execute the movement. Physiological and molecular genetic experiments in this preparation have started to unravel the basic circuit organization responsible for walking in mammals. Here, we review these experiments with a focus on the functional role of excitatory V2a interneurons in the mammalian locomotor network. With regard to these neurons and other network structures we also discuss similarities and differences between the mammalian walking central pattern generator (CPG) and the fish swimming CPG.

Keywords: spinal cord; Chx10; locomotion; interneurons; transcription factors

Introduction

Central pattern generators (CPGs) are neuronal networks that generate rhythmic motor outputs, including walking, breathing, chewing, and swimming. The walking CPG in mammals is located in the ventral horn of the lumbar and lower thoracic spinal cord and contains the three main elements required for locomotion: rhythm generation, left–right alternation, and flexor-extensor alternation.[1] The isolated rodent spinal cord preparation has been widely used to study mammalian locomotion, as the spinal cord can be separated from descending inputs and retain the capability to produce coordinated locomotor-like activity when appropriately stimulated.

Despite the laminar structure of the spinal cord, many CPG neurons seem to be intermingled which makes it difficult to reliably target specific spinal interneuronal subpopulations in order to elucidate the CPG circuitry. One way in which subpopulations have been successfully identified is by the expression of developmentally related transcription factors. Interneurons in the ventral spinal cord can be divided into four major subgroups (V0–V3) based on their expression of early transcription factors.[2,3] These transcription factors have been used to identify subsets of interneurons and molecular genetics has been used to determine the roles these classes of neurons may play in locomotion in both the mouse[4–16] and the zebrafish.[17,18]

In this review we will discuss recent physiological and molecular genetic experiments designed to understand the function of excitatory V2a interneurons in the rodent spinal cord. Studying these neurons and how they project onto other known parts of the mammalian CPG circuit has started to give comprehensive insights into the locomotor network architecture. The V2a interneurons have molecular homologs in the swimming CPG, therefore they also provide an excellent vantage point to discuss generalities about the vertebrate CPG organization.

Model of CPG circuitry based on Chx10 ablation studies

V2 interneurons express Lhx3 early in development and are a mixed excitatory/inhibitory population located in lamina VII.[19–21] This class of interneurons is further subdivided based on transcription factor expression. V2a interneurons express Chx10 and are exclusively excitatory and project ipsilaterally,[19,20] while V2b interneurons express Gata2/3, are inhibitory, and project ipsilaterally.[19,20]

doi: 10.1111/j.1749-6632.2010.05502.x

The physiological function of spinal V2a interneurons in the locomotor network has been studied after genetically ablating Chx10 interneurons with diphtheria toxin A (DTA).[10] This approach resulted in almost total ablation of the Chx10 cell population in the spinal cord, without affecting V0, V1, V2b, and V3 interneurons or motor neurons (MNs). In the absence of Chx10 neurons it was still possible to elicit locomotor-like activity in spinal cords isolated from Chx10-DTA mice suggesting that Chx10 interneurons are not the main rhythm-generating neurons. The most striking locomotor defect in the Chx10-DTA mice was a disturbed left–right coordination as evidenced by drift and lack of coordination between activity on the left and right sides. However, flexor-extensor alternation remained unaffected. Because the deficit was in left–right coordination and the Chx10 cells only project ipsilaterally, the simplest explanation for the observed locomotor deficit is that Chx10 neurons activate commissural neurons responsible for left–right alternation. Previous work in our laboratory has identified the main elements in the segmental alternating pathways. This dual-inhibitory pathway is composed of direct inhibitory (CINi, "1," Fig. 1), and indirect inhibitory inputs (CINei, "2," Fig. 1) to MNs.[22] The indirect pathway is mediated through Renshaw cells[23] and other inhibitory interneurons possibly related to V1 interneurons expressing the early transcription factor Engrailed 1[24–26] ("3," Fig. 1). Based on these findings, we proposed a model in which the V2a (Chx10) spinal neurons ("4," Fig. 1) are part of the rodent CPG that drives the dual inhibitory pathway responsible for left–right alternation (Fig. 1). In this model Chx10 neurons are themselves driven by rhythm-generating neurons ("5," Fig. 1). The rhythm-generating core also provides excitation (directly or indirectly) to MNs ("6," Fig. 1) and drives inhibitory neurons projecting to MNs ("7," Fig. 1). The exact identity of these last order interneurons has not been defined but may include EphA4[27,28] or Hb9[4,6,8,29] positive excitatory neurons and Engrailed-1 positive inhibitory neurons.[24,25] In the absence of Chx10 neurons, both locomotor burst amplitude and frequency were significantly more variable as compared to control suggesting that Chx10 neurons contribute directly or indirectly to the excitation of both the MNs ("9," Fig. 1) and the rhythm-generating neurons ("8," Fig. 1). Another finding from Crone et al. 2008[10] was

that synchronous left–right activity was generated in Chx10-DTA spinal cords when all fast GABAergic and glycinergic transmission was blocked, similar to what is seen in wild-type mice. Therefore, commissural pathways involved in this coordination are unlikely to be driven by Chx10 neurons but rather they are driven directly from the rhythm-generating core ("10," Fig. 1).

Neither sensory afferent stimulation ("12," Fig. 1) nor stimulation in the lower brainstem ("13," Fig. 1) was capable of eliciting locomotor-like activity in the Chx10-DTA cords.[10] The inability of sensory inputs to produce locomotor rhythms suggests that Chx10 neurons may serve as a sensory gateway into the CPG, while the inability to evoke locomotion from brainstem stimulation suggests either that Chx10 neurons mediate supraspinal inputs to the CPG or that Chx10 neurons expressed in the lower brainstem are generating locomotor signals to the spinal CPG. The model presented in Crone et al. (2008)[10] places the Chx10 interneurons in a key position within the mammalian CPG, integrating sensory, possibly supraspinal, and rhythm-generator inputs and influencing both ipsilateral and contralateral circuitries.

The function of Chx10 neurons may vary with locomotor speed

The zebrafish homolog of Chx10, Alx, is expressed in a distinguishable class of neurons, the circumferential descending interneurons (CiDs[17]). Work in the zebrafish has shown that there is a locomotor-related speed-ordered recruitment of two excitatory classes of interneurons in the spinal cord. The commissural class (MCoDs) is recruited at the lowest speed, followed by the recruitment of CiDs at higher speeds.[30,31] This recruitment is not only ordered by class but also by dorsal–ventral positioning, with more dorsal cells becoming active as the speed increases. At higher speeds, the activation of MCoDs is not simply bypassed, but these cells become actively inhibited by inhibitory interneurons that seem to follow a similar, but reverse, ordered recruitment.[30,31] Similar speed-ordered recruitment has been extrapolated to encompass Chx10 neurons in mice.[11]

In the initial Chx10-DTA experiments[10] the mutant mice died within a day of birth because of respiratory problems. In a subsequent study it was

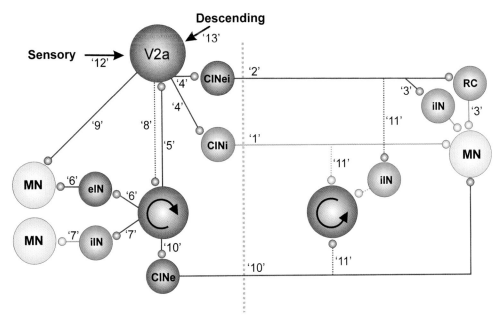

Figure 1. Organization of V2a segmental spinal locomotor networks in rodent diagram that shows the segmental ipsilateral flexor-extensor network connected to left–right coordinating networks. This diagram only shows connectivity at the segmental level and only accounts for activity in one locomotor phase (*e.g.,* flexor MNs). Left–right alternating networks are mediated by a dual inhibitory commissural system that comprises two commissural interneuron (CINs) populations: (i) a set of glycinergic/GABAergic commissural interneurons (CINi) ("1") that inhibit contralateral MNs directly, and (ii) a set of excitatory commissural interneurons that inhibit motor neurons indirectly (CINei) ("2") by acting on contralateral inhibitory interneurons (IN) that include Renshaw cells (RC) ("3") and other inhibitory neurons (iIN) ("3"). A group of excitatory neurons expressing the transcription factor Chx10, called V2a interneurons, provides inputs to the dual inhibitory pathway ("4") and is driven by the rhythm-generating core ("5") (indicated as one neuronal population). The rhythm-generating core also provides excitation (directly or indirectly (eIN)) to MNs ("6") and drives inhibitory neurons (iIN) projecting to MNs ("7") (only one module is included in this drawing). Chx10 neurons also contribute to the excitation of both the motor neurons ("9") and the rhythm-generating neurons ("8"). The rhythm-generating core drives the commissural interneuron systems responsible for left–right synchrony ("10"). Possible connections of CINs to rhythm-generating neurons on the contralateral side are indicated by *dotted lines* ("11"). V2a interneurons also seem to be a gate for sensory signals that evoke locomotion ("12") and for descending locomotor commands ("13"). *Vertical dotted line* indicates midline (adapted from Ref. 10).

found that if the original BL6/C57 mice were backcrossed into females of another strain (ICR mice), 40% of the Chx10-DTA mice survived into adulthood in this different genetic background.[11] Using these mice Crone *et al.* 2009[11] reconfirmed the findings that left–right alternation was drifting at moderate locomotor speeds both in the isolated spinal cord from newborns and during actual walking in adults. However, at low speeds (<0.4 Hz isolated newborn cord; <5 Hz intact adult), left–right alternation was intact and at higher speeds (>0.7 Hz isolated newborn cord; >8 Hz intact adult), left–right ventral root bursts became synchronous re-

sulting in a rabbit-like gate.[11] These findings led Crone *et al.* 2009[11] to propose that: (1) the Chx10 neurons are important for left–right alternation but only at moderate and high speeds and (2) Chx10 neurons are likely to be recruited only at moderate speeds, while at lower speeds other non-V2a neurons are active to ensure the left–right alternation. These experiments would endorse the speed-ordered recruitment as found in the zebrafish. Although such a model is attractive, it is not compatible with the firing properties seen in Chx10 cells during low speeds of locomotion. Recordings from Chx10 positive neurons in the isolated spinal cord of newborn mice during drug-evoked locomotion at low speeds (<0.4 Hz) have shown that 2/3 of Chx10 neurons in L2–L5 segments are rhythmically active[12] with 40% of them spiking rhythmically.[12,13] These findings clearly exclude a scenario where Chx10 cells are recruited only at moderate frequencies. In contrast, the Chx10 neurons seem to be active already at low locomotor speeds where they contribute, along with other neurons, to the left–right alternation. As the locomotor speed increases into the moderate frequency range it appears that more Chx10 cells are recruited and their tuning of firing becomes tighter although this increase in recruitment is modest at best.[13] However, the tighter tuning may contribute to a stronger influence on left–right alternation at moderate frequencies.

The intracellular recordings have also shown that the Chx10 neurons receive rhythmic excitatory drive during their active phase and that potential rhythmogenic properties (such as rebound and persistent inward currents) have no obvious relation to cell rhythmicity.[12,13] These findings support our model that Chx10 neurons are downstream of the rhythmogenic core in the rodent CPG.

Taken together, these studies suggest a complex role for the Chx10 neurons in the mammalian CPG. The model in which Chx10 neurons project to both pathways in the dual inhibitory left–right alternating system (Fig. 1) is unable to account for speed-related changes in left–right coordination. Moreover, the fact that Chx10 cells are rhythmically active at low locomotor speeds also excludes the model proposed by Crone et al. 2009.[11] In the next section, we will attempt to encompass these new findings in a modified model.

Updated CPG model

We propose a model in which Chx10 interneurons activate only one of the two paths in the dual inhibitory commissural pathways. The other alternating pathway is driven directly by the rhythm-generating core (Fig. 2). In this updated model, Chx10 neurons are active during locomotion at all speeds. The drive to the Chx10 neurons increases at higher speeds as does the drive to the other non-V2a driven left–right alternating pathway. At low speeds both of the dual inhibitory pathways are active but with a dominance in the non-V2a driven pathway. At moderate speeds the V2a pathway re-

ceives a stronger drive and becomes the dominating path, possibly by switching off activity in the non-V2a inhibitory crossed pathway.

Which of the two parts of the dual inhibitory pathway is the Chx10 population driving? At the moment we do not have any conclusive data to resolve this issue. Crone et al. 2008[10] have shown that V2a interneurons project to Evx1-positive commissural excitatory interneurons (EIN).[10,15,32–34] Moreover, a shorter latency crossed reflex is seen in the absence of Chx10 neurons.[10] This may suggest that the Chx10 neurons activate the indirect inhibitory pathway via excitatory commissural interneurons (Fig. 2). If this is the case, this pathway must inhibit the direct inhibitory pathway (not shown in Fig. 2), thus resulting in a shorter latency inhibition when the Chx10/indirect pathway is abolished. At low speeds the dominating left–right alternating circuits are therefore the direct crossed pathways involving inhibitory commissural interneurons. Aside from activating the indirect inhibitory commissural pathway, Chx10 neurons may also activate an unidentified inhibitory interneuron population that inhibits the direct inhibitory pathway and the crossed excitatory pathway mediating synchrony, therefore shutting them off at moderate frequencies, leaving the Chx10 crossed pathway as the dominant one (connections not shown in Fig. 2).

When Chx10 cells are lost, the alternating pathway is dominant at low frequencies, drifting at modest frequencies and a hopping gait is the result at higher frequencies. Chx10-DTA mice are able to maintain stable locomotion at low speeds because the direct inhibition is sufficient to balance the excitation. At higher speeds, the deficit in the crossed inhibitory pathway is exacerbated by the dis-inhibition of the crossed excitatory pathway. Excitation exceeds inhibition resulting in synchrony between right and left sides.

What is the molecular identity of the direct inhibitory pathway? These CINs can be either dI6 neurons or $Evx1^-/Dbx1^+$ neurons, both of which are GABAergic and/or glycinergic.[15,34] Altered left–right coordination is indeed seen in Dbx1 knockouts[15] and when Dbx1 neurons are ablated during development the alternating pattern is switched into a synchronous one[35,36] possibly because the entire dual inhibitory pathway is ablated (Fig. 2). Using Cre mice that target either Vglut2 positive neurons[37] or VIAAT positive neurons, it should be

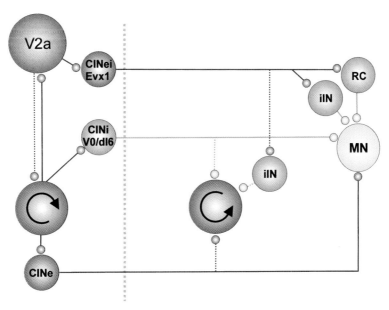

Figure 2. Updated model of left–right segmental V2a circuits diagram that shows the proposed V2a connections to the left–right coordinating networks. As in Fig. 1, the diagram only shows connectivity at the segmental level and only accounts for activity in one locomotor phase (*e.g.*, flexor motor neurons). The left–right alternating networks are mediated by a dual inhibitory commissural system (also shown in Fig. 1). In this model the V2a interneurons connect to only one path in the dual inhibitory system, namely the excitatory commissural interneurons that inhibit motor neurons indirectly (CINei). Molecularly, these CINs are the Evx1 positive V0 neurons. The other part of the alternating pathway, a set of glycinergic/GABAergic commissural interneurons that inhibit motor neurons directly (CINi), is driven directly by non-V2a rhythm-generating neurons, which also drive the V2a positive neurons. These neurons are either the Evx1 negative V0 neurons or dI6 neurons. The crossed circuits involved in segmental synchronous activity (CINe) are also driven by non-V2a interneurons. At low speeds both of the pathways of the dual inhibitory system are active while at moderate to higher speeds the indirect pathway dominates, possibly by inhibiting the direct inhibitory pathway (see text for details).

possible to selectively test the contribution from the indirect and direct pathways in the V0 population to left–right alternation in relationship to the V2a deficits. The prediction is that the selective deletion of the excitatory V0-pathway will mimic the V2a deficit while selective deletion of the inhibitory V0-pathway should only affect left–right alternation at low speeds. The V2a population can be further subdivided by the expression of transcription factors other than Chx10.[12,38] It will be important to determine the connectivity of these more refined V2a subpopulations and their role in the locomotor CPG.

Segmental V2a organization

Recordings of V2a interneuron activity along the cord showed that both flexor-related and extensor-related Chx10 interneurons coexist in the same segment, be it a flexor-related or extensor-related segment.[12] This may not be too surprising given the observation that although flexor MN activity dominates in the L2/L3 segments and extensor activity dominates in the L4/L5 segments, a substantial number of extensor MNs and extensor-related Renshaw cells are found in L2 and similarly a significant number of flexor MNs and flexor-related Renshaw cells are found in L5.[23,39] It remains unknown whether the Chx10 neurons that are out of phase with the local ventral roots (~1/3) are coordinated with the antagonist MNs in the same segment or with MNs in more rostral or caudal segments. Possibly coincidentally, about the same percentage (30%) of Chx10 neurons have long projections, whereas the rest of the Chx10 neurons have only local projections.[12] However, Chx10 ablation experiments

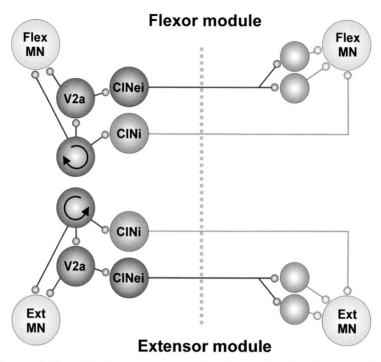

Figure 3. Modular organization of V2a interneuron connections diagram that shows the segmental flexor-related and extensor-related V2a connectivity. Flexor-related and extensor-related V2a interneurons provide inputs to ipsilateral motor neurons (flexors, "Flex" or extensors "Ext") and drive the indirect crossed pathways (CINei) in a coordinated fashion. Non-V2a interneurons drive the direct crossed pathway (CINi) and motor neurons. The flexor and extensor modules are reciprocally connected and the segmental organization is repeated along the cord (not shown).

did not lead to changes in flexor-extensor co-ordination.[10] The presence of both flexor- and extensor-related Chx10 neurons in each segment is compatible with a modular organization of the V2a neurons along the cord providing in-phase synaptic drive to segmental flexor- and extensor-related motor neurons[12] (Fig. 3). The activity of the flexor- and extensor-related Chx10 neurons observed along the lumbar cord is also well suited to drive the segmental commissural interneuron system involved in controlling left–right alternation[10,12,22] (Fig. 3).

Fish and rodent locomotor CPGs: how similar are they?

Descending excitatory interneurons (dEIN) in lamprey and tadpole are proposed to generate the rhythm and identified excitatory CPG interneurons have been shown to be interconnected synaptically.[40–45] These neurons share similarities with Alx-expressing CiDs in the zebrafish. However, based on the ablation experiments[10,11] and intracellular

recordings during locomotion,[12,13] it appears that Chx10 neuron activity is not the primary source of rhythm-generation in mammals. Rather, Chx10 activity is driven by convergent in-phase excitatory input from rhythm-generating CPG neurons.[12,13] Moreover, the Chx10 cells differ morphologically from the CiD neurons and the ipsilateral excitatory CPG neurons in the tadpole and lamprey. These latter neurons all have long descending axons[17,30,45–47] in contrast to most of the Chx10 cells that have short segmental axons while only a small proportion have long projecting axons.[12]

If Chx10 interneurons are homologous to CiD interneurons in zebrafish, which themselves correspond to dEINs in the lamprey and tadpole, the available data sets suggest significant differences in the CPG organization in swimming and walking animals. Alternatively, similar to rodents, the rhythm-generating circuitry in the zebrafish, lamprey, and tadpole has yet to be completely defined. Ipsilaterally-projecting, EIN have been strongly implicated[40–44] but there has not yet been a direct causal link between any cell population and rhythm generation in the zebrafish, lamprey, or tadpole. Now that technologies exist for ablation and activation of single cell populations, they should be used to establish this link directly.

Differential recruitment of CiD interneurons has been shown in the zebrafish.[30,31] One possible source of differential recruitment is differential membrane properties (such as input resistance and rheobase), similar to what has been well established in MNs.[48] Similarly, input resistance of EINs decreases more dorsally in zebrafish.[30,31] However, it remains unclear how this differential recruitment is established. It is conceivable that recruitment of additional cells or additional cell populations would not be necessary for an increase in speed. Thus, an increase in tonic descending drive would increase the depolarization of rhythm-generating neurons, thereby increasing the frequency of oscillations without the need to recruit new populations of cells.

Another difference between the mouse and zebrafish CPG is the proposed projection from V2a to Evx1 positive commissural interneurons. In the zebrafish MCoDs are excitatory, commissural and Evx positive.[30,31,49] MCoDs are thought to be responsible for the left–right alternation and rhythm-generation at low speeds. Finally, the swimming CPG has been described as a more simplistic circuitry than the dual inhibitory pathway and seemingly multi-layered organization (Figs. 1 and 2[1,29,39,50]) of the walking CPG.

Our analysis of the available data lends support to the suggestion that the swimming and walking CPGs share many similarities in their basic organization presumably resulting from their common phylogenetic origin. However, the CPGs also appear to display distinct differences in their overall organizations, possibly as a consequence of the different motor functions they support.[1,36]

What generates the rhythm?

Pharmacological experiments in the rodent spinal cord suggest that the rhythmicity is generated by glutamatergic neurons, similar to what has been proposed for the swimming CPG.[1,36] It is therefore interesting that none of the genetic manipulation experiments that have been used in the mouse to knock out neuronal fate-determining genes, chronically ablate or acutely silence major groups of glutamatergic neurons in the ventral spinal cord have been able to kill the *rhythm*. However, elimination of these glutamatergic neuronal populations, that include the V0, V2a, and V3 population do cause specific changes in the *pattern* of locomotion.[10,11,15,16] These findings suggest that classes of neurons other than the V0, V2a, and V3 neurons are primarily involved in the rhythm-generation, that the population of rhythm-generating neurons spans more than one class, or that glutamatergic neurons are not involved in rhythm generation. It is unlikely that the latter is the case because acute photoactivation of channelrhodopsin2 positive glutamatergic neurons in the lumbar mouse spinal cord is sufficient to evoke locomotion.[51] These findings suggest that glutamatergic neurons in the mammalian CPG indeed contribute to rhythm generation. Future experiments using acute photostimulation and inactivation of specific neuronal groups in the spinal cord will provide the details of the functional organization of rhythm-generating networks in the mammalian spinal cord.

Acknowledgments

This work was supported by NIH R01NS040795-08, EU-grant (SPINAL CORD REPAIR), Wings for Life, NSF 0701166 (KJD), Swedish Medical Research Council, Friends of Karolinska Institutet, and Hjärnfonden. The authors wish to thank Keith Sillar for comments on a previous version of the manuscript.

Conflicts of interest

The authors declare no conflicts of interest.

References

1. Kiehn, O. 2006. Locomotor circuits in the mammalian spinal cord. *Annu. Rev. Neurosci.* **29:** 279–306.

2. Jessell, T.M. 2000. Neuronal specification in the spinal cord: inductive signals and transcriptional codes. *Nat. Rev. Genet.* **1:** 20–29.

3. Goulding, M. & S.L. Pfaff. 2005. Development of circuits that generate simple rhythmic behaviors in vertebrates. *Curr. Opin. Neurobiol.* **15:** 14–20.

4. Hinckley, C.A. *et al.* 2005. Locomotor-like rhythms in a genetically distinct cluster of interneurons in the mammalian spinal cord. *J. Neurophysiol.* **93:** 1439–1449.

5. Hinckley, C.A. & L. Ziskind-Conhaim. 2006. Electrical coupling between locomotor-related excitatory interneurons in the mammalian spinal cord. *J. Neurosci.* **26:** 8477–8483.

6. Kwan, A.C. *et al.* 2009. Activity of Hb9 interneurons during fictive locomotion in mouse spinal cord. *J. Neurosci.* **29:** 11601–11613.

7. Wilson, J.M., A.I. Cowan & R.M. Brownstone. 2007. Heterogeneous electrotonic coupling and synchronization of rhythmic bursting activity in mouse Hb9 interneurons. *J. Neurophysiol.* **98:** 2370–2381.

8. Wilson, J.M. *et al.* 2005. Conditional rhythmicity of ventral spinal interneurons defined by expression of the Hb9 homeodomain protein. *J. Neurosci.* **25:** 5710–5719.

9. Ziskind-Conhaim, L., L. Wu & E.P. Wiesner. 2008. Persistent sodium current contributes to induced voltage oscillations in locomotor-related hb9 interneurons in the mouse spinal cord. *J. Neurophysiol.* **100:** 2254–2264.

10. Crone, S.A. *et al.* 2008. Genetic ablation of V2a ipsilateral interneurons disrupts left-right locomotor coordination in mammalian spinal cord. *Neuron* **60:** 70–83.

11. Crone, S.A. *et al.* 2009. In mice lacking V2a interneurons, gait depends on speed of locomotion. *J. Neurosci.* **29:** 7098–7109.

12. Dougherty, K. & O. Kiehn. 2010. Firing properties and cellular properties of V2a interneurons in the rodent spinal cord. *J. Neurosci.* **30:** 24–37.

13. Zhong, G. *et al.* 2010. Electrophysiological characterization of the V2a interneurons and their locomotor-related activity in the neonatal mouse spinal cord. *J. Neurosci.* **30:** 170–182.

14. Gosgnach, S. *et al.* 2006. V1 spinal neurons regulate the speed of vertebrate locomotor outputs [see comment]. *Nature* **440:** 215–219.

15. Lanuza, G.M. *et al.* 2004. Genetic identification of spinal interneurons that coordinate left-right locomotor activity necessary for walking movements. *Neuron* **42:** 375–386.

16. Zhang, Y. *et al.* 2008. V3 spinal neurons establish a robust and balanced locomotor rhythm during walking. *Neuron* **60:** 84–96.

17. Kimura, Y., Y. Okamura & S. Higashijima. 2006. alx, a zebrafish homolog of Chx10, marks ipsilateral descending excitatory interneurons that participate in the regulation of spinal locomotor circuits. *J. Neurosci.* **26:** 5684–5697.

18. Higashijima, S. *et al.* 2004. Engrailed-1 expression marks a primitive class of inhibitory spinal interneuron. *J. Neurosci.* **24:** 5827–5839.

19. Al-Mosawie, A., J.M. Wilson & R.M. Brownstone. 2007. Heterogeneity of V2-derived interneurons in the adult mouse spinal cord. *Eur. J. Neurosci.* **26:** 3003–3015.

20. Lundfald, L. *et al.* 2007. Phenotype of V2-derived interneurons and their relationship to the axon guidance molecule EphA4 in the developing mouse spinal cord. *Eur. J. Neurosci.* **26:** 2989–3002.

21. Peng, C.Y. *et al.* 2007. Notch and MAML signaling drives Scl-dependent interneuron diversity in the spinal cord. *Neuron* **53:** 813–827.

22. Quinlan, K.A. & O. Kiehn. 2007. Segmental, synaptic actions of commissural interneurons in the mouse spinal cord. *J. Neurosci.* **27:** 6521–6530.

23. Nishimaru, H., C.E. Restrepo & O. Kiehn. 2006. Activity of Renshaw cells during locomotor-like rhythmic activity in the isolated spinal cord of neonatal mice. *J. Neurosci.* **26:** 5320–5328.

24. Sapir, T. *et al.* 2004. Pax6 and engrailed 1 regulate two distinct aspects of Renshaw cell development. *J. Neurosci.* **24:** 1255–1264.

25. Wenner, P., M.J. O'Donovan & M.P. Matise. 2000. Topographical and physiological characterization of interneurons that express engrailed-1 in the embryonic chick spinal cord. *J. Neurophysiol.* **84:** 2651–2657.

26. Gosgnach, S. *et al.* 2006. V1 spinal neurons regulate the speed of vertebrate locomotor outputs. *Nature* **440:** 215–219.

27. Butt, S.J., L. Lundfald & O. Kiehn. 2005. EphA4 defines a class of excitatory locomotor-related interneurons. *Proc. Natl. Acad. Sci. USA* **102:** 14098–14103.

28. Kullander, K. *et al.* 2003. Role of EphA4 and EphrinB3 in local neuronal circuits that control walking. *Science* **299:** 1889–1892.

29. Brownstone, R.M. & J.M. Wilson. 2008. Strategies for delineating spinal locomotor rhythm-generating networks and the possible role of Hb9 interneurones in rhythmogenesis. *Brain Res. Rev.* **57:** 64–76.

30. McLean, D.L. *et al.* 2007. A topographic map of recruitment in spinal cord. *Nature* **446:** 71–75.

31. McLean, D.L. *et al.* 2008. Continuous shifts in the active set of spinal interneurons during changes in locomotor speed. *Nat. Neurosci.* **11:** 1419–1429.

32. Pierani, A. *et al.* 1999. A sonic hedgehog-independent, retinoid-activated pathway of neurogenesis in the ventral spinal cord. *Cell* **97:** 903–915.

33. Moran-Rivard, L. *et al.* 2001. Evx1 is a postmitotic determinant of v0 interneuron identity in the spinal cord. *Neuron* **29:** 385–399.

34. Goulding, M. 2009. Circuits controlling vertebrate locomotion: moving in a new direction. *Nat. Rev. Neurosci.* **10:** 507–518.

35. Talpalar, A.E. *et al.* 2007. Ablation of Dbx1-genrated commissural interneurons leads to hopping gate. *Society for Neuroscience* [Abstract].

36. Kiehn, O. *et al.* 2008. Excitatory components of the mammalian locomotor CPG. *Brain. Res. Rev.* **57:** 56–63.

37. Borgius, L. *et al.* 2009. BAC-Vglut2: Cre mouse, a new transgenic mouse line for molecular genetic analysis of excitatory glutamatergic interneurons in the brain and spinal cord. *Society for Neuroscience* [*Abstract*].

38. Dougherty, K.J. *et al.* 2009. Rhythmogenic properties and connectivity of a transcriptionally-defined subset of ipsilateral excitatory interneurons in mouse spinal cord. *Society for Neuroscience* [Abstract].

39. Endo, T. & O. Kiehn. 2008. Asymmetric operation of the locomotor central pattern generator in the neonatal mouse spinal cord. *J. Neurophysiol.* **100:** 3043–3054.

40. Cangiano, L. & S. Grillner. 2003. Fast and slow locomotor burst generation in the hemispinal cord of the lamprey. *J. Neurophysiol.* **89:** 2931–2942.

41. Cangiano, L. & S. Grillner. 2005. Mechanisms of rhythm generation in a spinal locomotor network deprived of crossed connections: the lamprey hemicord. *J. Neurosci.* **25:** 923–935.

42. Grillner, S. 1985. Neurobiological bases of rhythmic motor acts in vertebrates. *Science* **228:** 143–149.

43. Grillner, S. 2003. The motor infrastructure: from ion channels to neuronal networks. *Nat. Rev. Neurosci.* **4:** 573–586.

44. Li, W.C., A. Roberts & S.R. Soffe. 2009. Locomotor rhythm maintenance: electrical coupling among premotor excitatory interneurons in the brainstem and spinal cord of young Xenopus tadpoles. *J. Physiol.* **587:** 1677–1693.

45. Buchanan, J.T. & S. Grillner. 1987. Newly identified 'glutamate interneurons' and their role in locomotion in the lamprey spinal cord. *Science* **236:** 312–314.

46. Buchanan, J.T. *et al.* 1989. Identification of excitatory interneurons contributing to generation of locomotion in lamprey: structure, pharmacology, and function. *J. Neurophysiol.* **62:** 59–69.

47. Roberts, A. *et al.* 2008. Origin of excitatory drive to a spinal locomotor network. *Brain. Res. Rev.* **57:** 22–28.

48. Powers, R.K. & M.D. Binder. 2001. Input-output functions of mammalian motoneurons. *Rev. Physiol. Biochem. Pharmacol.* **143:** 137–263.

49. Satou, C., Y. Kimura & S. Higashijima. 2008. Analysis of spinal V0 neurons in zebrafish. *Society for Neuroscience* [*Abstract*].

50. McCrea, D.A. & I.A. Rybak. 2008. Organization of mammalian locomotor rhythm and pattern generation. *Brain. Res. Rev.* **57:** 134–146.

51. Hagglund, M. *et al.* 2010. Activation of groups of excitatory neurons in the mammalian spinal cord or hindbrain evokes locomotion. *Nature Neurosci.* **13:**1–7.

Ann. N.Y. Acad. Sci. ISSN 0077-8923

ANNALS OF THE NEW YORK ACADEMY OF SCIENCES
Issue: *Neurons and Networks in the Spinal Cord*

Some principles of organization of spinal neurons underlying locomotion in zebrafish and their implications

Joseph R. Fetcho[1] and David L. McLean[2]

[1]Department of Neurobiology and Behavior, Cornell University, Ithaca, New York. [2]Department of Neurobiology and Physiology, Northwestern University, Chicago, Illinois

Address for correspondence: Joseph R. Fetcho, Department of Neurobiology and Behavior, W103 Mudd Hall, Cornell University, Ithaca, NY 14853. jrf49@cornell.edu

Recent studies of the spinal motor system of zebrafish, along with work in other species, are leading to some principles that appear to underlie the organization and recruitment of motor networks in cord: (1) broad neuronal classes defined by a set of transcription factors, key morphological features, and transmitter phenotypes arise in an orderly way from different dorso-ventral zones in spinal cord; (2) motor behaviors and both motoneurons and interneurons differentiate in order from gross, often faster, movements and the neurons driving them to progressively slower movements and their underlying neurons; (3) recruitment order of motoneurons and interneurons is based upon time of differentiation; (4) different locomotor speeds involve some shifts in the set of active interneurons. Here we review these principles and some of their implications for other parts of the brain, other vertebrates, and limbed locomotion.

Keywords: motoneurons; spinal interneurons; transcription factors; locomotion; motor pattern

Introduction

Studies of spinal motor networks have focused in a concerted way on identifying neurons involved in rhythmic motor behaviors with an aim toward unraveling the network responsible for generating the rhythmic movements that underlie much of locomotion.[1–5] This admirable, though sometimes elusive, goal has left other, no less important, avenues of study less well populated. Our recent work has been focused on one of these: the patterns of recruitment of motoneurons and interneurons in the spinal cord.[6–14] While there is a long-standing body of important studies of how motoneurons are recruited,[15] with a few exceptions, the interneurons have been much less studied, probably because of the difficulties of studying identified populations active in rhythmic locomotion. The zebrafish model has allowed us to attack questions of the functional organization of interneurons (and motoneurons) in ways that are not feasible in other species.

Our results have revealed some simple underlying patterns to the organization of the spinal neurons that link their development and structural organization to their functional roles. This has allowed us to formulate some initial principles of the organization of spinal networks that might extend to networks in the brain. The patterns also allow for predictions about possible features of organization of the mammalian locomotor central pattern generator. Here we articulate the principles and review evidence supporting them from zebrafish, along with other evidence suggesting that they may apply broadly in vertebrate nervous systems. Finally, we also consider their implications for the construction of mammalian central pattern generators.

The generation of cell types

The already classic studies of the transcription factor code in chick and mouse spinal cord have revealed the way in which broad classes/categories of spinal neurons are generated.[5,16,17] Different categories of neurons arise from different dorso-ventral zones in spinal cord that express unique combinations of transcription factors. This patterning has been extensively reviewed by others.[5] What is important here is that the patterning represents a

doi: 10.1111/j.1749-6632.2010.05539.x

Ann. N.Y. Acad. Sci. 1198 (2010) 94–104 © 2010 New York Academy of Sciences.

fundamental underlying organization that, based upon studies of zebrafish, frog tadpoles, chicks, and mice, is shared by all vertebrates. The underlying set of core cell types is therefore much the same in all vertebrates.

This key assertion leads to important broader implications, so a brief account of some of the evidence for it is warranted. The transcription factor expression pattern in tetrapods is one in which the factors are expressed during development in bands across spinal cord at different dorso-ventral locations. These are arranged in a particular order from ventral to dorsal in mice and chicks. While not all of the tetrapod transcription factors have been examined in zebrafish, those that have been studied occupy the same relative positions along the dorso-ventral axis of spinal cord.[18–21] The similarity in the order of the bands in the distantly related zebrafish and mice (and some corroborating work in frogs[22]), suggests a very primitive origin of the patterning.

The parallels among chicks, mice, zebrafish, and frogs extend beyond the expression domains to the morphology, connectivity, and even some aspects of the functional roles of the cells arising from particular domains in these divergent species. The two best documented examples of this are the neurons marked by the transcription factors Engrailed and Chx10 (called Alx in zebrafish). These mark similar neurons in zebrafish and mice. Engrailed neurons are inhibitory neurons (Glycine/GABA) with ipsilateral ascending axons in both species.[12,23,24] This is also the case in frog tadpoles and chicks.[22,25] In all of these, the neurons not only share the primary axonal trajectory, but also share at least one synaptic output, as they all directly connect to motoneurons. The Chx10 (Alx) neurons, in contrast, are glutamatergic excitatory interneurons with a primary ipsilateral, descending axon in mice and zebrafish.[19,26] These neurons directly connect to motoneurons and probably other cell types as well. These are the best examples of the parallels between the different species because they have been examined in some detail, but there is preliminary evidence for a similar overall patterning of other neuronal types as well.

One interesting feature of the code is that neurons arising from particular regions share some phenotypic features, but differ in others. For example, cells with ipsilateral descending axons arising from a domain called V2 diverge into excitatory and inhibitory types, each marked by a different transcription factor.[18,26] Recent work shows that these arise via a terminal cell division that produces one excitatory and one inhibitory cell.[18] This developmental pattern could provide a mechanism for establishing a rough excitatory and inhibitory balance in spinal cord that might be important for circuit function based upon systems biology work that indicates such a balance enhances control. In addition, a fine tuning of the balance might also occur via switches in transmitter phenotype between the two types, given other evidence that switches can occur after alterations in the level of activity in spinal cord.[27] Such switches might allow a fine tuning of the balance of excitation and inhibition without gross morphological changes in the neurons because they represent switches in transmitter phenotype of otherwise morphologically similar cell types.

The implications of the shared transcription factor code are substantial. Until the code was revealed, there was no clear link between cell types in the spinal cord of aquatic animals and those in tetrapods. The code bridges that gap and has immediately allowed for predictions about the likely functional roles of neuronal types in mice based upon their functional role of cells in fish and frogs, where the connectivity and behavioral contributions have historically been easier to study. The engrailed neurons in frogs and fish were implicated in burst termination that might be important for high-speed swimming.[12,22] Subsequent studies in mice showed that genetic inactivation of the neurons led to a slowing of locomotor rhythms, at least consistent with what one might expect based upon swimming vertebrates.[28] Since not only the spinal cord, but much of the brain as well, is built using some of the same code, explorations of the classes of neuronal types arising from transcription factor domains and their functional organization has implications for structural and functional patterning throughout the nervous system that will be reviewed later in this article.

While the parallels in the code are striking across vertebrates, this does not mean that the cell types and networks in different species are identical. There is good evidence that specialization of neurons arising from within particular transcription factor domains gives rise to different neuronal types with somewhat divergent functions.[23] This specialization may not take the same form in different species, just as it might take different forms along the neuraxis in individual animals. Nonetheless, the transcription factor code represents a major unifying principle of organization across vertebrates, which suggests that specialized networks in different species arise by divergence from a common shared neuronal ground plan. Understanding that ground plan and the core wiring and activity patterns at its foundation is therefore an important goal.

Functional order within and across transcription factor domains

While the transcription factor code and its link to major classes of neurons was first defined in studies in mammals and chicks, the functional organization within the classes is more difficult to reveal in those animals because their spinal cords are more complex than in fishes. Evidence that there is clear functional order within and between the transcription factor domains comes from studies of larval zebrafish, where obtaining data about the patterns of activity during behavior is easier because of the ability to image activity with calcium indicators *in vivo* and to more easily target patch recordings from neurons because of the transparency of the fish. These data have revealed a remarkable order to the recruitment of neurons within and between transcription factor zones that ties together their development, location, and functional properties.

The evidence for a functional organization came not from a directed attack on the question of functional order within neurons sharing transcription factor expression, but rather from studies of the pattern of recruitment of neurons during behaviors of different speeds. While much was known about neurons that contributed to motor behaviors in both swimming and walking vertebrates, questions of how the neurons were recruited during different speeds or strengths of movement were mostly confined to recruitment of motoneurons. We set out to explore how both motoneurons and interneurons of known classes were recruited during changes in the frequency of bending of swimming zebrafish, which is correlated with how fast they move.

Both electrophysiological recordings and calcium imaging of motoneurons in paralyzed fish in which the "fictive" swimming frequency was monitored by recordings from spinal nerves revealed a striking relationship between where a motoneuron was located and the frequency of swimming at which it was recruited.[10] Motoneurons were recruited from the bottom of the motor column to its top as the frequency of swimming increased. Measures of input resistance and size showed that, like the recruitment frequency, both were also correlated with position, with the high resistance smaller motoneurons located ventrally and progressively lower resistance and larger motoneurons stacked above them. Earlier work had shown that some of the fastest motoneurons were in the dorsal part of the motor column, with slower ones below them,[29–31] but the more recent work showed that there is an overall orderly relationship between location, cellular properties, size, and recruitment.

Remarkably, electrophysiological and optical studies of spinal interneuron recruitment patterns showed that excitatory interneurons followed the same order of recruitment based on location and cellular properties.[10,11,32] The most ventral excitatory interneurons were recruited at the lowest swimming frequencies and progressively more dorsal ones were engaged as the frequency increased, just like the motoneurons. This pattern was not related to interneuron size, but rather to location and, to some extent, to properties such as input resistance. The order was evident both within a transcription factor class (the ipsilateral descending excitatory CiD interneurons marked by Alx—the zebrafish version of Chx10 in mammals), and across transcription factor classes, with both ventral Alx neurons and the ventral MCoD interneurons (a commissural excitatory class arising from an Evx domain) recruited at lower swimming frequencies than the more dorsal neurons. Inhibitory interneurons in contrast were recruited in the opposite direction, from dorsal down with increasing swimming frequency.

Importantly, there was no overall relationship between recruitment and soma size for either inhibitory and excitatory neurons, as there was in motoneurons. This may have important implications for principles of organization that extend across neuronal types in spinal cord. The well-known size principle of recruitment of motoneurons applies broadly across all species,[15,33,34] including the motoneurons in zebrafish. The evidence based upon soma size, however, indicates that it does not apply to interneurons. Interestingly, there are better predictors of recruitment that do apply to both motoneurons and interneurons.[33,34] These include both location and input resistance (which is not always well correlated with soma size among interneurons), and, even more importantly, time of differentiation, which is explored below. Thus, the size principle may be a subset of a broader pattern of organization that links time of differentiation, connectivity, and cellular properties to recruitment.

The best predictor of recruitment patterns is the time of differentiation of the neuron in spinal cord, whether the cell is a motoneuron, or excitatory or inhibitory interneuron. Studies using color change proteins to time stamp neurons that have differentiated at particular times indicate that the neurons differentiating first drive the higher frequency, larger and faster movements in older animals, with neurons driving progressively lower frequency and slower movements added later.[6] This age-related order underlies the orderly recruitment of all the neurons based upon location because the neurons are lined up dorsoventrally in cord roughly by when they differentiated. Indeed the pattern of age-related stacking can account for the opposite directions of recruitment of excitatory and inhibitory interneurons because they are stacked in opposite directions based upon age. Thus, there appears to be a very systematic organization that links the time of differentiation of a neuron to its location, cellular properties, and, importantly, the frequency of swimming at which it is recruited. The recruitment based upon age parallels the pattern of development of the animal because the first embryonic movements are large amplitude and fast movements and progressively weaker, and slower movements appear during development as neurons involved in progressively slower movements later in life are added to the differentiating population.[6] We know for the motoneurons and some of the interneurons that the link between recruitment and time of differentiation is retained even into adulthood, suggesting that it is not simply an early pattern that is linked to the gradual addition of ion channels as the neurons differentiate.[29,35,36]

Shifts in interneurons with locomotor speed

There is one major difference in how motoneurons are recruited as compared to excitatory interneurons. As frequency rises, more and more motoneurons are added to the active pool, with those active at low frequencies remaining active at higher ones. Among excitatory interneurons, those active at low frequency are removed from the active pool by inhibition as those involved in higher frequencies of movements are recruited.[7] This pattern occurs both within a cell type because ventral CiD interneurons involved in slow swimming are shut off as more dorsal CiD interneurons are recruited, and between cell types because the commissural, excitatory premotor MCoDs, which are active in slow swimming, are turned off as the CiD neurons active in faster swimming are recruited. The implications of this for motor control are significant as they indicate that the populations of neurons driving different speeds of movement change with speed, suggesting possible changes in the networks (maybe even the central pattern generating networks) with speed of locomotion. In the zebrafish, this switch also involves a change in premotor cell type from a commissural excitatory cell type to an ipsilateral descending one. This observation leads to some important potential implications, outlined in a later section, that could shed light on some puzzles in studies of mammalian limb control networks.

Summary of principles of the zebrafish organization, also presented in Figure 1:

Principle 1: ***Broad neuronal classes defined by a set of transcription factors, key morphological features, and transmitter phenotypes arise in an orderly way from different dorso-ventral zones in spinal cord.*** This core pattern appears to lie at the developmental and phylogenetic base of the construction of spinal networks in all vertebrates. Neurons arising from the zones that define the basic ground plan diversify further in their morphological and functional details to give rise to specialized cell types during development and evolution. For example, neurons arising from the engrailed domain in mammals share a common inhibitory phenotype and ipsilateral axonal projection, but give rise to several cell types including Renshaw cells and Ia inhibitory neurons.[23] Distinctions within the engrailed class are less obvious in larval zebrafish (which are free swimming and therefore functional from a motor control perspective), suggesting that they may have diversified during evolution to give rise to several types in mammals. They may, however, even diversify later in the development of zebrafish when the circuits have been more difficult to study (but see Ref. 37).

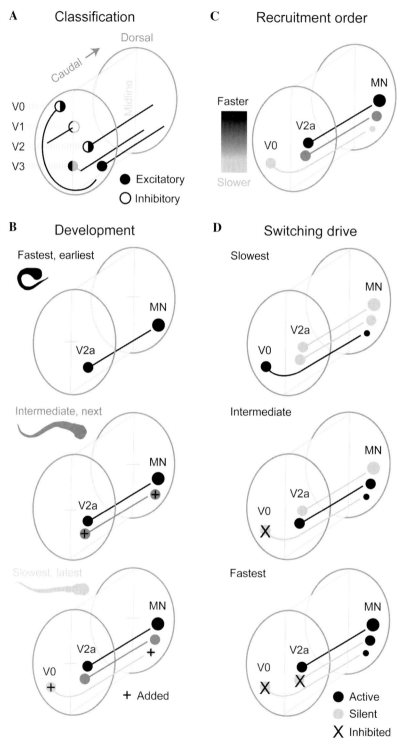

Figure 1. Summary of principles of organization of spinal neurons. (**A**) Spinal neurons of particular transmitter phenotypes and morphologies are specified in a dorso-ventral fashion by the combination of transcription factors activated by gradients of diffusible morphogens. V0 interneurons are a mixture of excitatory and inhibitory cells, all with commissural axons; V1 cells are inhibitory with a primary ascending ipsilateral axon; V2 interneurons are a

Principle 2: ***Motor behaviors and both motoneurons and interneurons differentiate in order from gross, often faster, movements and the neurons driving them to progressively slower movements and their underlying neurons.*** Gross movements such as escape-like bends and whole body swimming movements and the neurons producing them develop first, with slower movements and the neurons underlying them differentiating later. In zebrafish, much of this differentiation occurs in the egg, or just after hatching, but before the animal is free swimming. Once free swimming, as the speed of swimming gets faster and faster, both motoneurons and interneurons are activated in order from those differentiating last to those that differentiated first. Thus, the fast networks differentiate first, and the slow ones last.

Principle 3: ***Recruitment order of motoneurons and interneurons is based upon time of differentiation.*** In zebrafish, one consequence of principle 2 is a topographic map of neuronal recruitment in cord that arises because the neurons remain arranged in the spinal cord largely by the time at which they differentiated. In addition to position, other neuronal features such as input resistance are also correlated with time of differentiation, but are not as good a predictor of recruitment as when the neurons differentiated. Notably, the size principle of motoneurons does not apply in its simplest form to interneurons, as there is no simple relationship between at least soma size and recruitment. The best indicator of when a neuron is recruited as speed increases is when it differentiated, with neurons recruited from youngest to oldest as speed rises.

Principle 4: ***Different locomotor speeds involve some shifts in the set of active interneurons.*** Some interneurons active at slow speeds are silenced at faster ones and this pattern occurs both within and between excitatory classes. Thus, the interneurons behave differently from the motoneurons with respect to recruitment because the motoneurons only add neurons to the active pool as speed increases, while the interneurons add new ones while removing others that were active at slower speeds. The networks for slow and fast swimming are not the same and appear to constantly shift as speed increases.

How broad are these principles across species and in the nervous system?

The patterns observed in zebrafish are not unique to this species. As described earlier in this paper, the transcription factor code of cell types in principle 1 was first worked out in other species, but seems present among vertebrates generally. The broad classes of neurons appear to be generated via a similar developmental pattern in every vertebrate studied so far including fish, frogs, chicks, and mice. Other work indicates that development via a transcription factor code like that in spinal cord extends to hindbrain networks in zebrafish (unpublished work) and other species.[38,39]

The observation in principle 2 that motor behaviors develop from gross and fast to refined and slow is supported by behavioral observations from several species.[1,6,40–46] Even data from studies of human movements *in utero* show that fast, whole body movements such as the startle response are present early and more refined movements of, for example, the limbs come later.[41] The behavioral order implies that circuits for gross movements arise before those for refined movements, but there is less information matching cell types to time of differentiation in spinal systems of other species. Old data indicate that hindbrain neurons that drive the fastest movements in zebrafish, such as the Mauthner cell, develop very early, and our more recent studies provide evidence that neurons differentiate from fast to slow in hindbrain as in spinal cord.[47] While there is less neuronal-level evidence from mammals, coarse coding neurons with broad effects develop before finer

---

mixture of excitatory and inhibitory cells with a primary descending axon; (**B**) A summary schematic of the developmental order of spinal circuitry and the associated movement in larval zebrafish. Neurons responsible for progressively slower movements in larvae are added as zebrafish develop. (**C**) Schematic summarizing the recruitment order of interneurons and motoneurons, which occurs from the bottom of spinal cord up. (**D**) Schematic summarizing the switch in premotor interneuron activity responsible for driving the progressive dorso-ventral activation of motoneurons as larvae swim faster and faster.

resolution cells in parts of the mammalian nervous system, with, for example, the magnocellular parts of the visual pathways differentiating before the parvocellular ones[48–50] and the reticulospinal neurons in the startle response developing early.[51,52]

Less is known about how age-related order of recruitment of the spinal neurons in zebrafish (Principle 3) applies to other species, but there is increasing evidence that there is considerable age-related functional order in nervous systems. Neurons arising at different times in mammals have different properties, and it may well be that neuronal subpopulations arise at different times during development from individual transcription factor zones in spinal cord.[23,53] More direct studies of recruitment and its links to age in mammals and other species will help to resolve the generality of the pattern observed in fish. We do have evidence that there is an orderly recruitment by age in the hindbrain networks, suggesting that such patterns extend beyond spinal cord.[54]

The details of recruitment within classes of interneurons, and particularly assessment of switches in cell types, as articulated in principle 4, are more difficult to study in other species. Earlier studies of interneuron recruitment in dogfish spinal cord and in Xenopus tadpoles did not find such switches, but they were not done in a way that would be likely to reveal such switches either.[55,56] In both cases, the recorded neurons were not identified, so their transmitter phenotype and premotor status is unknown. The relevant premotor neurons might simply have not been studied due to sampling problems. In addition, the Xenopus work was early in the animal's development, at a stage corresponding to one in zebrafish before the slowest networks have even developed, so one would not expect to find such a pattern at that stage. We predict that studies of premotor excitatory interneurons in Xenopus after the slower tail driven swimming movements have developed will show the same pattern as we found in zebrafish.

Mammals are even harder to study than fishes and amphibians. Nonetheless there are hints that may point to speed-related changes in the involvement of neuronal types even in mammals. Genetic destruction of ipsilateral excitatory neurons in the Alx domain leads to mice that move with a normal gait at slow speeds, but that switch at higher speeds to a galloping type gait that they never use normally.[57]

This speed-related disruption, which also occurs in spinal preparations, is consistent with the possibility of at least partially different networks being engaged at different speed in mammalian spinal cord. Very recent observations from human walking are also consistent with the possibility of speed-related network switches,[58] suggesting that it might be a very broad feature of organization.

Total speculation arising from the patterns in fish, but with some predictions

While the breath of the relevance of some features of the simple axial motor patterns in fish remains to be revealed, they nonetheless prompt some more speculative considerations about other aspects of motor organization as well as possible arrangements of networks for limbed locomotion, which are derivatives of primitive axial networks. Of course, limbed locomotion is not identical to axial locomotion, so we cannot expect that everything will be the same.[59] Nonetheless, the two are related by evolution and it can be instructive to consider the possible implications of the organization of axial networks for the construction of limb circuits.[60,61]

Neuromodulation

One striking feature of motor systems is the ability to shape their output by neuromodulation.[62–64] The effects of neuromodulators are complex, without an obvious overall pattern in the neuromodulatory changes in features like synaptic strength and excitability.[64,65] Perhaps this complexity is in part a consequence of the fact that studies of the neurons are typically done after development is complete, and even after neurons arising from different transcription factor zones and of different ages have migrated to intermingle in the spinal cord or brain. One testable hypothesis is that there will be orderly effects of neuromodulators on neurons and synapses based upon the time of differentiation of the cells. Such an orderly pattern could be obscured later in life as neurons move around. This simple, although untested, idea has some appeal because we know that recruitment patterns are ordered by age. One could imagine that a change in the slope of recruitment (e.g., a more rapid recruitment of more potent interneurons and motoneurons that might be important for a fish in a cold environment) could be achieved by a systematic alteration of the properties of neurons in the population by a neuromodulator. This change could accomplish a more rapid recruitment, while maintaining a smooth recruitment order to allow for a graded movement. If so, we might predict that neuromodulatory effects might be comparable on neurons that differentiated around the same time and change systematically with the time of differentiation of the neuron. It remains to be seen whether there are such age-related patterns in neuromodulatory effects, but they can be explored with relative ease in the zebrafish model.

Limbed locomotion

Fin and limb muscles are derived from somites that primitively gave rise to axial muscles, so we might expect that axial motor organization could inform us about at least some aspects of limb control.[66] While there are some likely candidates for neurons in the central pattern generators for axial motor circuits based upon work in lampreys and frog embryos (still not tested by cell specific perturbations because of their difficulty in these non-genetic models),[67,68] the mammalian central pattern generating networks have proved more elusive.[17] Surprisingly, genetic perturbations of a variety of known neuronal classes—even large groups of neurons—have failed to disrupt the ability of the networks to produce a rhythm. This has led to speculation that there are other critical neurons that have been missed and, along with observations of motor pattern deletions, to the development of ideas about multilevel CPGs.[69] A consideration of evidence from axial networks may shed some light on some of these more mysterious results concerning mammalian central pattern generators.

The interpretation of mammalian perturbation experiments depends heavily on an assumption that there is a network that contains a discrete set of neurons that forms the central pattern generator and that the same neuronal classes (while maybe not the exact same population of neurons) contribute to that CPG over the range of possible locomotor speeds. Our studies of axial motor circuits in zebrafish, however, indicate that there can be switches in cell types at different speeds, raising the possibility that the contributors to the rhythm might change with speed. In particular, there are premotor commissural excitatory interneurons active at slow speeds that are silenced at higher speeds. Most of the mammalian work (and even axial work), while

acknowledging the presence of commissural excitatory interneurons, has focused on a conceptual organization in which coordination between the two sides is accomplished largely by crossed inhibitory interneurons (but see Ref. 17). The data from mouse perturbation experiments are typically interpreted in light of assumptions that (1) there are not cell type changes in the CPG with speed and (2) crossed inhibitory neurons are always critical for side to side coordination. Both assumptions may be wrong, and if they are, so might be the interpretations of the genetic perturbation experiments and ideas about the role of cell types in generating the motor output.

For example, work by the Goulding lab concluded that commissural inhibitory neurons are essential for coordination between the two sides of the body.[70] This was based upon modern experimental genetic manipulations. In the first, perturbations of Dbx positive neurons, which included all commissural cells, both excitatory and inhibitory, led to disruptions of coordination between the two sides of the body, pointing to an important role for commissural neurons. In the second experiment, only the excitatory commissural neurons were perturbed, and they did not eliminate coordination between the two sides. This led to the inference that commissural inhibitory neurons are critical for normal bilateral coordination. These experiments could be interpreted differently if there are switches in the commissural interneurons used at different speeds. Suppose, for example, that commissural excitatory interactions (between extensor interneurons on one side and flexor interneurons on the other) are more important than commissural inhibitory neurons for coordinating the two sides of the body at low speeds. These could phase flexor and extensors properly on the two sides, with ipsilateral inhibitory neurons being critical for proper phasing between extensors and flexors on the same side at the slow speeds. Suppose further that as speed rises, commissural inhibitory neurons replace the commissural excitatory cells as the primary commissural coordination system, with the interaction changing to one between flexor and flexor pairs (or extensor/extensor) on opposite sides, rather than flexor/extensor pairs (this idea has parallels with that of Crone *et al.* 2008, but is somewhat different from the change in commissural inhibitory neurons with normal changes in speed that they suggest).[57]

If this happened, the earlier Dbx perturbations might be interpreted differently. We would expect that the disruption of all commissural neurons would indeed affect bilateral coordination. The switch model would suggest that disrupting excitatory commissural neurons would affect coordination at slow speeds of locomotion. There were no disruptions in the DBx experiments, which on the face of it would seem to refute the switch idea. The absence of effects could, however, be a consequence of the approach used to elicit locomotion. In the Dbx experiments, bath application of drugs was used to activate spinal cord. This massive excitation would not necessarily allow for the normal speed-related changes in the networks and could easily mask the contribution of the excitatory cells by disrupting proper speed-related network shifts.

This is all very speculative, but there is one clear prediction that would at least be consistent with the idea of such speed-related switches. If the commissural inhibitory interneurons were selectively perturbed and the locomotion was assessed in the intact animal, the idea of a switch would predict that bilateral coordination would be normal at slower speeds and disrupted at higher ones. This is akin to the pattern observed for descending excitatory Chx10 neurons, which are involved in higher speeds in fish and whose disruption in mice results in changes in bilateral coordination at higher speeds of locomotion. We are not at all wedded to this hypothesis, but rather want to emphasize that even the interpretation of existing experiments depends on assumptions about the network construction. While the previous discussion focused on side to side coordination rather than rhythm generation itself, it could be that the actual rhythm-generating network changes with speed, which might underlie conclusions that neurons so far identified are not part of the rhythm generator.

In thinking about limb control it is important to keep in mind that in the primitive axial system that gave rise to limbs, the coordination of ipsilateral body segments was no more important than the coordination between the two sides. Without both, swimming is problematic. A focus on single limbs and flexor and extensor coordination between them can to lead to a de-emphasis on the possibility that neurons from one side of the body might, as they were primitively, be critical to normal rhythm generation and patterning of output on the opposite

side and that their roles might change with changes in speed. The derivation of limbs from axial muscles increases the possibility that some of rules that underlie axial locomotor circuits in zebrafish presented here may also appear in limb motor networks. This is not to say that there will not be differences (there must be!), but rather that the evolutionary history makes it likely that there may be core similarities as well.

Conflicts of interest

The authors declare no conflicts of interest.

References

1. Roberts, A. *et al.* 1981. Neural control of swimming in a vertebrate. *Science* **213:** 1032–1034.
2. Grillner, S. 2006. Biological pattern generation: the cellular and computational logic of networks in motion. *Neuron* **52:** 751–766.
3. Grillner, S. & M.J. Thomas. 2009. Measured motion: searching for simplicity in spinal locomotor networks. *Curr. Opin. Neurobiol.* **19:** 572–586.
4. Kozlov, A. *et al.* 2009. Simple cellular and network control principles govern complex patterns of motor behavior. *Proc. Natl. Acad. Sci. USA* **106:** 20027–20032.
5. Goulding, M. 2009. Circuits controlling vertebrate locomotion: moving in a new direction. *Nat. Rev. Neurosci.* **10:** 507–518.
6. McLean, D.L. & J.R. Fetcho. 2009. Spinal interneurons differentiate sequentially from those driving the fastest swimming movements in larval zebrafish to those driving the slowest ones. *J. Neurosci.* **29:** 13566–13577.
7. McLean, D.L. *et al.* 2008. Continuous shifts in the active set of spinal interneurons during changes in locomotor speed. *Nat. Neurosci.* **11:** 1419–1429.
8. McLean, D.L. & J.R. Fetcho. 2008. Using imaging and genetics in zebrafish to study developing spinal circuits *in vivo*. *Dev. Neurobiol.* **68:** 817–834.
9. Liao, J.C. & J.R. Fetcho. 2008. Shared versus specialized glycinergic spinal interneurons in axial motor circuits of larval zebrafish. *J. Neurosci.* **28:** 12982–12992.
10. McLean, D.L. *et al.* 2007. A topographic map of recruitment in spinal cord. *Nature* **446:** 71–75.
11. Bhatt, D.H. *et al.* 2007. Grading movement strength by changes in firing intensity versus recruitment of spinal interneurons. *Neuron* **53:** 91–102.
12. Higashijima, S. *et al.* 2004. Engrailed-1 expression marks a primitive class of inhibitory spinal interneuron. *J. Neurosci.* **24:** 5827–5839.

13. Ritter, D.A., D.H. Bhatt & J.R. Fetcho. 2001. *In vivo* imaging of zebrafish reveals differences in the spinal networks for escape and swimming movements. *J. Neurosci.* **21:** 8956–8965.

14. Hale, M.E., D.A. Ritter & J.R. Fetcho. 2001. A confocal study of spinal interneurons in living larval zebrafish. *J. Comp. Neurol.* **437:** 1–16.

15. Cope, T.C. & M.J. Pinter. 1995. The size principle: still working after all these years. *NIPS* **10:** 280–286.

16. Briscoe, J. *et al.* 2000. A homeodomain protein code specifies progenitor cell identity and neuronal fate in the ventral neural tube. *Cell* **101:** 435–445.

17. Kiehn, O. 2006. Locomotor circuits in the mammalian spinal cord. *Annu. Rev. Neurosci.* **29:** 279–306.

18. Kimura, Y., C. Satou & S. Higashijima. 2008. V2a and V2b neurons are generated by the final divisions of pair-producing progenitors in the zebrafish spinal cord. *Development* **135:** 3001–3005.

19. Kimura, Y., Y. Okamura & S. Higashijima. 2006. alx, a zebrafish homolog of Chx10, marks ipsilateral descending excitatory interneurons that participate in the regulation of spinal locomotor circuits. *J. Neurosci.* **26:** 5684–5697.

20. Thaeron, C. *et al.* 2000. Zebrafish evx1 is dynamically expressed during embryogenesis in subsets of interneurones, posterior gut and urogenital system. *Mech. Dev.* **99:** 167–172.

21. Colombo, A. *et al.* 2006. Zebrafish BarH-like genes define discrete neural domains in the early embryo. *Gene Expr. Patterns.* **6:** 347–352.

22. Li, W.C. *et al.* 2004. Primitive roles for inhibitory interneurons in developing frog spinal cord. *J. Neurosci.* **24:** 5840–5848.

23. Alvarez, F.J. *et al.* 2005. Postnatal phenotype and localization of spinal cord V1 derived interneurons. *J. Comp. Neurol.* **493:** 177–192.

24. Saueressig, H., J. Burrill & M. Goulding. 1999. Engrailed-1 and netrin-1 regulate axon pathfinding by association interneurons that project to motor neurons. *Development* **126:** 4201–4212.

25. Wenner, P., M.J. O'Donovan & M.P. Matise. 2000. Topographical and physiological characterization of interneurons that express engrailed-1 in the embryonic chick spinal cord. *J. Neurophysiol.* **84:** 2651–2657.

26. Lundfald, L. *et al.* 2007. Phenotype of V2-derived interneurons and their relationship to the axon guidance molecule EphA4 in the developing mouse spinal cord. *Eur. J. Neurosci.* **26:** 2989–3002.

27. Borodinsky, L.N. *et al.* 2004. Activity-dependent homeostatic specification of transmitter expression in embryonic neurons. *Nature* **429:** 523–530.

28. Gosgnach, S. *et al.* 2006. V1 spinal neurons regulate the speed of vertebrate locomotor outputs. *Nature* **440:** 215–219.

29. Liu, D.W. & M. Westerfield. 1988. Function of identified motoneurones and co-ordination of primary and secondary motor systems during zebra fish swimming. *J. Physiol.* **403:** 73–89.

30. Westerfield, M., J.V. McMurray & J.S. Eisen. 1986. Identified motoneurons and their innervation of axial muscles in the zebrafish. *J. Neurosci.* **6:** 2267–2277.

31. Myers, P.Z., J.S. Eisen & M. Westerfield. 1986. Development and axonal outgrowth of identified motoneurons in the zebrafish. *J. Neurosci.* **6:** 2278–2289.

32. Fetcho, J.R. 1992. Excitation of motoneurons by the Mauthner axon in goldfish: complexities in a "simple" reticulospinal pathway. *J. Neurophysiol.* **67:** 1574–1586.

33. Gustafsson, B. & M.J. Pinter. 1984. An investigation of threshold properties among cat spinal alpha-motoneurones. *J. Physiol.* **357:** 453–483.

34. Gustafsson, B. & M.J. Pinter. 1984. Relations among passive electrical properties of lumbar alpha-motoneurones of the cat. *J. Physiol.* **356:** 401–431.

35. Fetcho, J.R. 1990. Morphological variability, segmental relationships, and functional-role of a class of commissural interneurons in the spinal-cord of goldfish. *J. Comp. Neurol.* **299:** 283–298.

36. Gao, B.X. & L. Ziskind-Conhaim. 1998. Development of ionic currents underlying changes in action potential waveforms in rat spinal motoneurons. *J. Neurophysiol.* **80:** 3047–3061.

37. Gabriel, J.P. *et al.* 2008. Locomotor pattern in the adult zebrafish spinal cord *in vitro*. *J. Neurophysiol.* **99:** 37–48.

38. Cepeda-Nieto, A.C., S.L. Pfaff & A. Varela-Echavarria. 2005. Homeodomain transcription factors in the development of subsets of hindbrain reticulospinal neurons. *Mol. Cell Neurosci.* **28:** 30–41.

39. Moreno, N. *et al.* 2005. LIM-homeodomain genes as territory markers in the brainstem of adult and developing *Xenopus laevis*. *J. Comp. Neurol.* **485:** 240–254.

40. Bradley, N.S. & A. Bekoff. 1990. Development of coordinated movement in chicks: I. Temporal analysis of hindlimb muscle synergies at embryonic days 9 and 10. *Dev. Psychobiol.* **23:** 763–782.

41. de Vries, J.I., G.H. Visser & H.F. Prechtl. 1982. The emergence of fetal behaviour. Part I. Qualitative aspects. *Early Hum. Dev.* **7:** 301–322.

42. Hamburger, V. *et al.* 1965. Periodic motility of normal and spinal chick embryos between 8 and 17 days of incubation. *J. Exp. Zool.* **159:** 1–13.

43. Westerga, J. & A. Gramsbergen. 1990. The development of locomotion in the rat. *Brain Res. Dev. Brain Res.* **57:** 163–174.

44. Tunstall, M.J. & K.T. Sillar. 1993. Physiological and developmental aspects of intersegmental coordination in Xenopus embryos and tadpoles. *Sem. Neurosci.* **5:** 29–40.

45. van Mier, P., J. Armstrong & A. Roberts. 1989. Development of early swimming in *Xenopus laevis* embryos: myotomal musculature, its innervation and activation. *Neuroscience* **32:** 113–126.

46. von Seckendorff-Hoff, K. & R.J. Wassersug. 1986. The kinematics of swimming in larvae of the clawed frog, *Xenopus laevis. J. Exp. Biol.* **122:** 1–12.

47. Mendelson, B. 1986. Development of reticulospinal neurons of the zebrafish. Part I. Time of origin. *J. Comp. Neurol.* **251:** 160–171.

48. Livingstone, M. & D. Hubel. 1988. Segregation of form, color, movement, and depth: anatomy, physiology, and perception. *Science* **240:** 740–749.

49. Rakic, P. 1977. Genesis of the dorsal lateral geniculate nucleus in the rhesus monkey: site and time of origin, kinetics of proliferation, routes of migration and pattern of distribution of neurons. *J. Comp. Neurol.* **176:** 23–52.

50. Rakic, P. 1974. Neurons in rhesus monkey visual cortex: systematic relation between time of origin and eventual disposition. *Science* **183:** 425–427.

51. Lingenhohl, K. & E. Friauf. 1994. Giant neurons in the rat reticular formation: a sensorimotor interface in the elementary acoustic startle circuit? *J. Neurosci.* **14:** 1176–1194.

52. Altman, J. & S.A. Bayer. 1980. Development of the brain stem in the rat. Part IV. Thymidine-radiographic study of the time of origin of neurons in the pontine region. *J. Comp. Neurol.* **194:** 905–929.

53. Butt, S.J. *et al.* 2005. The temporal and spatial origins of cortical interneurons predict their physiological subtype. *Neuron* **48:** 591–604.

54. Riley, M.R. *et al.* 2009. A topographic map of function along the axis of stripes in the hindbrain of zebrafish. *Soc. Neuro. Abstr.* **366:** 591.

55. Sillar, K.T. & A. Roberts. 1993. Control of frequency during swimming in Xenopus embryos: a study on interneuronal recruitment in a spinal rhythm generator. *J. Physiol.* **472:** 557–572.

56. Mos, W., B.L. Roberts & R. Williamson. 1990. Interneuronal activity patterns during fictive locomotion of spinal dogfish. *Phil. Trans. R. Soc. Lond. B.* **330:** 341–349.

57. Crone, S.A. *et al.* 2008. Genetic ablation of V2a ipsilateral interneurons disrupts left-right locomotor coordination in mammalian spinal cord. *Neuron* **60:** 70–83.

58. Vasudevan, E.V. & A.J. Bastian. 2010. Split-belt treadmill adaptation shows different functional networks for fast and slow human walking. *J. Neurophysiol.* **103:** 183–191.

59. Combes, D. *et al.* 2004. Developmental segregation of spinal networks driving axial- and hindlimb-based locomotion in metamorphosing *Xenopus laevis. J. Physiol.* **559:** 17–24.

60. Fetcho, J.R. 1987. A review of the organization and evolution of motoneurons innervating the axial musculature of vertebrates. *Brain Res.* **434:** 243–280.

61. Fetcho, J.R. 1992. The spinal motor system in early vertebrates and some of its evolutionary changes. *Brain Behav. Evol.* **40:** 82–97.

62. McLean, D.L., S.D. Merrywest & K.T. Sillar. 2000. The development of neuromodulatory systems and the maturation of motor patterns in amphibian tadpoles. *Brain Res. Bull.* **53:** 595–603.

63. Sillar, K.T. *et al.* 2008. Neuromodulation and developmental plasticity in the locomotor system of anuran amphibians during metamorphosis. *Brain Res. Rev.* **57:** 94–102.

64. Marder, E. & D. Bucher. 2007. Understanding circuit dynamics using the stomatogastric nervous system of lobsters and crabs. *Annu. Rev. Physiol.* **69:** 291–316.

65. Parker, D. & S. Grillner. 1998. Cellular and synaptic modulation underlying substance P-mediated plasticity of the lamprey locomotor network. *J. Neurosci.* **18:** 8095–8110.

66. Neyt, C. *et al.* 2000. Evolutionary origins of vertebrate appendicular muscle. *Nature* **408:** 82–86.

67. Grillner, S. *et al.* 2007. Modeling a vertebrate motor system: pattern generation, steering and control of body orientation. *Prog. Brain Res.* **165:** 221–234.

68. Roberts, A. *et al.* 1998. Central circuits controlling locomotion in young frog tadpoles. *Ann. N. Y. Acad. Sci.* **860:** 19–34.

69. Rybak, I.A. *et al.* 2006. Modelling spinal circuitry involved in locomotor pattern generation: insights from deletions during fictive locomotion. *J. Physiol.* **577:** 617–639.

70. Lanuza, G.M. *et al.* 2004. Genetic identification of spinal interneurons that coordinate left-right locomotor activity necessary for walking movements. *Neuron* **42:** 375–386.

Ann. N.Y. Acad. Sci. ISSN 0077-8923

ANNALS OF THE NEW YORK ACADEMY OF SCIENCES

Issue: *Neurons and Networks in the Spinal Cord*

Alternation of agonists and antagonists during turtle hindlimb motor rhythms

Paul S.G. Stein

Biology Department, Washington University, St. Louis, Missouri

Address for correspondence: Paul S.G. Stein, Professor of Biology, Washington University Biology Department, Campus Box 1137, One Brookings Drive, St. Louis, Missouri 63130. stein@wustl.edu

In a variety of vertebrates, including turtle, many classical and contemporary studies of spinal cord neuronal networks generating rhythmic motor behaviors emphasize a Reciprocal Model with alternation of agonists and antagonists, alternation of excitatory postsynaptic potentials (EPSPs) and inhibitory postsynaptic potentials (IPSPs), and reciprocal inhibition. Some studies of spinal cord neuronal networks, including some in turtle during scratch motor rhythms, describe a Balanced Model with concurrent EPSPs and IPSPs. The present report reviews turtle spinal cord studies and concludes that there is support for a Combined Model with both alternating and concurrent excitation and inhibition, that is, characteristics of both the Reciprocal and the Balanced Models, in the same spinal cord neuronal network for scratch reflex in turtle. Studies of spinal cord neuronal networks for locomotion in a variety of vertebrates also support a Combined Model.

Keywords: turtle; scratch reflex; spinal cord; central pattern generator; reciprocal inhibition; balanced excitation and inhibition

Introduction

Agonist-antagonist alternation is a fundamental feature of the motor neuron patterns responsible for generating vertebrate rhythmic limb motor behaviors.[1–19] These rhythmically alternating motor patterns are generated within the spinal cord by neuronal networks, termed central pattern generators (CPGs), without movement-related sensory inputs and without information from supraspinal structures.[2–19] Hypotheses about the organization of these CPGs incorporate reciprocal inhibition between agonist and antagonist modules (also termed half-centers or unit-burst-generators, UBGs) as one of the fundamental mechanisms responsible for the generation of agonist-antagonist alternation.[1–19] This reciprocal inhibitory organization is also termed the Reciprocal Model.[20]

Concurrent excitation and inhibition is another important feature of neuronal networks.[5–8,10,13,20–28] Some of the experimental support for this feature in spinal cord utilizes intracellular recordings (REC) from turtle hindlimb motor neurons during fictive scratch motor rhythms.[7,20,26,27] During these rhythms, each motor neuron has an active phase during which the neuron fires action potentials and a quiet phase during which the motor neuron does not fire. For each motor neuron, there are concurrent excitatory postsynaptic potentials (EPSPs) and inhibitory postsynaptic potentials (IPSPs): this coactivation is termed Balanced Excitation and Inhibition, that is, the Balanced Model.[20,26,27] The Reciprocal Model is contrasted with the Balanced Model in Figure S1 of Berg, Alaburda, and Hounsgaard:[20] one interpretation of this contrast is that these two Models represent divergent points of view with features that do not coexist in the same network.

The present review summarizes data obtained in studies of turtle scratch reflex[7,18,29–66] that support the point of view that features of the Reciprocal Model characterize turtle spinal cord CPGs for scratch. The review further discusses studies that support the point of view that features of the Balanced Model also characterize these turtle scratch CPGs.[7,20,26,27] The review concludes with the point

doi: 10.1111/j.1749-6632.2010.05500.x
Ann. N.Y. Acad. Sci. 1198 (2010) 105–118 © 2010 New York Academy of Sciences.

of view that features of both the Reciprocal and the Balanced Models are characteristics of the same neuronal network in the turtle spinal cord. The Combined Model is the term for a network with features of both the Reciprocal Model and the Balanced Model. The Combined Model is supported by experiments with turtle scratch neuronal networks that demonstrate in the same network that there is: some inhibition that alternates with excitation (Reciprocal Model); other inhibition that is concurrent with excitation during the active phase of that motor neuron's motor pool (Balanced Model during Motor Pool's Active Phase); and still other inhibition that is concurrent with excitation during the quiet phase of that motor neuron's motor pool (Balanced Model during Motor Pool's Quiet Phase).

Chance, Abbott, and Reyes[23] and Abbott and Chance[25] provide important perspectives in support of a neuronal network characterized by a Combined Model. They use the term "driving inputs" to describe a Reciprocal Model with excitation and inhibition acting in a push-pull manner and the term "modulatory inputs" to describe a Balanced Model with concurrent excitation and inhibition. They state "Sets of balanced inputs that have excitatory and inhibitory rates rising and falling together comprise modulatory inputs, and those for which excitation and inhibition vary in opposite directions act as driving inputs. This arrangement has the advantage that individual excitatory inputs can rapidly switch between driving and modulatory functions, depending upon whether they are varying in parallel with or in opposition to changes in inhibition."[23] Additional data supporting a Combined Model perspective that both alternating and concurrent excitation and inhibition are present in the same neuronal network are described in studies of the CPGs for *Aplysia* feeding,[28] lamprey swimming,[5,21] zebrafish swimming,[19,24] tadpole swimming,[6,10] turtle scratching,[7] and rodent locomotion.[8,13]

The reciprocal model in turtle

Agonist-antagonist rhythmic alternation during normal scratch

A fundamental feature of turtle normal hindlimb scratch is rhythmic alternation between hip-flexor motor activity and quiescence:[7,30,34,40,47,48,54] hip-extensor motor activity occurs during hip flexor quiescence (Fig. 1A). Another feature of turtle nor-

mal scratch is rhythmic alternation between knee-extensor motor activity and quiescence. These features have been described during all three forms of scratch: rostral, pocket, and caudal.[34] The most studied form of turtle scratch is the rostral scratch in which knee-extensor motor activity occurs during the latter portions of the hip-flexor motor neuron burst (Fig. 1A). In this form of scratch, knee-flexor motor activity occurs during knee-extensor quiescence[30,56,57] (Fig. 2A) and the duration of knee-flexor motor activity is related to the duration of knee-extensor quiescence.[57] Thus, turtle normal scratch motor patterns demonstrate both hip and knee agonist-antagonist rhythmic alternations: these alternations are consistent with Reciprocal Models for hip modules as well as for knee modules. Figure 3A is a schematic of some of the possible synaptic connections in the turtle rostral scratch CPG that includes reciprocal relationships between flexor and extensor neurons related to hip motor outputs and reciprocal relationships between flexor and extensor neurons related to knee motor outputs.

Studies with many neuronal networks have demonstrated that reciprocal inhibitory networks are well suited to produce agonist-antagonist rhythmic alternation.[4,9,11,12,14–18,67] The sketch in Figure 3A shares reciprocal inhibitory features with sketches for mammalian stepping CPGs presented by Grillner[4,11] in his UBG hypothesis, by McCrea and Rybak[17] in their two-layer CPG model, and by Endo and Kiehn[14] in their CPG model. Agonist-antagonist rhythmic alternation when both agonists and antagonists are activated is a prediction of these Reciprocal Models.

Agonist quiescence between successive agonist bursts

Motor pattern variations of rostral scratch provide considerable insights into the underlying structure of the turtle scratch CPG. The most studied variation is hip-extensor deletion rostral scratch.[7,18,29,31,40,47,48,50,54,57,60,66] During a hip-extensor deletion rostral scratch, there is no activity in hip-extensor motor neurons and no quiescence between successive bursts of hip-flexor motor neuron activity (Figs. 1B and 2B). During a hip-extensor deletion rostral scratch, there is rhythmic alternation between knee-extensor and knee-flexor activity (last 2 cycles with unfilled diamonds in Fig. 2B).

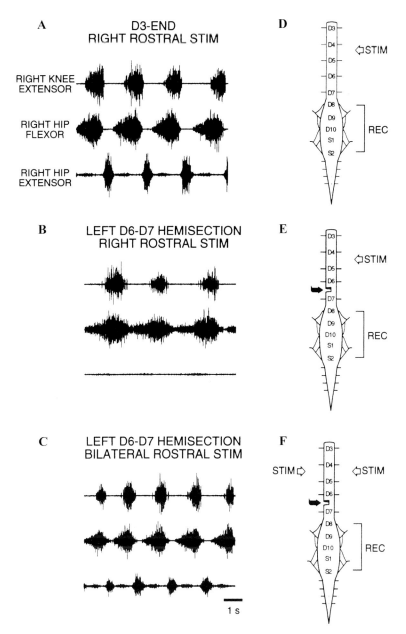

Figure 1. Rostral scratch motor neuron activity patterns in the spinal immobilized turtle. Electroneurographic (ENG) recordings from the right biarticular knee-extensor nerve (*top trace*), the right hip-flexor nerve (*middle trace*), and the right hip-extensor nerve (*bottom trace*). (**A**) Right rostral scratch stimulation (STIM) in the D3-end preparation elicits normal rostral scratch with rhythmic right hip-flexor and hip-extensor alternation. (**B**) Right rostral scratch stimulation in the D3-end with left D6–D7 hemisection preparation elicits hip-extensor deletion rostral scratch with right hip-flexor rhythms. (**C**) Bilateral stimulation of mirror-image rostral scratch sites in the D3-end with left D6–D7 hemisection preparation elicits reconstructed normal rostral scratch with rhythmic right hip-flexor and hip-extensor alternation. (**D**) Sketch of the spinal cord in the D3-end preparation with a complete transection between the second and third postcervical spinal segments (D2–D3). (**E** and **F**) Sketches of the spinal cord in the D3-end with left D6–D7 hemisection preparation. All ENG REC are from nerves on the right-hand side. From Ref. 48 and used with permission of and copyright 1998 by the New York Academy of Sciences and Wiley-Blackwell.

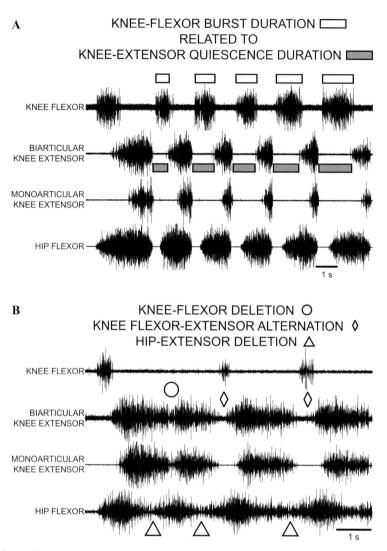

Figure 2. Rostral scratch motor neuron activity patterns in response to stimulation of a site in the right rostral scratch receptive field in a D3-end preparation. ENG REC from the right knee-flexor nerve, the right biarticular knee-extensor nerve, the right monoarticular knee-extensor nerve, and the right hip-flexor nerve. (**A**) Normal rostral scratch. Knee-flexor activity marked with *unfilled rectangles*; biarticular knee-extensor quiescence marked with *gray-filled rectangles*. (**B**) Rostral scratch with hip-extensor deletions. Hip-extensor deletions marked with *unfilled triangles*; knee-flexor deletion marked with *unfilled circle*; rhythmic knee-flexor bursts during knee-extensor quiescence marked with unfilled diamonds. From Ref. 57 and used with permission of and copyright 2004 by the American Physiological Society.

Hip-extensor deletions occur in a small percentage of rostral scratch cycles in preparations with a single complete transection of the spinal cord, for example, D3-end preparations (Fig. 1D).[40,47] Preparations with additional removals of spinal circuitry (Fig. 1E) demonstrate higher percentages of hip-extensor deletions in response to one-site stimu-lation (Fig. 1B).[36,40,47,48,50] A candidate neuronal network with quiescence of hip-extensor interneurons and motor neurons during hip-extensor deletions is sketched in Figure 3B. The sketch emphasizes that knee-related flexor and extensor neurons are still alternately active along with each burst of hip-flexor neurons during a hip-extensor deletion.

A

Hip and Knee UBGs for
Normal Rostral Scratch

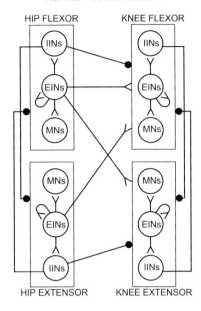

B

Hip and Knee UBGs for
Hip-Extensor Deletion Rostral Scratch

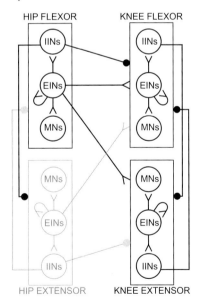

Figure 3. Schematic of a hypothesis describing a portion of the spinal neuronal network responsible for the production of the turtle rostral scratch as described in the modular UBG hypothesis. Only ipsilateral hip and knee UBGs are shown; only a subset of the possible synaptic connections are included in the sketch. EINs, excitatory interneurons; IINs, inhibitory interneurons; MNs,

Data from hip-extensor deletion rostral scratch support the following Reciprocal Model concepts: certain subcomponents of a neuronal network, for example, knee-flexor module and knee-extensor module, demonstrate rhythmic alternation that is a characteristic of many Reciprocal Models; other subcomponents of the same neuronal network, for example, hip-flexor module and hip-extensor module, demonstrate continuous hip-flexor activity and no hip-extensor activity as predicted when one module in a Reciprocal Model completely inhibits its antagonist module (Fig. 3B).

More recently, two distinct knee-related deletions of rostral scratch motor patterns have been recognized.[57] In a knee-flexor deletion, there is no activity in knee-flexor motor neurons and no quiescence between successive bursts of knee-extensor motor neuron activity (unfilled circle in Fig. 2B). In a knee-extensor deletion, there is no activity in knee-extensor motor neurons and no quiescence between successive bursts of knee-flexor motor neuron activity. In a deletion variation with no antagonist activity in a cycle, the Reciprocal Model predicts an absence of agonist quiescence between two successive agonist bursts due to the absence of reciprocal inhibition from the antagonist module during the deletion cycle. The knee-related deletion results therefore provide additional support for the Reciprocal Model.

Reconstruction of normal agonist-antagonist alternation

In most studies of turtle rostral scratch hip-extensor deletions, the experimenter does not have direct control in a given episode over whether a variation

---

motor neurons. Reciprocal inhibition between agonist and antagonist UBGs at each degree of freedom is a fundamental characteristic of organization of this network. Active neurons shown in **black**; quiet neurons shown in **light gray**. (A) During normal rostral scratch, all hip and knee UBGs are rhythmically active. (B) During hip-extensor deletion variation of rostral scratch, the hip-flexor, the knee-flexor, and the knee-extensor UBGs are rhythmically active. Neurons in the hip-extensor UBG are quiet. This schematic emphasizes that neurons in the hip-flexor UBG are rhythmic even when neurons in the hip-extensor UBG are quiet. From Ref. 18 and used with permission of and copyright 2008 by Elsevier B.V.

is produced or whether a normal motor pattern is produced. In contrast, a preparation with a complete D2–D3 spinal cord transection just posterior to the second postcervical segment with an additional transverse D6–D7 hemisection one segment anterior to the hindlimb enlargement (Fig. 1E) displays high percentages of hip-extensor deletions with one-site stimulation.[47,48] The side of the hemisection is termed lesion-side; the side opposite the hemisection is termed intact-side. Intact-side one-site stimulation in the rostral scratch receptive field results mainly in hip-extensor deletion rostral scratches in intact-side motor neurons (Figs. 1B and E). Reconstruction of normal rostral scratch motor patterns in intact-side motor neurons occurs with two-site bilateral stimulation of rostral scratch receptive fields (Figs. 1C and F). In this preparation, intact-side stimulation favors rhythmic activation of intact-side hip-flexor neurons and lesion-side stimulation favors activation of intact-side hip-extensor neurons and inhibition of intact-side hip-flexor neurons. Bilateral stimulation activates intact-side hip-flexor and hip-extensor neurons rhythmically in alternation. The rhythmic alternation between hip-flexor and hip-extensor motor activities in this preparation in response to two-site stimulation is termed reconstruction.[47,48] There are several experimental situations in which the presence of hip-extensor activity is associated with quiescence of hip-flexor activity.[47] This reconstruction of agonist-antagonist alternation when both hip-flexor and hip-extensor neurons are activated is consistent with reciprocal inhibitory connections between hip-flexor and hip-extensor interneurons as described by a Reciprocal Model (Fig. 3A).

IPSPs during motor neuron quiescence

Additional experimental support for a Reciprocal Model comes from intracellular REC from turtle motor neurons[7,31,55,58] during rhythmic scratch motor patterns. Intracellular REC from a hip-flexor motor neuron (top trace marked VP-HP in Fig. 4A) and from a hip-extensor motor neuron (top trace marked HR-KF in Fig. 4B) are shown along with electoneurograms (ENGs) from three motor nerves: monoarticular knee-extensor (FT-KE), hip-flexor (VP-HP), and hip-extensor (HR-KF). In the last three cycles of Figure 4A, there is rhythmic alternation between hip-flexor and hip-extensor motor activities characteristic of normal rostral scratch.

Note the large negative-going IPSPs in the intracellular REC of the hip-flexor motor neuron during each burst of extracellular hip-extensor motor neuron activity. These large IPSPs during normal rostral scratch provide support for a Reciprocal Model (Fig. 3A).

In the first 2 cycles of Figure 4A marked with filled triangles, there is a hip-extensor deletion rostral scratch. Note the absence of the large IPSPs in the hip-flexor motor neuron associated with the absence of hip-extensor motor activities. (See section later, however, on "Concurrent Excitation and Inhibition in a Motor Neuron during Activity of Its Motor Pool" for a discussion that notes that some inhibition in the hip-flexor motor neuron still remains in the first two cycles of Fig. 4A.) Similarly, intracellular REC from a hip-extensor motor neuron (Fig. 4B) display large EPSPs during the extracellular hip-extensor motor neuron activity in normal rostral scratch cycles; these EPSPs are absent during rostral scratch cycles with a hip-extensor deletion shown with filled triangles in Figure 4B. The absence of the large IPSPs in hip-flexor motor neurons and the absence of large EPSPs in hip-extensor motor neurons during hip-extensor deletion rostral scratch provide further support for a Reciprocal Model (Fig. 3B).

Robertson and Stein[7] provide additional evidence for the presence of IPSPs in hip-flexor motor neurons during the phase of the cycle in which hip-flexor motor neurons are quiet. In their Figure 3,[7] they demonstrate a reversal of the IPSPs by DC hyperpolarization of the motor neuron. In their Figure 4A,[7] they demonstrate a high conductance during the quiet phase of the motor neuron's cycle. This high-conductance state during the quiet phase of motor neuron rhythmic activity is also described by Alaburda et al.[58] in their Figures 1C and 2A. In addition, their Figure 4[58] describes reduced excitability of the motor neuron during its quiet phase of the scratch cycle in response to depolarizing current pulses: this reduced excitability is consistent with inhibition due to IPSPs during this phase of the cycle. In Figure 4B of Robertson and Stein,[7] chloride injection into the motor neuron is used to demonstrate a depolarizing IPSP during the quiet phase of the motor neuron. Figure 5 here is a summary sketch of the synaptic potentials recorded from motor neurons during turtle rostral scratch.[7] There is a portion of the scratch cycle in which the motor neuron receives

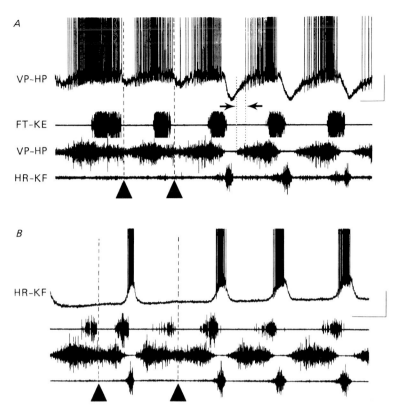

Figure 4. Comparison of voltage trajectories recorded intracellularly from hip-flexor (VP-HP) motor neuron (*top trace* in A) and hip-extensor (HR-KF) motor neuron (*top trace* in B) during normal rostral scratch and during hip-extensor deletion rostral scratch. In (A) and (B) ENG REC from monoarticular knee-extensor nerve (FT-KE; *second trace*), hip-flexor nerve (VP-HP; *third trace*) and hip-extensor nerve (HR-KF; *bottom trace*). (A) Hip-extensor motor neuron activity is deleted in first two cycles (marked with filled triangles). Hip-flexor motor neuron intracellular REC shows corresponding deletion of hyperpolarization normally associated with hip-extensor activity (compare with last three cycles showing hip-extensor nerve activity). (B) Hip-extensor nerve activity is deleted in the first and third cycles (marked with *filled triangles*) and is associated with a complete absence of depolarization in the hip-extensor motor neuron intracellular REC (compare with cycles with hip-extensor nerve activity). Calibrations: 1 s, 20 mV. From Ref. 7 and used with permission of and copyright 1988 by The Physiological Society and Wiley-Blackwell.

inhibition (designated "I") and the motor neuron is not firing. These experimental results are consistent with a Reciprocal Model in which turtle motor neurons receive significant IPSPs during their quiescent phase of the scratch cycle.

Antagonist single-unit interneuron activity during normal and deletion rostral scratch

In the Reciprocal Model, hip-extensor motor neurons and interneurons are active during the quiet phase of hip-flexor motor activity (Fig. 3A). A prediction of the Reciprocal Model is that hip-extensor interneurons will be quiet during hip-extensor deletion rostral scratch (Fig. 3B). The lack of IPSPs in

hip-flexor motor neurons and the lack of EPSPs in hip-extensor motor neurons described in the prior section provide evidence in support of this prediction.

This prediction is tested further using single-unit extracellular axonal REC from propriospinal interneurons with descending axons during normal rostral scratch and during hip-extensor deletion rostral scratch.[54] Interneurons that fire during hip-flexor quiescence and/or hip-extensor activity during normal rostral scratch cycles are termed "hip-extensor interneurons." Figure 6A is an example of a hip-extensor interneuron active during hip-flexor quiescence of normal rostral scratch (last

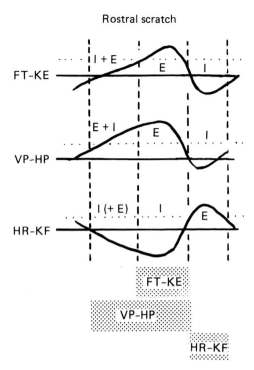

Figure 5. Diagram comparing intracellularly recorded voltage changes in monoarticular knee-extensor (FT-KE), hip-flexor (VP-HP), and hip-extensor (HR-KF) motor neurons during rostral scratch. ENG motor patterns depicting timing of corresponding motor pools shown at the bottom. Firing threshold shown as *dotted line.* I (IPSPs) and E (EPSPs) indicate synaptic inputs to motor neurons derived from data.[7] Note there is at least one phase of reciprocal inhibition for each motor neuron and at least one phase of balanced inhibition for knee-extensor and hip-flexor motor neuron. The phase of balanced inhibition for the hip-extensor motor neuron is based upon preliminary observations. From Ref. 7 and used with permission of and copyright 1988 by the Physiological Society and Wiley-Blackwell.

five cycles in Fig. 6A) and quiet during a hip-extensor deletion (cycle ending with filled diamond in Fig. 6A). Recordings[54] from 18 hip-extensor interneurons produced a total of 9465 action potentials during 767 cycles of normal rostral scratch and a total of 24 action potentials during 167 cycles of hip-extensor deletion rostral scratch. These hip-extensor interneurons are mainly quiet during hip-extensor deletion rostral scratch: this provides further support for the Reciprocal Model hypothesis that neurons in the hip-extensor module (or UBG

or half-center) are mainly quiet during hip-extensor deletion rostral scratch (Fig. 3B).

ON-units are interneurons whose start-phases are positively correlated with the start-phases of knee-extensor motor neuron activity during normal rostral scratch.[56] ON-units are candidate members of a knee-extensor module. OFF-units are interneurons whose end-phases are positively correlated with the start-phases of knee-extensor motor activity during normal rostral scratch.[56] OFF-units are candidate members of a knee-flexor module. Both ON-units and OFF-units fire in bursts during hip-extensor deletions.[56] ON-units are usually quiet during knee-extensor deletions and OFF-units are usually quiet during knee-flexor deletions.[66] These data provide support for the Reciprocal Model hypotheses that: ON-units are members of the knee-extensor module, OFF-units are members of the knee-flexor module, and that there is reciprocal inhibition between the knee-extensor module and the knee-flexor module (Fig. 3).

Intracellular interneuronal REC during normal scratch

Additional support for the Reciprocal Model has been obtained with direct intracellular REC during fictive scratch from turtle interneurons.[58,59,61,62,64] Berkowitz[59,61,62,64] recorded from interneurons during each of the three forms of scratch and characterized the morphology of each of the interneurons. He used averaging techniques to characterize the average membrane potential of each interneuron during each phase of the scratch cycle. The membrane voltage during each interneuron's quiet phase displayed a significant trough. He also recorded intracellularly from turtle interneurons during fictive swim as well as during each of the three forms of fictive scratch.[64] Most interestingly, he found that the phase of minimum of the membrane voltage during swim was strongly correlated with the phase of its minimum during scratch. This differed from measurements obtained with respect to the phases of maximum voltage during swim compared with scratch. Berkowitz[64] suggested that this indicated the importance of reciprocal inhibition in interneurons not only during rhythmic scratch but also during rhythmic swim motor patterns. These data provide additional support for the Reciprocal Model hypothesis.

A

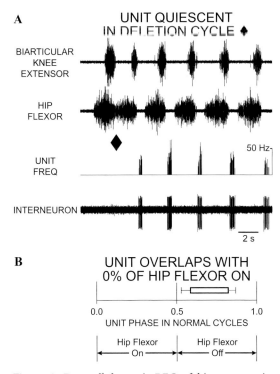

UNIT QUIESCENT
IN DELETION CYCLE ◆

BIARTICULAR
KNEE
EXTENSOR

HIP
FLEXOR

UNIT
FREQ

50 Hz

INTERNEURON

2 s

B

UNIT OVERLAPS WITH
0% OF HIP FLEXOR ON

0.0   0.5   1.0
UNIT PHASE IN NORMAL CYCLES

Hip Flexor
— On —

Hip Flexor
— Off —

Figure 6. Extracellular unit REC of hip-extensor interneuron with 0% overlap with the hip-flexor burst was active in a burst during hip-flexor quiescence of normal rostral scratch and was quiet during rostral scratch with a hip-extensor deletion. (**A**) ENG REC of the biarticular knee-extensor motor nerve (*top trace*); ENG REC of the hip-flexor motor nerve (*second trace*); instantaneous frequency of unit (*third trace*); and interneuron unit activity (*bottom trace*). The first cycle is an example of rostral scratch with a hip-extensor deletion (end of cycle marked with *filled diamond*). The other cycles are examples of normal rostral scratch. (**B**) Start and end of bar represent mean ON-phase and mean OFF-phase, respectively, of unit firing during normal rostral scratch. *Bar is unfilled* to represent unit quiescence during hip-extensor deletion rostral scratch. From Ref. 54 and used with permission of and copyright 2002 by the Society for Neuroscience.

Reciprocal model conclusions

Evidence described above supports Reciprocal Model concepts that agonist-antagonist alternation, alternation of excitatory and inhibitory postsynaptic potentials, and reciprocal inhibition are fundamental features of the spinal CPG for scratch in turtle spinal cord.[7,18,29–66] Turtle scratch CPGs therefore

share Reciprocal Model characteristics that are well established in other vertebrate CPGs.[1,6,8,17,19]

The next section summarizes support for the Balanced Model of Concurrent Excitation and Inhibition in these same turtle scratch CPGs. Some of the evidence for the Balanced Model is obtained in the same turtle experimental preparation that also provides support for the Reciprocal Model.[7] The positive evidence for the Reciprocal Model presented in the aforementioned sections is therefore compatible with the positive evidence for the Balanced Model presented in the following sections.

The balanced model in turtle

This section describes evidence for concurrent excitation and inhibition in turtle motor neurons during scratch motor rhythms in the work of Robertson and Stein[7] and Berg et al.[20] This evidence is gathered from adult turtles with intracellular REC from motor neurons during scratch motor rhythms produced in response to natural mechanical stimulation of cutaneous sensory neurons.

Concurrent excitation and inhibition in a motor neuron during activity of its motor pool

There is a distinct recruitment order[68] observed in the extracellular REC from the axons of the nerve innervating the hip-flexor muscle during each burst of a rostral scratch motor rhythm (third trace in Fig. 4A, labeled VP-HP). Axons with the smallest extracellular action potentials are recruited first, then those with medium-sized action potentials are recruited at intermediate phases, and finally those with the largest-sized action potentials are recruited during the highest amplitude part of the ENG burst. De-recruitment occurs in reverse order.

Robertson and Stein[7] characterized the synaptic drive in medium-recruited hip-flexor motor neurons during rostral scratch (Fig. 4A). Using a variety of techniques, they established that medium-recruited hip-flexor motor neurons received concurrent excitation and inhibition during the early portion of the hip-flexor nerve burst when only small early-recruited hip-flexor motor axons are firing. This concurrent excitation and inhibition is present during normal rostral scratch (last three cycles of Fig. 4A) and also during hip-extensor deletion rostral scratch (first two cycles of Fig. 4A: note that reciprocal inhibition is absent during these cycles of hip-extensor deletion rostral scratch). The inhibition that is concurrent with excitation during normal rostral scratch is sensitive to strychnine.[43] This supports the Balanced Model.

Concurrent excitation and inhibition in hip-flexor motor neurons (VP-HP) during normal rostral scratch is diagrammed as "E + I" in Figure 5. Balanced excitation and inhibition may be a major contributor to the generation of motor neuron recruitment order: it may prevent medium- and late-recruited motor neurons from firing at the early phases of its motor pool's activity. Importantly, positive data supporting both a Balanced Model and a Reciprocal Model are obtained during the same episode of rostral scratch.

Concurrent excitation and inhibition in a motor neuron during quiescence of its motor pool

The monoarticular knee-extensor (FT-KE) nerve fires during the latter portion of the hip-flexor motor burst during normal rostral scratch. Intracellular REC from monoarticular knee-extensor motor neurons during normal rostral scratch reveal concurrent excitation and inhibition during the early portion of the hip-flexor burst when the monoarticular knee-extensor motor pool is quiet.[7] This is diagrammed as "I + E" for monoarticular knee-extensor motor neurons (FT-KE) during rostral scratch (Fig. 5). Thus balanced excitation and inhibition prevents knee-extensor motor neurons from firing during an inappropriate phase of the rostral scratch motor pattern. This may be especially important since a major difference between the motor pattern for rostral scratch and the motor patterns for other forms of scratch is the timing of knee-extensor motor neurons in the cycle of hip motor neuron activity. These observations support the Balanced Model and suggest that balanced excitation and inhibition may be an important contributor to the selection and production of the appropriate motor pattern for each form of scratch.

Knee-extensor motor neurons are inhibited during flexion reflex produced by a brief mechanical stimulus to the dorsum of the foot.[7] The hip-flexor ENG serves as a monitor of flexion reflex. There are strong chloride-dependent IPSPs in knee-extensor motor neurons during flexion reflex.[7] The voltage trajectories of these IPSPs provide an index of the relative position of the chloride equilibrium potential relative to the resting membrane potential.

Robertson and Stein[7] presented synaptic potentials of knee-extensor motor neurons during both rostral scratch and flexion reflex in their Figure 7A in three different situations: the chloride equilibrium potential was more negative than, equal to, and more positive than the resting potential. Based on these REC, they concluded that, during rostral scratch, there was balanced excitation and inhibition (with inhibition dominating) during the early portion of the hip-flexor burst and reciprocal inhibition during the hip-extensor burst. These observations provide data that support both a Balanced Model and a Reciprocal Model in the same episode of rostral scratch.

Concurrent excitation and inhibition in knee-extensor motor neurons is present in the early portion of the hip-flexor burst during a hip-extensor deletion rostral scratch (Fig. 6A of Ref. 7). This balanced excitation and inhibition in the knee-extensor motor neuron is present even though the reciprocal inhibition normally present during the hip-extensor phase of a normal rostral scratch is absent during the hip-extensor deletion. This observation invites future work to examine the potential sources of inhibitory drives in motor neurons during Balanced Excitation and Inhibition and during Reciprocal Inhibition. An interesting hypothesis is that there may be one population of interneurons responsible for the inhibition characterized by the Balanced Model and a different population of interneurons responsible for the inhibition characterized by the Reciprocal Model.

Concurrent excitation and inhibition during action potential firing in motor neurons during scratch

Berg et al.[20] measure the total excitatory conductance and the total inhibitory conductance in turtle motor neurons during scratch motor rhythms.[69] This technique allows the evaluation of how much inhibitory conductance is present when there is a sufficient excitatory conductance to drive action potential firing during the scratch motor pattern. Interestingly, the peak of excitatory conductance occurs in-phase with the peak of inhibitory conductance. Additional support for their conclusion of concurrent excitation and inhibition is obtained by blocking inhibitory glycinergic receptors with strychnine and observing an increased depolarization during the motor neuron's on-phase and a decreased variability of successive interspike intervals. These observations[20] support the Balanced Model, establish that concurrent excitation and inhibition occur in turtle motor neurons in a much larger portion of the scratch cycle than described previously, and considerably extend the prior work.[7]

The observations of Berg et al.[20] are obtained from motor neuron cell bodies in the D10 spinal segment, the third segment of the five-segment turtle hindlimb enlargement.[70] Peripheral axons of D10 spinal segment motor neurons run mainly in the hip-extensor nerve or the sciatic nerve. Berg et al.[20] do not type-identify the specific muscle that each recorded motor neuron cell body innervates. Different motor neuron types have different patterns of synaptic inputs for rostral scratch (Fig. 5). Differences between these patterns are more pronounced when other forms of scratch, for example, pocket and caudal, are also examined (see Figs. 1, 6–8 of Ref. 7). Future experiments that characterize concurrent excitation and inhibition[69] in type-identified motor neurons during each of several forms of scratch will add additional information to our knowledge of turtle spinal cord neuronal networks.

Balanced model conclusions

Concurrent excitation and inhibition and support for the Balanced Model occur in turtle motor neurons during scratch motor patterns.[7,20] Observations of concurrent excitation and inhibition are obtained in the same preparations that also demonstrate alternation of agonists and antagonists, alternation of excitatory and inhibitory potentials, and reciprocal inhibition.[7] Thus, turtle scratch motor circuitry exhibits aspects of both the Reciprocal and the Balanced Models, that is, the Combined Model.

Considerable work is now needed in turtles to characterize fully the extent of both concurrent and alternating excitation and inhibition. In particular, it will be important to see additional work in preparations that display (1) strong agonist-antagonist rhythmic alternation, for example, normal rostral scratch, and (2) antagonist deletion variations, for example, hip-extensor deletion variations of rostral scratch. Such work can evaluate the relative contributions of both the Reciprocal Model and the Balanced Model under each of these conditions. We are only starting to appreciate the true complexity of the turtle spinal cord CPGs that generate these complex behaviors.

The combined model

This review describes evidence and concludes that the CPG neuronal circuitry that generates scratch motor patterns in turtle spinal cord has Combined Model features, that is, the same spinal circuit has features of both the Reciprocal Model (inhibition that alternates with excitation) and the Balanced Model (inhibition that is concurrent with excitation).[7]

The evidence described here for the Combined Model for the turtle scratch CPG adds to the considerable evidence for Combined Model circuitry with both Reciprocal and Balanced Model features in many vertebrate locomotion CPGs, for example, lamprey,[5,21] zebrafish,[19,24] tadpole,[6,10] and rodent.[8,13] Thus, concurrent and alternating excitation and inhibition are fundamental features of the spinal cord neuronal networks responsible for the production of rhythmic vertebrate behaviors.

Summary

The turtle spinal cord CPG that produces the motor patterns for scratch reflex is an excellent model system for the study of the mechanisms for spinal cord motor control. It displays many of the fundamental principles of organization of other vertebrate spinal CPGs. It offers the technical advantage that responses of an adult nervous system can be obtained with natural cutaneous stimulation: robust rhythms with complex coordination patterns are produced without the need for stimulation with electrical impulses or bath application of neuroactive agents. The network driving the scratch rhythms can be studied in a wide variety of preparations: (1) in vivo preparations with moving limbs,[29,30,34,44,45,51,52,60] (2) in vivo preparations without movement-related sensory input,[7,29,34,36,38,39,54,60,61] and (3) in vitro preparations without muscles.[20,26,27,32,41,49,55,58] Considerable work is now required by future experimentalists to reveal all the molecular, synaptic, cellular, and systems mechanisms in the spinal cord responsible for orchestrating the elegant coordinated movements of the turtle hindlimb when it successfully rubs against a site on the turtle body surface that has received a gentle mechanical stimulus.

Acknowledgments

Studies on turtle spinal cord in the Stein Laboratory have been supported by grants to PSGS from the NIH (1979–1989, 1992–2010) and from the NSF (1972–1979, 1989–1992). Most recent support for the Stein Laboratory is provided by NIH Grant NS-30786. I thank Drs. Ari Berkowitz, Scott Currie, Ole Kiehn, and Gail Robertson for their editorial comments.

Conflicts of interest

The author declares no conflicts of interest.

References

1. Sherrington, C.S. 1906. *The Integrative Action of the Nervous System.* Yale University Press. New Haven, CT.

2. Brown, T.G. 1911. The intrinsic factors in the act of progression in the mammal. *Proc. R. Soc. Lond. Biol.* **84:** 308–319.

3. Brown, T.G. 1914. On the nature of the fundamental activity of the nervous centres; together with an analysis of the conditioning of rhythmic activity in progression, and a theory of evolution of function in the nervous system. *J. Physiol. (London)* **48:** 18–46.

4. Grillner, S. 1981. Control of locomotion in bipeds, tetrapods, and fish. In *Handbook of Physiology, Sect. 1, The Nervous System, Vol. 2, Motor Control.* V.B. Brooks, Ed.: 1179–1236. American Physiological Society. Bethesda, MD.

5. Kahn, J.A. 1982. Patterns of synaptic inhibition in motoneurons and interneurons during fictive swimming in the lamprey, as revealed by Cl injections. *J. Comp. Physiol. A* **147:** 189–194.

6. Dale, N. 1985. Reciprocal inhibitory interneurones in the *Xenopus* embryo spinal cord. *J. Physiol. (London)* **363:** 61–70.

7. Robertson, G.A. & P.S.G. Stein. 1988. Synaptic control of hindlimb motoneurones during three forms of the fictive scratch reflex in the turtle. *J. Physiol. (London)* **404:** 101–128.

8. Raastad, M., B.R. Johnson & O. Kiehn. 1997. Analysis of EPSCs and IPSCs carrying rhythmic, locomotor-related information in the isolated spinal cord of the neonatal rat. *J. Neurophysiol.* **78:** 1851–1859.

9. Stein, P.S.G., S. Grillner, A.I. Selverston, *et al.*, Eds. 1997. *Neurons, Networks, and Motor Behavior.* MIT Press. Cambridge, MA.

10. Li, W.C., S. Higashijima, D.M. Parry, *et al.* 2004. Primi-tive roles for inhibitory interneurons in developing frog spinal cord. *J. Neurosci.* **24:** 5840–5848.

11. Grillner, S. 2006. Biological pattern generation: the cellular and computational logic of networks in motion. *Neuron* **52:** 751–766.

12. Kiehn, O. 2006. Locomotor circuits in the mammalian spinal cord. *Annu. Rev. Neurosci.* **29:** 279–306.

13. Nishimaru, H., C.E. Restrepo & O. Kiehn. 2006. Activity of Renshaw cells during locomotor-like rhythmic activity in the isolated spinal cord of neonatal mice. *J. Neurosci.* **26:** 5320–5328.

14. Endo, T. & O. Kiehn. 2008. Asymmetric operation of the locomotor central pattern generator in the neonatal mouse spinal cord. *J. Neurophysiol.* **100:** 3043–3054.

15. Grillner, S., A. El Manira, O. Kiehn, *et al.*, Eds. 2008. Networks in motion. *Brain Res. Rev.* **57:** 1–270.

16. Kiehn, O., K.A. Quinlan, C.E. Restrepo, *et al.* 2008. Excitatory components of the mammalian locomotor CPG. *Brain Res. Rev.* **57:** 56–63.

17. McCrea, D.A. & I.A. Rybak. 2008. Organization of mammalian locomotor rhythm and pattern generation. *Brain Res. Rev.* **57:** 134–146.

18. Stein, P.S.G. 2008. Motor pattern deletions and modular organization of turtle spinal cord. *Brain Res. Rev.* **57:** 118–124.

19. Gabriel, J.P., R. Mahmood, A. Kyriakatos, *et al.* 2009. Serotonergic modulation of locomotion in zebrafish: endogenous release and synaptic mechanisms. *J. Neurosci.* **29:** 10387–10395.

20. Berg, R.W., A. Alaburda & J. Hounsgaard. 2007. Balanced inhibition and excitation drive spike activity in spinal half-centers. *Science* **315:** 390–393.

21. Buchanan, J.T. & S. Grillner. 1988. A new class of small inhibitory interneurones in the lamprey spinal cord. *Brain Res.* **438:** 404–407.

22. Parkis, M.A., X. Dong, J.L. Feldman, *et al.* 1999. Concurrent inhibition and excitation of phrenic motoneurons during inspiration: phase-specific control of excitability. *J. Neurosci.* **19:** 2368–2380.

23. Chance, F.S., L.F. Abbott & A.D. Reyes. 2002. Gain modulation from background synaptic input. *Neuron* **35:** 773–782.

24. Higashijima, S., M.A. Masino, G. Mandel, *et al.* 2004. Engrailed-1 expression marks a primitive class of inhibitory spinal interneuron. *J. Neurosci.* **24:** 5827–5839.

25. Abbott, L.F. & F.S. Chance. 2005. Drivers and modulators from push-pull and balanced synaptic input. *Prog. Brain Res.* **149:** 147–155.

26. Berg, R.W., S. Ditlevsen & J. Hounsgaard. 2008. Intense synaptic activity enhances temporal resolution in spinal motoneurons. *PLoS One.* **3:** e3218.

27. Berg, R.W. & J. Hounsgaard. 2009. Signaling in large-scale neural networks. *Cogn Process.* **10**(Suppl 1): S9–S15.

28. Sasaki, K., V. Brezina, K.R. Weiss, *et al.* 2009. Distinct inhibitory neurons exert temporally specific control over activity of a motoneuron receiving concurrent excitation and inhibition. *J. Neurosci.* **29:** 11732–11744.

29. Stein, P.S.G. & M.L. Grossman. 1980. Central program for scratch reflex in turtle. *J. Comp. Physiol. A* **140:** 287–294.

30. Bakker, J.G.M. & A. Crowe. 1982. Multicyclic scratch reflex movements in the terrapin *Pseudemys scripta elegans*. *J. Comp. Physiol. A* **145:** 477–484.

31. Stein, P.S.G., G.A. Robertson, J. Keifer, *et al.* 1982. Motor neuron synaptic potentials during fictive scratch reflex in turtle. *J. Comp. Physiol. A* **146:** 401–409.

32. Keifer, J. & P.S.G. Stein. 1983. *In vitro* motor program for the rostral scratch reflex generated by the turtle spinal cord. *Brain Res.* **266:** 148–151.

33. Mortin, L.I., J. Keifer & P.S.G. Stein. 1985. Three forms of the scratch reflex in the spinal turtle: movement analyses. *J. Neurophysiol.* **53:** 1501–1516.

34. Robertson, G.A., L.I. Mortin, J. Keifer, *et al.* 1985. Three forms of the scratch reflex in the spinal turtle: central generation of motor patterns. *J. Neurophysiol.* **53:** 1517–1534.

35. Currie, S.N. & P.S.G. Stein. 1989. Interruptions of fictive scratch motor rhythms by activation of cutaneous flexion reflex afferents in the turtle. *J. Neurosci.* **9:** 488–496.

36. Mortin, L.I. & P.S.G. Stein. 1989. Spinal cord segments containing key elements of the central pattern generators for three forms of scratch reflex in the turtle. *J. Neurosci.* **9:** 2285–2296.

37. Mortin, L.I. & P.S.G. Stein. 1990. Cutaneous dermatomes for the initiation of three forms of the scratch reflex in the spinal turtle. *J. Comp. Neurol.* **295:** 515–529.

38. Berkowitz, A. & P.S.G. Stein. 1994. Activity of descending propriospinal axons in the turtle hindlimb enlargement during two forms of fictive scratching: broad tuning to regions of the body surface. *J. Neurosci.* **14:** 5089–5104.

39. Berkowitz, A. & P.S.G. Stein. 1994. Activity of descending propriospinal axons in the turtle hindlimb enlargement during two forms of fictive scratching: phase analyses. *J. Neurosci.* **14:** 5105–5119.

40. Stein, P.S.G., J.C. Victor, E.C. Field, *et al.* 1995. Bilateral control of hindlimb scratching in the spinal turtle: contralateral spinal circuitry contributes to the normal ipsilateral motor pattern of fictive rostral scratching. *J. Neurosci.* **15:** 4343–4355.

41. Currie, S.N. & S. Lee. 1996. Sensory-evoked pocket scratch motor patterns in the *in vitro* turtle spinal cord: reduction of excitability by an *N*-methyl-ᴅ-aspartate antagonist. *J. Neurophysiol.* **76:** 81–92.

42. Currie, S.N. & G.G. Gonsalves. 1997. Right–left interactions between rostral scratch networks generate rhythmicity in the preenlargement spinal cord of the turtle. *J. Neurophysiol.* **78:** 3479–3483.

43. Currie, S.N. & S. Lee. 1997. Glycinergic inhibition contributes to the generation of rostral scratch motor patterns in the turtle spinal cord. *J. Neurosci.* **17:** 3322–3333.

44. Field, E.C. & P.S.G. Stein. 1997. Spinal cord coordination of hindlimb movements in the turtle: intralimb temporal relationships during scratching and swimming. *J. Neurophysiol.* **78:** 1394–1403.

45. Field, E.C. & P.S.G. Stein. 1997. Spinal cord coordination of hindlimb movements in the turtle: interlimb temporal relationships during bilateral scratching and swimming. *J. Neurophysiol.* **78:** 1404–1413.

46. Stein, P.S.G. & J.L. Smith. 1997. Neural and biomechanical control strategies for different forms of vertebrate hindlimb motor tasks. In *Neurons, Networks, and Motor Behavior*. P.S.G. Stein, S. Grillner, A.I. Selverston, *et al.* Eds.: 61–73. MIT Press. Cambridge, MA.

47. Stein, P.S.G., M.L. McCullough & S.N. Currie. 1998. Reconstruction of flexor/extensor alternation during fictive rostral scratching by two-site stimulation in the spinal turtle with a transverse spinal hemisection. *J. Neurosci.* **18:** 467–479.

48. Stein, P.S.G., M.L. McCullough & S.N. Currie. 1998. Spinal motor patterns in the turtle. *Ann. N.Y. Acad. Sci.* **860:** 142–154.

49. Currie, S.N. 1999. Fictive hindlimb motor patterns evoked by AMPA and NMDA in turtle spinal cord-hindlimb nerve preparations. *J. Physiol. (Paris)* **93:** 199–211.

50. Currie, S.N. & G.G. Gonsalves. 1999. Reciprocal interactions in the turtle hindlimb enlargement contribute to scratch rhythmogenesis. *J. Neurophysiol.* **81:** 2977–2987.

51. Earhart, G.M. & P.S.G. Stein. 2000. Scratch-swim hybrids in the spinal turtle: blending of rostral scratch and forward swim. *J. Neurophysiol.* **83:** 156–165.

52. Earhart, G.M. & P.S.G. Stein. 2000. Step, swim, and scratch motor patterns in the turtle. *J. Neurophysiol.* **84:** 2181–2190.

53. Juranek, J. & S.N. Currie. 2000. Electrically evoked fictive swimming in the low-spinal immobilized turtle. *J. Neurophysiol.* **83:** 146–155.

54. Stein, P.S.G. & S. Daniels-McQueen. 2002. Modular organization of turtle spinal interneurons during normal and deletion fictive rostral scratching. *J. Neurosci.* **22:** 6800–6809.

55. Alaburda, A. & J. Hounsgaard. 2003. Metabotropic modulation of motoneurons by scratch-like spinal network activity. *J. Neurosci.* **23:** 8625–8629.

56. Stein, P.S.G. & S. Daniels-McQueen. 2003. Timing of knee-related spinal neurons during fictive rostral scratching in the turtle. *J. Neurophysiol.* **90:** 3585–3593.

57. Stein, P.S.G. & S. Daniels-McQueen. 2004. Variations in motor patterns during fictive rostral scratching in the turtle: knee-related deletions. *J. Neurophysiol.* **91:** 2380–2384.

58. Alaburda, A., R. Russo, N. MacAulay, *et al.* 2005. Periodic high-conductance states in spinal neurons during scratch-like network activity in adult turtles. *J. Neurosci.* **25:** 6316–6321.

59. Berkowitz, A. 2005. Physiology and morphology indicate that individual spinal interneurons contribute to diverse limb movements. *J. Neurophysiol.* **94:** 4455–4470.

60. Stein, P.S.G. 2005. Neuronal control of turtle hindlimb motor rhythms. *J. Comp. Physiol. A Neuroethol. Sens. Neural. Behav. Physiol.* **191:** 213–229.

61. Berkowitz, A., G.L. Yosten & R.M. Ballard. 2006. Somatodendritic morphology predicts physiology for neurons that contribute to several kinds of limb movements. *J. Neurophysiol.* **95:** 2821–2831.

62. Berkowitz, A. 2007. Spinal interneurons that are selectively activated during fictive flexion reflex. *J. Neurosci.* **27:** 4634–4641.

63. Samara, R.F. & S.N. Currie. 2007. Crossed commissural pathways in the spinal hindlimb enlargement are not necessary for right left hindlimb alternation during turtle swimming. *J. Neurophysiol.* **98:** 2223–2231.

64. Berkowitz, A. 2008. Physiology and morphology of shared and specialized spinal interneurons for locomotion and scratching. *J. Neurophysiol.* **99:** 2887–2901.

65. Samara, R.F. & S.N. Currie. 2008. Electrically evoked locomotor activity in the turtle spinal cord hemi-enlargement preparation. *Neurosci. Lett.* **441:** 105–109.

66. Stein, P.S.G. 2009. Modules for rostral scratch pattern generation in the turtle spinal cord. In *Proceedings of the Conference on Cellular and Network Functions in the Spinal Cord.* p. 4. Madison, WI.

67. Marder, E. & R.L. Calabrese. 1996. Principles of rhythmic motor pattern generation. *Physiol. Rev.* **76:** 687–717.

68. Stuart, D.G. 1999. The segmental motor system—advances, issues, and possibilities. *Prog. Brain Res.* **123:** 3–28.

69. Borg-Graham, L.J., C. Monier & Y. Fregnac. 1998. Visual input evokes transient and strong shunting inhibition in visual cortical neurons. *Nature* **393:** 369–373.

70. Ruigrok, T.J.H. & A. Crowe. 1984. The organization of motoneurons in the turtle lumbar spinal cord. *J. Comp. Neurol.* **228:** 24–37.

Ann. N.Y. Acad. Sci. ISSN 0077-8923

Multifunctional and specialized spinal interneurons for turtle limb movements

Ari Berkowitz

Department of Zoology, University of Oklahoma, Norman, Oklahoma

Address for correspondence: Ari Berkowitz, Department of Zoology, University of Oklahoma, 730 Van Vleet Oval, Norman, OK 73019. Voice: 405-325-3492; fax: 405-325-6202. ari@ou.edu

The turtle spinal cord can help reveal how vertebrate central nervous system (CNS) circuits select and generate an appropriate limb movement in each circumstance. Both multifunctional and specialized spinal interneurons contribute to the motor patterns for the three forms of scratching, forward swimming, and flexion reflex. Multifunctional interneurons, activated during all of these motor patterns, can have axon terminal arborizations in the ventral horn, where they likely contribute to limb motor output. Specialized interneurons can be specialized for a behavior, as opposed to a phase or motor synergy. Interneurons specialized for scratching can be hyperpolarized throughout swimming. Interneurons specialized for flexion reflex can be hyperpolarized throughout scratching and swimming. Some structure–function correlations have been revealed: flexion reflex-selective interneurons had somata exclusively in the dorsal horn, in contrast to scratch-activated interneurons. Transverse interneurons, defined by quantitative morphological criteria, had higher peak firing rates, narrower action potentials, briefer afterhyperpolarizations, and larger membrane potential oscillations than scratch-activated interneurons with different dendritic morphologies. Future investigations will focus on how multifunctional and specialized spinal interneurons interact to generate each motor output.

Keywords: locomotion; scratching; swimming; flexion reflex; dedicated; central pattern generator

Introduction

How does the central nervous system (CNS) select and generate an appropriate behavior for each circumstance an animal faces? This question has received increasing experimental attention in diverse contexts. Foci have included how the primate forebrain mediates perceptual decision making,[1,2] how diverse animals make behavioral choices,[2,3] and how CNS networks generate multiple rhythmic motor patterns.[4–6]

Understanding mechanisms underlying behavioral choice or motor pattern selection ultimately requires cellular analysis. Thus, there are advantages to studying smaller and more accessible nervous systems or components to test circuit-level hypotheses.[5,7–9] One simple hypothesis is that a separate set of dedicated CNS neurons produces each type of movement. An opposing hypothesis is that a single set of multifunctional CNS neurons produces all movements of a given body part.

There is experimental support for both dedicated and multifunctional circuits, especially from invertebrates. Pioneering work in crayfish and mollusks revealed inhibition between specialized neurons or circuits for competing behaviors.[3,10] Also, separate groups of specialized interneurons are rhythmically activated during walking and flying in locusts[11] and during stridulation and flying in crickets.[12] However, different forms of rhythmic crustacean digestive movements are generated largely by multifunctional neurons that are reconfigured by neuromodulators.[5,6,13–15] Distinct rhythmic behaviors of leeches are produced by a combination of multifunctional and specialized neurons.[8,16]

Studies of vertebrate brainstem and spinal cord have also addressed these issues. For example, multifunctional brainstem interneurons are rhythmically activated during different forms of mammalian

doi: 10.1111/j.1749-6632.2009.05428.x

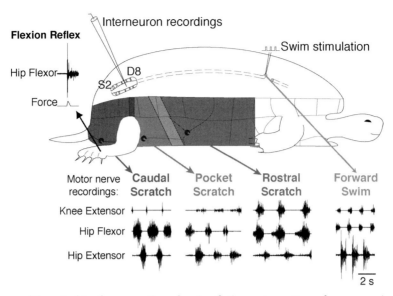

Figure 1. Diagram of the spinal turtle preparation, showing fictive motor patterns from one animal. Scratching is evoked by mechanical stimulation of the body surface; color-coded regions indicate the three scratch form receptive fields and transition zones between forms. Flexion reflex (limb withdrawal) is evoked by a tap to the dorsal foot. Forward swimming is evoked by electrical stimulation in the contralateral dorsal funiculus rostrally. Interneurons are recorded in the hindlimb enlargement segments, dorsal (D) 8–10 and sacral (S) 1–2.

respiration and oromotor movements.[17–24] Different forms of axial locomotion in larval fish and tadpoles are produced by a combination of multifunctional and specialized neurons.[25–30]

We have focused on spinal cord interneurons activated during limb motor patterns in the adult turtle spinal cord *in vivo*. We can thus investigate at a cellular level how an adult CNS mediates selection and generation of distinct naturalistic motor patterns for a multi-jointed limb. The adult turtle spinal cord, without input from the brain and movement-related sensory feedback, can appropriately generate the hindlimb motor patterns for forward swimming, three forms of scratching, and withdrawal or flexion reflex[31] (Fig. 1).

In vivo studies of limb movements are more feasible in adult turtles than in adult mammals, partly because turtles (being diving animals) resist hypoxia much better than mammals.[32] Also, groundwork has been laid for these studies by detailed descriptions of muscle and nerve activity patterns underlying several behaviors.[33–37] Findings from turtle spinal cord likely have counterparts in mammals because spinal cord mechanisms are largely conserved.[38–40] Moreover, spinal interneurons are involved not only in rhythmic limb movements and

reflexive movements, but also in voluntary movements.[41] In this review, I will highlight recent evidence that a combination of multifunctional and specialized turtle spinal interneurons contributes to scratching, swimming, and flexion reflex.

Results and discussion

Spinal interneurons and the three forms of scratching

Mechanical stimulation of a site on a spinalized turtle's body surface evokes scratching, in which the ipsilateral hindlimb rubs repeatedly and rhythmically against the site.[34] Three forms of scratching—rostral, pocket, and caudal—are used to reach three regions of the body surface (Fig. 1). Sites within narrow transition zones can elicit either of two scratch forms or a blend of the two. The three forms differ in the part of the limb that rubs against the body and the relative timing of knee and hip movements. Fictive scratching motor patterns in immobilized animals are very similar to muscle motor patterns in moving animals.[35]

In principle, each form of scratching could be produced by a separate group of dedicated spinal interneurons. Such neurons would be activated whenever one form of scratching occurs and not at all during the other two. We searched for such interneurons using extracellular single-neuron and intracellular recordings.[42–44] Out of approximately 200 scratch-activated interneurons studied, only two had excitatory receptive fields similar to a scratch form receptive field (both for caudal scratching).[43] This was true using white matter recordings of descending axons[42] as well as gray matter somatic recordings,[43] so it is unlikely to be due to the recording method. Thus, spinal interneurons dedicated to one form of scratching appear to be rare.

Instead, most scratch-activated spinal interneurons were activated during all three forms. Their firing rates during scratching typically varied systematically according to the site stimulated, with a peak at one rostrocaudal region (Fig. 2).[42,43] In other words, each neuron was coarsely or broadly tuned to a region of the body surface. Different interneurons in the same animal were broadly tuned to different regions. This suggests the hypothesis that scratch form selection is mediated by a large population of multifunctional and broadly tuned neurons (rather than dedicated neurons), as has been shown in several other systems.[45,46]

Most scratch-activated interneurons were also rhythmically modulated with scratching[44,47–49] (Figs. 3A and B). Thus, some interneurons may contribute to both selection and generation of a scratch form. The degree of rhythmic modulation a neuron displayed for different sites was often negatively correlated with its mean firing rate.[47] This suggests that rhythmic inhibition plays an important role in sculpting scratch motor patterns. Firing tends to occur in a particular phase of the hip flexor activity cycle for each interneuron, regardless of which form of scratching is produced (e.g., Fig. 3A), although a small number do shift phase depending on the site stimulated.[44,47,48]

Scratch-activated interneurons were often multifunctional in additional ways. Many were activated during ipsilateral fictive flexion reflex[44] (Fig. 3A). Moreover, many were rhythmically activated during fictive scratching of either hindlimb[42–44,47,48] (Fig. 3B). This surprising finding suggested that contralateral interneurons contribute to ipsilateral scratching. This suggestion was strongly supported by studies in which the hindlimb enlargement spinal cord was ablated on one side.[50] This lesion eliminated the hip extensor phase of rostral scratching on the intact side, even though the hip flexor rhythm remained.

Of course, a temporal correlation between an interneuron's activity and motor output cannot demonstrate a causal role for the interneuron. An alternative hypothesis is that these interneurons send corollary discharge signals to the brain but have no direct effect on motor output. This is unlikely for many interneurons studied, however, for two reasons. First, such interneurons recorded via their spinal descending axons[47] almost certainly terminate within the spinal cord. Second, intracellular recordings and dye injections of such interneurons revealed axon terminal arborizations in the ventral horn of the hindlimb enlargement (e.g., Fig. 3C), suggesting that they affect hindlimb motor output relatively directly.[44]

Spinal interneurons during scratching and swimming

Given that scratch-activated interneurons are often multifunctional, do they also contribute to swimming? Hindlimb swimming movements[33] and fictive motor patterns[37] can be evoked in a spinalized turtle by electrical stimulation of descending axons in the contralateral lateral funiculus (Fig. 1). We recorded from spinal interneurons extracellularly and intracellularly during fictive scratching and fictive forward swimming.

Most scratch-activated interneurons were also activated during swimming; they often showed a similar degree of rhythmic modulation and a similar phase preference within the hip cycle (Fig. 4).[51,52] The phases of their membrane potential oscillation troughs were significantly correlated between scratching and swimming, although the phases of their oscillation peaks were not, which again suggests the importance of rhythmic inhibition in sculpting scratching and swimming motor patterns.[52] Another subset of cells was rhythmically activated during scratching but tonically activated during swimming.[51]

Surprisingly, though, a subset of rhythmic, scratch-activated interneurons was not activated during swimming.[51,52] Some had their activity suppressed during swimming.[51] These scratch-specialized interneurons could receive hyperpolarizing inhibition during swimming[52] (Fig. 5). This hyperpolarization could outlast by several seconds

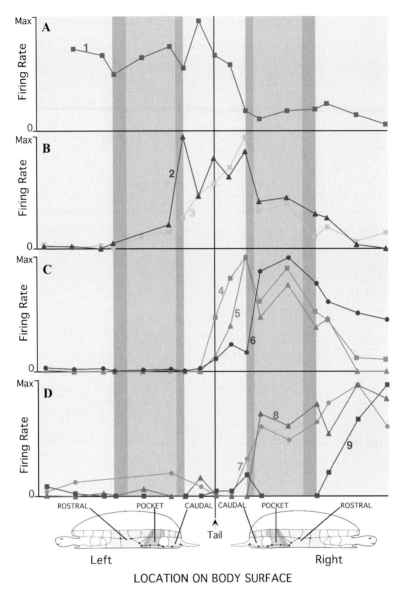

Figure 2. Scratch-activated spinal interneurons are often broadly tuned to a region of the body surface. Tuning curves are shown for nine interneurons recorded on the right side of one animal (A–D). (From *J. Neurophysiol.* 86: 1017–1025, 2001; used with permission of the American Physiological Society.)

the electrical stimulation that evoked swimming, indicating that the inhibition was closely associated with the swimming motor pattern itself, not simply with the electrical stimulation used to evoke it.

One might hypothesize that specialized, rhythmic interneurons would be specialized for a particular motor synergy. This appears not to be the case, however, at least for scratch-activated interneurons.

Forward swimming and rostral scratching share a knee-hip synergy in which the monoarticular knee extensor bursts during the latter portion of each hip flexor burst;[37,53–55] the knee-hip synergies for pocket scratching and caudal scratching differ.[53–55] Nonetheless, rhythmic, scratch-activated interneurons tend to be activated during all three forms of scratching (which have different knee-hip synergies), while scratch-specialized interneurons are

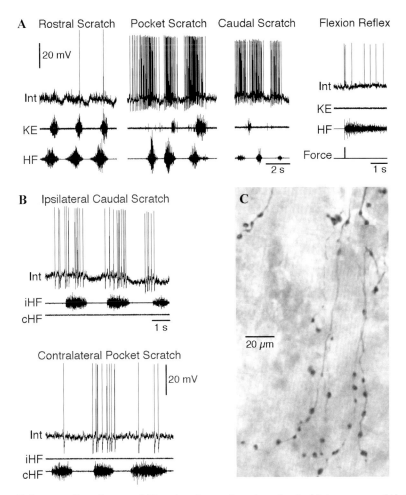

Figure 3. Intracellular recordings from multifunctional scratch-activated spinal interneurons. (A) An interneuron that was rhythmically activated during all forms of ipsilateral fictive scratching, plus fictive flexion reflex. (B) An interneuron that was rhythmically activated during ipsilateral and contralateral fictive scratching. (C) Ventral horn axon terminal arborizations for the interneuron shown in B. Int, interneuron; KE, knee extensor; HF, hip flexor; i, ipsilateral; c, contralateral. (B-C from *J. Neurophysiol.* 94: 4455–4470, 2005; used with permission of the American Physiological Society.)

activated during rostral scratching but not forward swimming (which share a knee-hip synergy).[51] Thus, scratch-specialized interneurons are specialized for a particular behavior, not for a particular synergy.

The existence of multifunctional, scratch/swim interneurons is consistent with the hypothesis that a single central pattern generator (CPG) produces scratching and locomotion, as first proposed in a pioneering study of the cat spinal cord.[56] The existence of scratch-specialized interneurons, however, suggests additional complexity. Scratching and

swimming may be produced by a combination of multifunctional and specialized interneurons, as has been shown for feeding, withdrawal, and swimming in *Pleurobranchea*,[57] for crawling and swimming in leeches,[8,16] for feeding behaviors in *Aplysia*,[58] and for different forms of axial locomotion in larval zebrafish and tadpoles.[25–28,30,59] In at least some of these cases, it may be that distinct, rhythmic behaviors evolved at different times, and that the later-evolving behavior utilized some, but not all, of the existing CPG components.[8,16,51] This could give rise to an asymmetric

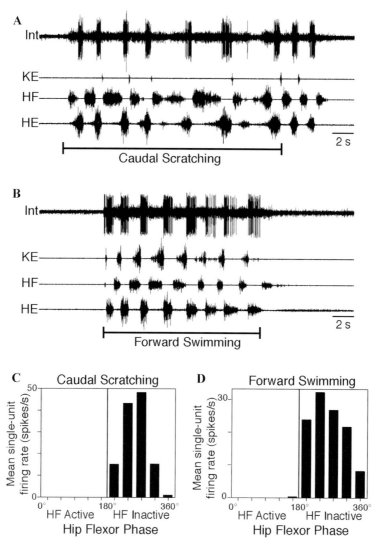

Figure 4. Example of a multifunctional scratch/swim spinal interneuron. Activity of the interneuron during (**A**) caudal scratching and (**B**) forward swimming. (**C, D**) Dual-referent phase histograms of the interneuron's firing rate during each motor pattern. Note that the neuron fired rhythmically in the same phase of the hip flexor activity cycle during scratching and swimming. (With kind permission from Springer Science + Business Media: *J. Comp. Physiol. A*, "Both shared and specialized spinal circuitry for scratching and swimming in turtles," Vol. 188, 2002, pp. 225–234, Ari Berkowitz, Figure 1.)

CPG organization, in which one behavior relies on a larger fraction of specialized neurons than the other behavior.

Correlations between morphology and physiology of interneurons

Are there structure–function correlations among scratch-activated interneurons? Using intracellular interneuron recording and Neurobiotin injection, we identified a morphological grouping of spinal interneurons that were strongly activated during limb motor patterns.[49] These transverse interneurons, or T neurons, had dendrites that were extensive in the transverse plane, but short rostrocaudally; they also tended to have mediolaterally elongated somata (Figs. 6 and 7A). T neurons were strongly activated during all forms of fictive scratching, forward swimming, and usually ipsilateral flexion

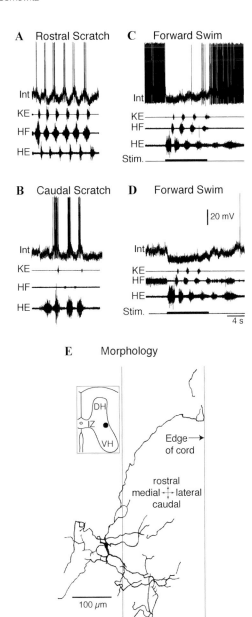

A Rostral Scratch

C Forward Swim

B Caudal Scratch

D Forward Swim

20 mV

4 s

E   Morphology

DH
IZ
VH

Edge
of cord

rostral
medial → ← lateral
caudal

100 μm

VH   LF

Figure 5. Example of a scratch-specialized spinal interneuron recorded intracellularly. Activity of the neuron during (**A**) rostral scratching, (**B**) caudal scratching, and (**C, D**) forward swimming. Note that the interneuron received hyperpolarizing inhibition during swimming. Int, interneuron; HE, hip extensor, Stim., stimulus. (**E**) Reconstruction of this neuron's morphology from horizontal sections; *inset* indicates soma location in cross section. DH, dorsal horn; IZ, intermediate zone; VH, ventral horn; LF, lateral funiculus. (From *J. Neurophysiol.* 99: 2887–2901, 2008; used with permission of the American Physiological Society.)

reflex.[49,52] T neurons are thus multifunctional and are a subset of scratch/swim neurons.

T neurons differed physiologically in several respects from scratch-activated interneurons with different dendritic morphologies ("non-T neurons").[49] T neurons on average displayed significantly higher peak firing rates during scratching than non-T neurons (Fig. 7B). We explored possible mechanisms for these higher firing rates using measurements of averaged action potentials (APs) (Figs. 7C–E) and of scratch phase-averaged membrane potential oscillations (with action potentials deleted; Fig. 7F). T neurons on average had significantly narrower APs (Fig. 7D) with briefer afterhyperpolarizations (AHPs) (Fig. 7E) than non-T neurons. T neurons also had significantly larger scratch membrane potential oscillations (Fig. 7F).

The strong and rhythmic activity of T neurons during scratching makes them good candidates to be pattern-generating neurons and/or last-order premotor interneurons. In favorable cases, we could follow T neuron axons to axon terminal arborizations, which could be found in the ventral horn of the hindlimb enlargement (Fig. 6D), consistent with their having relatively direct effects on limb motoneurons.[49]

Flexion reflex-selective interneurons

In addition to scratch-specialized neurons, we found a group of spinal interneurons specialized for flexion reflex.[60] These interneurons were strongly activated during a mechanically evoked fictive flexion reflex (Fig. 8A). Electrical stimulation of the dorsal foot skin evoked interneuron firing within 20 ms (fast for a turtle!), earlier than the onset of the hip flexor burst (Fig. 8B). One might hypothesize that such interneurons would also be activated during the hip flexor bursts of scratching and swimming. However, these interneurons were not activated during scratching or swimming. In fact, most received hyperpolarizing inhibition during scratching (Fig. 8C) and swimming (Fig. 8D). The hyperpolarization typically included a rhythmic component. The maximal hyperpolarization (i.e., the trough of the membrane potential) could occur during the hip flexor bursts (Fig. 8E). Thus, flexion reflex-selective interneurons (like scratch-specialized interneurons) are apparently specialized for a particular behavior, not a particular muscle or hip phase.

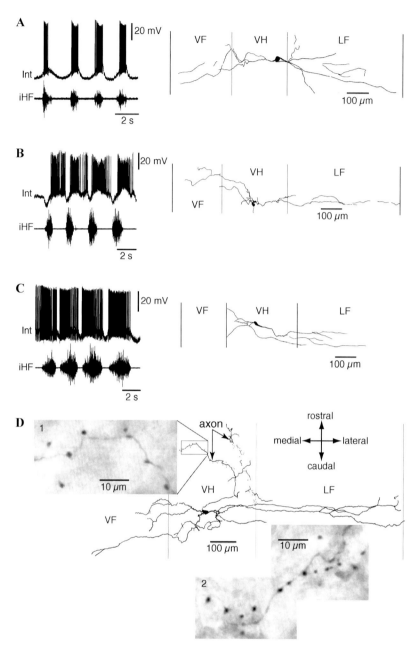

Figure 6. Examples of transverse interneurons (T neurons). (A–C) Three T neurons: *left*, activity during (A, B) caudal scratching and (C) rostral scratching; *right*, morphological reconstructions. (D) Morphological reconstruction of another T neuron (caudal axon truncated); *insets* show example ventral horn axon terminal arborizations (1) rostral and (2) caudal to the soma. VF, ventral funiculus. (B, C (right), and D from *J. Neurophysiol.* 95: 2821–2831, 2006; used with permission of the American Physiological Society.)

Flexion reflex-selective interneurons had somata in the dorsal horn, unlike most T neurons and other scratch-activated interneurons[60] (Fig. 8F). Thus, to some extent, there is anatomical segre-gation of this functional group of interneurons. Flexion reflex-selective interneurons also displayed a variety of somato-dendritic morphologies, which could include complex higher-order branching and

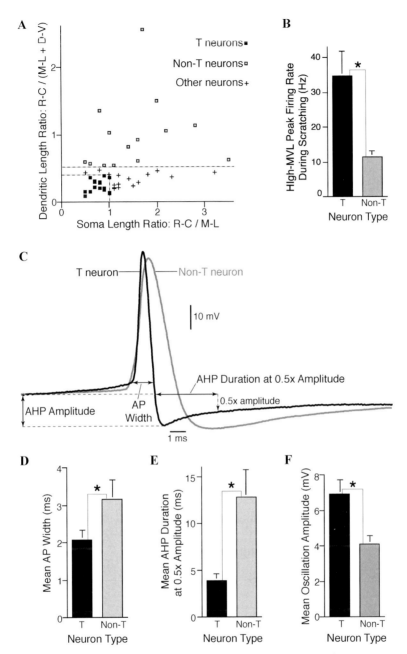

Figure 7. Physiological differences between T neurons and other scratch-activated interneurons. (A) T neurons were defined by quantitative somato-dendritic features. (B) T neurons fired at significantly higher peak rates during scratching than scratch-activated interneurons with different dendritic morphologies ("non-T neurons"). (C) Illustration of AP parameters measured from the averaged AP of each interneuron, with example T neuron and non-T neurons shown. (D–F) Significant differences between T neurons and non-T neurons in (D) mean AP width, (E) mean AHP duration, and (F) scratch phase-normalized membrane potential oscillation amplitude. (From *J. Neurophysiol.* 95: 2821–2831, 2006; used with permission of the American Physiological Society.)

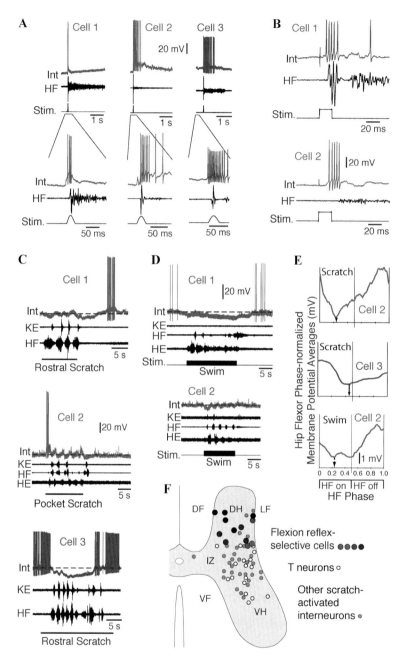

Figure 8. Examples of flexion reflex-selective interneurons. (**A**) Responses of three flexion reflex-selective interneurons to a dorsal foot tap; records below expand initial portions of records above. Note that each interneuron responded quickly and strongly, beginning before the hip flexor burst. (**B**) Responses of two of these cells to a dorsal foot skin electrical pulse. Note that the interneurons began firing within 20 ms, before the hip flexor burst. (**C, D**) Responses of the same interneurons during (**C**) scratching and (**D**) swimming. Note that these cells were hyperpolarized during scratching and swimming. (**E**) Phase-averaged membrane potentials for two of these cells. Note that maximal hyperpolarization could occur during the hip flexor burst of scratching and swimming even though these cells were activated during the hip flexor burst of flexion reflex. (**F**) Soma locations of all flexion reflex-selective interneurons recorded were in the dorsal horn, in contrast to T neurons. DF, dorsal funiculus. (From *J. Neurosci.* 27:4634–4641, 2007; used with permission of the Society for Neuroscience.)

rostrocaudally oriented dendrites, in contrast to T neurons.[60]

Conclusions

A combination of multifunctional and specialized spinal interneurons appears to mediate selection and generation of limbed locomotion, scratching, and withdrawal in turtles. Future research will aim to decipher how each type of interneuron contributes to motor pattern selection and generation. One possibility is that multifunctional neurons are components of a rhythm- and/or pattern-generator, while specialized neurons are sensory interneurons that differentially trigger or modify the operation of a shared CPG. This would be consistent with the relatively dorsal location of flexion reflex-specialized and scratch-specialized neurons studied to date. This would also be consistent with recent findings that distinct classes of spinal interneurons provide the excitatory drive to the CPG during swimming and struggling in hatchling tadpoles.[27] Alternatively, some specialized neurons may be unshared CPG components. To distinguish these possibilities, it will be important to obtain physiological and/or morphological evidence of the postsynaptic targets of multifunctional and specialized interneurons. In particular, which, if any, of these types of interneurons are last-order premotor neurons? T neurons are multifunctional neurons that are good candidates to be premotor neurons, based on their large membrane potential oscillations and high peak firing rates.[49,52] It will also be important to determine whether each type of multifunctional and specialized interneuron is excitatory or inhibitory. Pharmacological and/or immunocytochemical approaches should allow us to address this issue.

Until recently, the idea that the vertebrate spinal cord and medulla use largely shared CPGs to generate distinct rhythmic motor patterns in common sets of muscles has been emphasized.[17–23,37,47,48,54,56,61–73] For example, it was hypothesized that cat locomotion and scratching use the same CPG[56] and that swimming and struggling in tadpoles use the same interneuron types (though more cells are recruited from each type during struggling).[68–70] However, during the past decade, new studies of larval zebrafish spinal cord,[25,26,29,30] hatchling tadpole spinal cord,[27] adult turtle spinal cord,[51,52,60] and cat medulla[24] have all identified behaviorally specialized interneurons, potentially including CPG components, that may play important roles selectively in one or another of these rhythmic motor patterns. These new findings necessitate a more complex and nuanced view of how distinct rhythmic movements of shared muscles are generated in vertebrates, involving combinations of multifunctional and specialized neurons.

The earlier emphasis on shared CPGs in vertebrates may have been strongly influenced by data from several intensively studied invertebrate systems, especially the crustacean stomatogastric nervous system (STNS), in which (unlike vertebrate CPGs) it is possible to obtain a complete circuit diagram of the CPG for each motor pattern. In the STNS, a variety of neuromodulators can reconfigure a single, or largely shared CPG, to produce distinct outputs for each situation.[5,6,13–15] There are reasons to think, however, that additional mechanisms of motor pattern selection may operate in the spinal cord. First, fast (electrical and chemical) synaptic inputs from distinct projection neurons contribute to behavior-specific circuit reconfiguration (in addition to neuromodulation), even in the STNS.[8] Thus, there are behaviorally specialized neurons associated with the STNS, even if they are not CPG components. Second, there are entirely separate CPGs for the control of shared muscles for some invertebrate behaviors, such as locust flight and walking[11] and cricket flight and stridulation.[12] Third, there is now evidence that combinations of multifunctional and specialized neurons select and generate behaviors for feeding, withdrawal, and swimming in *Pleurobranchea*,[57] for crawling and swimming in leeches,[8,16] and for feeding behaviors in *Aplysia*,[58] in addition to the vertebrate examples mentioned above. Fourth, reconfiguration via neuromodulators may occur too slowly to be the exclusive mechanism of motor pattern selection for behaviors that must be initiated quickly, such as those commonly used to escape from predators. In such cases, recruitment of specialized interneurons, perhaps in addition to differential secretion of neuromodulators, may allow the necessary behavior to be initiated in time to escape predation.

Conflicts of interest

The author declares no conflicts of interest.

References

1. Rushworth, M.F. & T.E. Behrens. 2008. Choice, uncertainty, and value in prefrontal and cingulate cortex. *Nat. Neurosci.* **11:** 389–397.

2. Kristan, W.B. 2008. Neuronal decision-making circuits. *Curr. Biol.* **18:** R928–R932.

3. Kupfermann, I. & K.R. Weiss. 2001. Motor program selection in simple model systems. *Curr. Opin. Neurobiol.* **11:** 673–677.

4. Marder, E. & R.L. Calabrese. 1996. Principles of rhythmic motor pattern generation. *Physiol. Rev.* **76:** 687–717.

5. Marder, E. *et al.* 2005. Invertebrate central pattern generation moves along. *Curr. Biol.* **15:** R685–R699.

6. Dickinson, P.S. 2006. Neuromodulation of central pattern generators in invertebrates and vertebrates. *Curr. Opin. Neurobiol.* **16:** 604–614.

7. Morton, D.W. & H.J. Chiel. 1994. Neural architectures for adaptive behavior. *Trends Neurosci.* **17:** 413–420.

8. Briggman, K.L. & W.B. Kristan. 2008. Multifunctional pattern-generating circuits. *Annu. Rev. Neurosci.* **31:** 271–294.

9. Kristan, W.B., Jr. & B.K. Shaw. 1997. Population coding and behavioral choice. *Curr. Opin. Neurobiol.* **7:** 826–831.

10. Edwards, D.H., W.J. Heitler & F.B. Krasne. 1999. Fifty years of a command neuron: the neurobiology of escape behavior in the crayfish. *Trends Neurosci.* **22:** 153–161.

11. Ramirez, J.M. & K.G. Pearson. 1988. Generation of motor patterns for walking and flight in motoneurons supplying bifunctional muscles in the locust. *J. Neurobiol.* **19:** 257–282.

12. Hennig, R.M. 1990. Neuronal control of the forewings in two different behaviours: stridulation and flight in the cricket, *Teleogryllus commodus*. *J. Comp. Physiol. A* **167:** 617–627.

13. Marder, E. & D. Bucher. 2001. Central pattern generators and the control of rhythmic movements. *Curr. Biol.* **11:** R986–R996.

14. Harris-Warrick, R.M. *et al.* 1992. *Dynamic Biological Networks: The Stomatogastric Nervous System*. The MIT Press. Cambridge, MA.

15. Stein, W. 2009. Modulation of stomatogastric rhythms. *J. Comp. Physiol. A Neuroethol Sens Neural Behav. Physiol.* **95:** 989–1009.

16. Briggman, K.L. & W.B. Kristan, Jr. 2006. Imaging dedicated and multifunctional neural circuits generating distinct behaviors. *J. Neurosci.* **26:** 10925–10933.

17. Grelot, L. *et al.* 1993. Respiratory interneurons of the lower cervical (C4-C5) cord: membrane potential changes during fictive coughing, vomiting, and swallowing in the decerebrate cat. *Pflugers Arch.* **425:** 313–320.

18. Oku, Y., I. Tanaka & K. Ezure. 1994. Activity of bulbar respiratory neurons during fictive coughing and swallowing in the decerebrate cat. *J. Physiol. (Lond.)* **480:** 309–324.

19. Gestreau, C. *et al.* 1996. Activity of dorsal respiratory group inspiratory neurons during laryngeal-induced fictive coughing and swallowing in decerebrate cats. *Exp. Brain Res.* **108:** 247–256.

20. Gestreau, C., L. Grelot & A.L. Bianchi. 2000. Activity of respiratory laryngeal motoneurons during fictive coughing and swallowing. *Exp. Brain Res.* **130:** 27–34.

21. Lieske, S.P. *et al.* 2000. Reconfiguration of the neural network controlling multiple breathing patterns: eupnea, sighs and gasps. *Nat. Neurosci.* **3:** 600–607.

22. Baekey, D.M. *et al.* 2001. Medullary respiratory neurones and control of laryngeal motoneurones during fictive eupnoea and cough in the cat. *J. Physiol. (Lond.)* **534:** 565–581.

23. Gestreau, C. *et al.* 2005. Activation of XII motoneurons and premotor neurons during various oropharyngeal behaviors. *Resp. Physiol. Neurobiol.* **147:** 159–176.

24. Shiba, K. *et al.* 2007. Multifunctional laryngeal premotor neurons: their activities during breathing, coughing, sneezing, and swallowing. *J. Neurosci.* **27:** 5156–5162.

25. Ritter, D.A., D.H. Bhatt & J.R. Fetcho. 2001. In vivo imaging of zebrafish reveals differences in the spinal networks for escape and swimming movements. *J. Neurosci.* **21:** 8956–8965.

26. Kimura, Y., Y. Okamura & S. Higashijima. 2006. alx, a zebrafish homolog of Chx10, marks ipsilateral descending excitatory interneurons that participate in the regulation of spinal locomotor circuits. *J. Neurosci.* **26:** 5684–5697.

27. Li, W.-C. *et al.* 2007. Reconfiguration of a vertebrate motor network: specific neuron recruitment and context-dependent synaptic plasticity. *J. Neurosci.* **27:** 12267–12276.

28. Liao, J.C. & J.R. Fetcho. 2008. Shared versus specialized glycinergic spinal interneurons in axial motor circuits of larval zebrafish. *J. Neurosci.* **28:** 12982–12992.

29. McLean, D.L. *et al.* 2008. Continuous shifts in the active set of spinal interneurons during changes in locomotor speed. *Nat. Neurosci.* **11:** 1419–1429.

30. Satou, C. *et al.* 2009. Functional role of a specialized class of spinal commissural inhibitory neurons during fast escapes in zebrafish. *J. Neurosci.* **29:** 6780–6793.

31. Stein, P.S.G. 2005. Neuronal control of turtle hindlimb motor rhythms. *J. Comp. Physiol. A* **191:** 213–229.

32. Lutz, P.L. & S.L. Milton. 2004. Negotiating brain anoxia survival in the turtle. *J. Exp. Biol.* **207:** 3141 3147.

33. Lennard, P.R. & P.S. Stein. 1977. Swimming movements elicited by electrical stimulation of turtle spinal cord. I. Low-spinal and intact preparations. *J. Neurophysiol.* **40:** 768–778.

34. Mortin, L.I., J. Keifer & P.S.G. Stein. 1985. Three forms of the scratch reflex in the spinal turtle: movement analyses. *J. Neurophysiol.* **53:** 1501–1516.

35. Robertson, G.A. *et al.* 1985. Three forms of the scratch reflex in the spinal turtle: central generation of motor patterns. *J. Neurophysiol.* **53:** 1517–1534.

36. Stein, P.S.G. *et al.* 1982. Motor neuron synaptic potentials during fictive scratch reflex in turtle. *J. Comp. Physiol.* **146:** 401–409.

37. Juranek, J. & S.N. Currie. 2000. Electrically evoked fictive swimming in the low-spinal immobilized turtle. *J. Neurophysiol.* **83:** 146–155.

38. Fetcho, J.R. 1992. The spinal motor system in early vertebrates and some of its evolutionary changes. *Brain Behav. Evol.* **40:** 82–97.

39. Kusuma, A., H.J. ten Donkelaar & R. Nieuwenhuys. 1979. Intrinsic organization of the spinal cord. In *Biology of the Reptilia,* Vol. 10. C. Gans, R.G. Northcutt & P. Ulinski, Eds.: 59–109. Academic Press. New York.

40. Nieuwenhuys, R. 1964. Comparative anatomy of the spinal cord. *Prog. Brain Res.* **11:** 1–55.

41. Prut, Y., S.I. Perlmutter & E.E. Fetz. 2001. Distributed processing in the motor system: spinal cord perspective. *Prog. Brain Res.* **130:** 267–278.

42. Berkowitz, A. & P.S. Stein. 1994. Activity of descending propriospinal axons in the turtle hindlimb enlargement during two forms of fictive scratching: broad tuning to regions of the body surface. *J. Neurosci.* **14:** 5089–5104.

43. Berkowitz, A. 2001. Broadly tuned spinal neurons for each form of fictive scratching in spinal turtles. *J. Neurophysiol.* **86:** 1017–1025.

44. Berkowitz, A. 2005. Physiology and morphology indicate that individual spinal interneurons contribute to diverse limb movements. *J. Neurophysiol.* **94:** 4455–4470.

45. Lee, C., W.H. Rohrer & D.L. Sparks. 1988. Population coding of saccadic eye movements by neurons in the superior colliculus. *Nature* **332:** 357–360.

46. Georgopoulos, A.P., A.B. Schwartz & R.E. Kettner. 1986. Neuronal population coding of movement direction. *Science* **233:** 1416–1419.

47. Berkowitz, A. & P.S. Stein. 1994. Activity of descending propriospinal axons in the turtle hindlimb enlargement

during two forms of fictive scratching: phase analyses. *J. Neurosci.* **14:** 5105–5119.

48. Berkowitz, A. 2001. Rhythmicity of spinal neurons activated during each form of fictive scratching in spinal turtles. *J. Neurophysiol.* **86:** 1026–1036.

49. Berkowitz, A., G.L. Yosten & R.M. Ballard. 2006. Somatodendritic morphology predicts physiology for neurons that contribute to several kinds of limb movements. *J. Neurophysiol.* **95:** 2821–2831.

50. Stein, P.S. *et al.* 1995. Bilateral control of hindlimb scratching in the spinal turtle: contralateral spinal circuitry contributes to the normal ipsilateral motor pattern of fictive rostral scratching. *J. Neurosci.* **15:** 4343–4355.

51. Berkowitz, A. 2002. Both shared and specialized spinal circuitry for scratching and swimming in turtles. *J. Comp. Physiol. A* **188:** 225–234.

52. Berkowitz, A. 2008. Physiology and morphology of shared and specialized spinal interneurons for locomotion and scratching. *J. Neurophysiol.* **99:** 2887–2901.

53. Field, E.C. & P.S. Stein. 1997. Spinal cord coordination of hindlimb movements in the turtle: intralimb temporal relationships during scratching and swimming. *J. Neurophysiol.* **78:** 1394–1403.

54. Robertson, G.A. *et al.* 1985. Three forms of the scratch reflex in the spinal turtle: central generation of motor patterns. *J. Neurophysiol.* **53:** 1517–1534.

55. Mortin, L.I., J. Keifer & P.S. Stein. 1985. Three forms of the scratch reflex in the spinal turtle: movement analyses. *J. Neurophysiol.* **53:** 1501–1516.

56. Berkinblit, M.B. *et al.* 1978. Generation of scratching. Part II. Nonregular regimes of generation. *J. Neurophysiol.* **41:** 1058–1069.

57. Kristan, W. & R. Gillette. 2007. Behavioral choice. In *Invertebrate Neurobiology.* G. North & R.J. Greenspan, Eds.: 533–553. Cold Spring Harbor Laboratory Press. Cold Spring Harbor, NY.

58. Jing, J. *et al.* 2004. The construction of movement with behavior-specific and behavior-independent modules. *J. Neurosci.* **24:** 6315–6325.

59. McLean, D.L. *et al.* 2008. Continuous shifts in the active set of spinal interneurons during changes in locomotor speed. *Nat. Neurosci.* **11:** 1419–1429.

60. Berkowitz, A. 2007. Spinal interneurons that are selectively activated during fictive flexion reflex. *J. Neurosci.* **27:** 4634–4641.

61. Jankowska, E. *et al.* 1967. The effect of DOPA on the spinal cord. Part 5. Reciprocal organization of pathways transmitting excitatory action to alpha motoneurones of flexors and extensors. *Acta Physiol. Scand.* **70:** 369–388.

62. Grillner, S. 1981. Control of locomotion in bipeds, tetrapods, and fish. In *Handbook of Physiology, Sect. 1, The Nervous System*, Vol. 2, Motor Control. V. Brooks, Ed.: 1179–1236. American Physiological Society. Bethesda, MD.

63. Grillner, S. 1985. Neurobiological bases of rhythmic motor acts in vertebrates. *Science* **228**: 143–149.

64. Carter, M.C. & J.L. Smith. 1986. Simultaneous control of two rhythmical behaviors. Part II. Hindlimb walking with the paw-shake response in spinal cat. *J. Neurophysiol.* **56**: 184–195.

65. Bekoff, A. *et al.* 1987. Neural control of limb coordination. Part I. Comparison of hatching and walking motor output patterns in normal and deafferented chicks. *J. Neurosci.* **7**: 2320–2330.

66. Gelfand, I.M., G.N. Orlovsky & M.L. Shik. 1988. Locomotion and scratching in tetrapods. In *Neural Control of Rhythmic Movements in Vertebrates*. A.H. Cohen, S. Rossignol & S. Grillner, Eds.: 167–199. John Wiley & Sons. New York.

67. Pearson, K.G. 1993. Common principles of motor control in vertebrates and invertebrates. *Annu. Rev. Neurosci.* **16**: 265–297.

68. Soffe, S.R. 1993. Two distinct rhythmic motor patterns are driven by common premotor and motor neurons in a simple vertebrate spinal cord. *J. Neurosci.* **13**: 4456–4469.

69. Soffe, S.R. 1996. Motor patterns for two distinct rhythmic behaviors evoked by excitatory amino acid agonists in the Xenopus embryo spinal cord. *J. Neurophysiol.* **75**: 1815–1825.

70. Green, C.S. & S.R. Soffe. 1996. Transitions between two different motor patterns in Xenopus embryos. *J. Comp. Physiol. A* **178**: 279–291.

71. Johnston, R.M. & A. Bekoff. 1996. Patterns of muscle activity during different behaviors in chicks: implications for neural control. *J. Comp. Physiol. A* **179**: 169–184.

72. Earhart, G.M. & P.S. Stein. 2000. Scratch-swim hybrids in the spinal turtle: blending of rostral scratch and forward swim. *J. Neurophysiol.* **83**: 156–165.

73. Marder, E. 2000. Motor pattern generation. *Curr. Opin. Neurobiol.* **10**: 691–698.

Ann. N.Y. Acad. Sci. ISSN 0077-8923

ANNALS OF THE NEW YORK ACADEMY OF SCIENCES

Issue: Neurons and Networks in the Spinal Cord

Defining rhythmic locomotor burst patterns using a continuous wavelet transform

Benjamin W. Gallarda,[1,3] Tatyana O. Sharpee,[2,3] Samuel L. Pfaff,[1,3] and William A. Alaynick[1,3]

[1]Howard Hughes Medical Institute and Gene Expression Laboratory. [2]Computational Neurobiology Laboratory. [3]The Salk Institute for Biological Studies, La Jolla, California

Address for correspondence: Samuel L. Pfaff, 10010 North Torrey Pines Rd. GEL-P, La Jolla, CA 92037. pfaff@salk.edu

We review an objective and automated method for analyzing locomotor electrophysiology data with improved speed and accuracy. Manipulating central pattern generator (CPG) organization via mouse genetics has been a critical advance in the study of this circuit. Better quantitative measures of the locomotor data will further enhance our understanding of CPG development and function. Current analysis methods aim to measure locomotor cycle period, rhythmicity, and left–right and flexor–extensor phase; however, these methods have not been optimized to detect or quantify subtle changes in locomotor output. Because multiple experiments suggest that development of the CPG is robust and that the circuit is able to achieve organized behavior by several means, we sought to find a more objective and sensitive method for quantifying locomotor output. Recently, a continuous wavelet transform (CWT) has been applied to spinal cord ventral root recordings with promising results. The CWT provides greater resolution of cycle period, phase, and rhythmicity, and is proving to be a superior technique in assessing subtle changes in locomotion due to genetic perturbations of the underlying circuitry.

Keywords: spinal cord; locomotion; central pattern generator; continuous wavelet transform

Introduction

In the study of locomotion, statistical and genetic techniques have been advanced in the past two decades to improve the understanding of the circuits underlying this ubiquitous behavior. Kjaerulff and Kiehn applied circular statistics to measure the strength of right and left motor burst phase relationships and by precisely lesioning the spinal cord, they located the rhythmic centers producing the coordinated locomotor output.[1] The application of mouse genetics to manipulate classes of spinal neurons involved in establishing locomotor circuitry has been similarly useful (Fig. 1). For example, the elimination of an axon-guidance factor, *EphA4*, results in left and right sides of the spinal cord operating synchronously to produce a hopping phenotype.[2] Targeting transcription factors that label broad, developmentally-defined interneuron populations has illuminated the role of interneuron classes. Specifically, Evx1-positive V0 interneurons are involved in contralateral coordination, En1-

positive V1 interneurons regulate the speed of locomotor output, and loss of Chx10-positive V2a interneurons causes greater variability in cycle period and burst amplitude as well as a loss of left–right coordination.[3–6]

Despite these advances in manipulating and recording locomotor activity, relatively little has been done to improve analysis of locomotor recordings since the seminal studies by Kjaerulff and Kiehn.[1] The most common method of extracting useful information from ventral root recordings of neonatal spinal cords during fictive locomotion involves band-pass filtering, rectifying, and smoothing or integrating the data. This is followed by identification of burst onsets and based on a small number of randomly selected bursts ($\sim$25), cycle period and phase information are calculated (Fig. 2).

Although these methods have proven well suited to detect gross changes in locomotor output, they are not well suited for analysis of trends in locomotion over longer time periods or the detection of subtle

doi: 10.1111/j.1749-6632.2010.05437.x

A

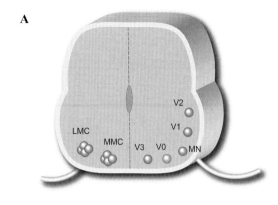

B

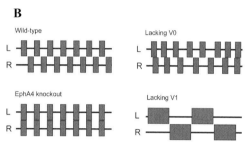

Figure 1. Classes of spinal neurons and locomotor output. (A) Diagram of a cross section of the lumbar spinal cord with medial and lateral motor pool divisions (MMC and LMC) and motor neurons; contralaterally projecting V0 interneurons, ipsilaterally projecting V1 interneurons; ipsilaterally projecting V2 interneurons, and contralaterally projecting V3 interneurons in their approximate locations in the ventral half of the spinal cord. (B) Diagrams of locomotor output in: wild-type showing normal left–right alternation; EphA4 knockout showing left-right synchrony; V0-deleted (*Dbx1* null) showing a perturbation of left-right coordination; and V1-deleted (*En1-DTA* or *Pax6* null) showing an increase in locomotor cycle period.

departures from control conditions. In light of this, several attempts have been made to introduce new analytical methods. For example, auto- and cross-correlation have been used as measures of rhythmicity[7,8] and power spectral analysis has been applied to determine frequencies of bursting (Fig. 3).[9] These analyses, however, are sensitive to changes in data set processing and selection, and none have significantly improved upon the traditional methods. To improve the analysis of CPG activity it is desirable to employ analytical tools that are: (1) easily automated; (2) objective and non-arbitrary; and (3) quantitative and sensitive, especially when applied to larger data sets, that is, longer recording sessions.

Results and discussion

Identification of rhythmic patterns using a continuous wavelet transform

A recent advance that meets the criteria needed for accurate quantification of CPG activity is the use of the continuous wavelet transform (CWT).[10] The CWT is a method of time-frequency analysis, localizing the dominant cycle periods or frequencies of the signal in time. It works by comparing the input signal across its length in time (for example, a ventral root recording—Fig. 4) to a wavelet basis—a function with zero mean, localized in time and frequency space—and plotting the resulting convolution.[11] The wavelet basis is then scaled and iteratively compared to the input signal (for example, 100 scales from 0.016 to 32 Hz—Figs. 4A and B). The resulting plot displays regions where the wavelet basis is best matched to the signal, with frequency as the *y*-axis (typically plotted in a logarithmic scale), time as the *x*-axis, and power as the color map (Fig. 4B). When using the Morlet wavelet, a complex function, phase and frequency information are determined simultaneously. By comparing the phase of one trace with that of another, a continuous phase relationship can be determined over time (Fig. 4C). Overall cycle period and phase can then be derived (as in Figs. 2C and D). One additional benefit to the CWT is that regions of significant power can be isolated relative to an appropriate noise simulation of the input data (for details, see References 10 and 11). These are plotted as dotted white contours in Figure 4B.

The time-frequency analysis accomplished by the CWT has several advantages over previous methods. First, the CWT can be entirely automated. Much of the previously reported analysis is done manually, or is only partially automated. Because the CWT derives its results from an entire data set, there is no need for user-intervention to select parts of the data set amenable to analysis. Furthermore, although the CWT is sensitive to abrupt fluctuations in the unprocessed data, the standard preprocessing of data to remove slow fluctuations and flatten the baseline has little effect on the results. This negates the need to preprocess data, improving automation and speed of analysis. Second, the

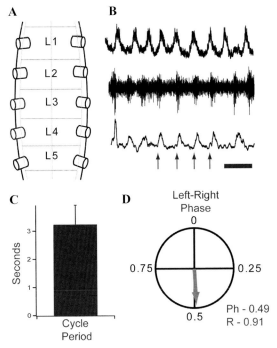

Figure 2. Conventional data analysis. (A) Diagram of the ventral surface of the lumbar spinal cord in which entire ventral roots are drawn into suction electrodes and fictive locomotion is elicited with 10 μM NMDA and 20 μM serotonin. (B) Conventional preprocessing of ventral root recording data for analysis. *Upper trace:* the unfiltered neurogram recorded from DC to 1 kHz, amplified 1000×, and digitized at 10 kHz. *Middle trace:* filtered with a 40 Hz high-pass filter. *Lower trace:* 40 Hz high-pass filter, then rectified and smoothed with a 5 Hz low-pass filter. The onset of randomly selected bursts (*arrows*) are then used to calculate cycle period (average of burst onset to next burst onset) and phase (average of burst onset of reference trace to average burst onset of comparison trace). (C) Average cycle period, mean ± SEM. (D) Average phase where the vector direction (Ph) indicates phase, 0.0 indicates synchrony, 0.5 indicates alternation, and vector length (R) indicates strength of phase. Scale bar equals 5 s.

CWT, being a continuous measure, is able to assess changes in locomotor output over time due to treatments or perturbations of the system. Whether traditional lesion studies or pharmacological treatments, or newer techniques such as allatostatin signaling or channelrhodopsin/light-based perturbation of neuronal activity,[5,12] the CWT can accommodate a dynamic measure of changes in output.

This is superior to a simple summary of pre- and posttreatment metrics. Third, the CWT is scalable in time, so that it extracts cycle period and phase information with appropriate temporal resolution. For example, one may be concerned with a change in cycle period of motor output from 1.0 to 1.2 s, but is less likely to be as concerned with a change from 20.0 to 20.2 s. The CWT addresses this, especially when using scales on power-of-2 intervals, by allowing the user to select only the desired scales with increasing intervals between them. This is superior to other time-frequency analyses such as a short-term Fourier transform, which uses a fixed interval based on the selected window size (see Reference 10, Fig. 2). In their paper, Mor and Lev-Tov point out that the CWT does not depend on burst detection to quantify cycle period or phase. However, should one desire to identify bursts for further analysis, the CWT is an excellent tool for burst detection as well. Instead of computing the complex transform, a real wavelet transform highlights peaks and valleys where the wavelet basis is in-phase and out-of-phase with the raw signal. By following the trend of the cycle period relevant to bursting, individual bursts can be identified and extracted for further analysis.

Statistical considerations

There are several ways to quantify the strength of the peaks in the wavelet transform. Monte-Carlo simulations, consisting of thousands of generated samples of noise with similar power spectra to the raw data (white noise being most appropriate for filtered and smoothed spinal cord ventral root recordings), can be averaged to produce a wavelet transform of random noise.[10] The wavelet transform of the raw data can then be compared to this and any peaks above the noise are considered significant. There are also equation-based approximations of noise spectra that can be used with similar results as Monte Carlo simulations that drastically reduce computation time.[11] Others have pointed out possible shortcomings in the noise-based detection of significant regions of the wavelet transform and have suggested other mathematical models for identifying these regions.[13,14] By selecting the appropriate method of assessing the strength of signal in the wavelet transform, quantification of regions of significant power can be automated. In sum, the CWT is an advance from previous methods as it

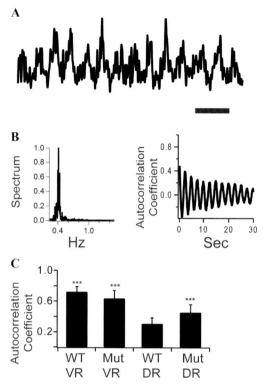

Figure 3. Other data analysis methods. (**A**) Raw data recorded and processed as in Figure 2 used in alternative analysis methods in *Panel B*; bar equals 5 s. (**B**) Power spectral analysis is a measure of the dominant frequencies in the data but does not provide timing information; power spectrum of data in A normalized to 1; autocorrelation is a measure of rhythmicity in the data generated by comparing the raw data to itself; autocorrelation plot normalized to 1 (at time equals 0 s, not shown). (**C**) Autocorrelation coefficient statistical analysis on ventral and dorsal root recordings in wild type and mutant mice. Mutant dorsal root recordings show significant increase in rhythmic output due to ectopic innervation of dorsal root ganglion with motor nerves; ✱✱✱indicates significantly greater than random, ANOVA followed by Dunnett's Test, $P < 0.001$. VR = ventral root; DR = dorsal root (Panel C adapted from Reference 8, used with permission).

demonstrates a more objective, sensitive, and quantitative analysis of electrophysiological signals that can be easily automated.

Defining flexor–extensor phase using CWT

What then are the results of applying the CWT to locomotor data from typical lumbar level record-

ings? The average cycle period and phase are indistinguishable from those obtained through conventional methods, in most instances (Figs. 4 and 5), and the CWT is achieving these values when applied to data sets 20 or more times as long as those used conventionally. Such an increase in the amount of data analyzed will improve statistical analysis of the results. Although most of the results of CWT-based analysis accurately reproduce those previously reported, an interesting difference appears when assessing flexor–extensor phase in late-embryonic/early-postnatal mice. Flexor–extensor phase has been generally defined by previous studies using previous methods as 0.5—exact alternation, similar to left–right phase (Figs. 2D and 5B). This value is calculated from data recorded at lumbar level 2 (L2) and lumbar level 5 (L5) ventral roots, which are thought to innervate predominantly flexor and extensor muscles, respectively. The CWT, however, reports a flexor–extensor phase value of 0.36, a significantly different result (Fig. 5B). This is not an artifact of the CWT, as left–right phase relationships calculated by the CWT are 0.5 (Fig. 2D). Rather, this discrepancy between the CWT and conventional methods is due to filtering, rectifying, and smoothing the raw data for conventional analysis (Fig. 2B). The result of preprocessing raw data in such a way is an effective integration of high-frequency motor bursting; whereas low-frequency phenomena such as the population of motor neuron membrane depolarizations, recorded in DC, are discarded.[15] Thus, when the onset of motor bursting is not aligned with the onset of DC depolarization, a phase shift can occur (Fig. 5C). Furthermore, conventional methods define a specific point, typically burst onset, in order to assess phase. In contrast, the CWT defines phase throughout the burst cycle, giving a more comprehensive measure of this relationship between the two signals. The cumulative effect of these two points is that the actual phase of L5 is obscured by preprocessing the data and using a single point for each burst to define phase. This effect is likely more significant in L5 data. A similar effect is not noticed in L2 because the onset of motor bursting aligns with the onset of DC depolarization in L2 output; and this shift in L5 with corresponding lack of shift in L2 explains the change in L2–L5 phase. Interestingly, the 0.36 flexor–extensor phase value detected at E18.5-P0 shifts to 0.5 at P2

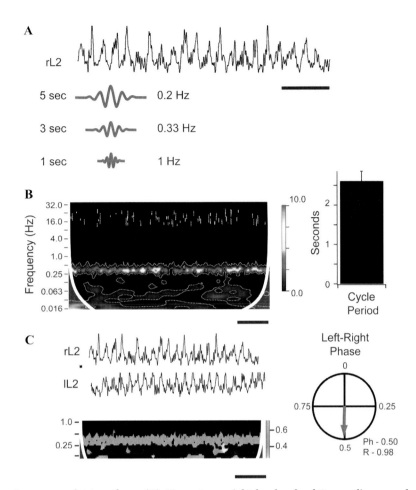

Figure 4. Continuous wavelet transform. (**A**) *Upper trace:* right lumbar level 2 recording recorded from DC to 1 kHz, high-pass filtered (40 Hz), rectified, and low pass filtered (5 Hz). *Lower traces:* examples of Morlet wavelet bases of three different scales. Data are convolved with similar wavelets of 100 different scales to produce the 2D plot in *Panel B*. Scale bar equals 10 s. (**B**) Wavelet transform of data in *Panel A* derived with 100 scales from 0.03 to 64 s or 0.016–32 Hz with cone of influence (*solid white line*, see text for details) denoting area not analyzed due to edge effects. Significance contour (*dotted white line*) indicates areas of significant power above white noise simulation (power is indicated by color-scale gradient that is normalized to standard deviations above white noise). The *y*-axis is presented in a logarithmic scale (log2). Average cycle period is calculated from region within significance contours of wavelet transform. Scale bar equals 50 s. (**C**) Left and right lumbar level 2 data and resulting phase of cross wavelet transform superimposed on significant regions of cross wavelet transform with cone of influence (*solid white line*; only scales from 0.125 to 1 Hz shown), color-scale gradient indicates direction of vector in phase plot from 0 to 1 (only 0.4–0.6 shown); average phase circular plot derived from phase of cross wavelet transform within significant regions (as in Fig. 2C). Scale bars equal 10 s (raw data) and 50 s (cross-wavelet transform).

(unpublished observation BWG, WAA). This suggests that the CWT is capable of detecting postnatal changes in flexor–extensor locomotor output. The basis for this postnatal phase shift remains to be defined.

Conclusions

In summary, the CWT improves upon previous methods in the following ways. First, the CWT is easily automated, objective, and quantitative. For

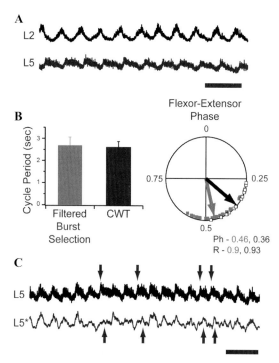

Figure 5. Continuous wavelet transform results. (A) Ipsilateral L2 and L5 recordings from DC to 1 kHz, not filtered. (B) Comparison of cycle period and phase calculated by conventional methods (*red squares* in phase plot offset slightly for clarity) or with CWT (*open squares*) using 800 s of data, a portion of which is shown in *Panel A*. Cycle period is mean + SEM; phase plot includes mean vector and 25 individual data points representing phase values at 25 bursts in the raw data. (C) *Upper trace*: DC to 1 kHz, not filtered. *Lower trace*: filtered, rectified, smoothed L5 data. *Arrows* indicate shifts due to processing that account for the change in phase between conventional methods and CWT in *Panel B*. Scale bars equal 5 s.

example, CWT produces quantitative measures of rhythmicity by virtue of detection of frequencies compared to noise-simulation cutoffs for statistical significance. This is a substantial improvement over autocorrelation that is dependent on both preprocessing and the length of data selected for analysis (Fig. 3B). Second, unlike previous methods that only provide a summary of important measures such as cycle period and phase, the CWT extracts this information continuously across the length of a recording, which can be averaged to produce conventional summary statistics or examined to see if measures

change over time. Unlike power spectral analysis, which is a measure of frequency only, and can change drastically based on differences in data processing and selection (Fig. 3B), the CWT measures frequencies or cycle periods in the data continuously. Third, the CWT is a more precise measure of electrophysiological data, uncovering a previously unappreciated flexor–extensor phase relationship obfuscated by conventional methods (Fig. 5). Some practical considerations related to application of the CWT follow. Instead of selecting subsets of bursts, only clearly aberrant artifacts need to be removed from the raw data. There are edge effects that need to be considered at the beginning and end of a CWT of raw data that are proportional to the size of the scale being applied. These are known as the cone of influence (COI),[11] but this region can be easily plotted with the CWT and these areas can be discounted from analysis (Fig. 4B). Finally, while electrophysiological recordings are typically processed according to the steps described in Figure 2, we have found that this preprocessing does not greatly improve the results of a CWT, and unprocessed data can be used for analysis. This matter of preprocessing data clearly alters the phase relationship when comparing the output from different lumbar levels (see Fig. 5).

Prospectively, use of the CWT will allow for additional analyses to be considered. For example, the CWT can be used to rapidly define hundreds of individual motor bursts in long data sets. Such large numbers of motor bursts could be extracted and subjected to other statistical analyses, such as principal component analysis (PCA).[16] As motor bursts are generally considered in an almost binary fashion—"on" or "off"—this added benefit of using the CWT may uncover new dynamics in locomotor output not previously appreciated. And because the data analyzed through the CWT need not be preprocessed, subsequent manipulations of the data are still available.

The study of locomotion will benefit tremendously from advances in data analysis. New standards for characterizing abnormal locomotor output that extend beyond summary statistics will be critical in defining the changes in circuitry produced by subtle genetic manipulations of the spinal cord. These findings may then serve to better inform computer models and interpretation of experimental results. The CWT appears to meet the necessary criteria for emerging analysis methods of electro-physiological data that offer a more comprehensive and informative view of locomotor activity.

Conflicts of interest

The authors declare no conflicts of interest.

References

1. Kjaerulff, O. & O. Kiehn. 1996. Distribution of networks generating and coordinating locomotor activity in the neonatal rat spinal cord *in vitro*: a lesion study. *J. Neurosci.: Off. J. Soc. Neurosci.* **16:** 5777–5794.

2. Kullander, K. *et al.* 2003. Role of EphA4 and EphrinB3 in local neuronal circuits that control walking. *Science* **299:** 1889–1892.

3. Lanuza, G.M., S. Gosgnach, A. Pierani, *et al.* 2004. Genetic identification of spinal interneurons that coordinate left-right locomotor activity necessary for walking movements. *Neuron* **42:** 375–386.

4. Crone, S. *et al.* 2008. Genetic ablation of V2a ipsilateral interneurons disrupts left-right locomotor coordination in mammalian spinal cord. *Neuron* **60:** 70–83.

5. Gosgnach, S. *et al.* 2006. V1 spinal neurons regulate the speed of vertebrate locomotor outputs. *Nature* **440:** 215–219.

6. Goulding, M. 2009. Circuits controlling vertebrate locomotion: moving in a new direction. *Nat. Rev. Neurosci.* **10:** 507–518.

7. Hinckley, C., B. Seebach & L. Ziskind-Conhaim. 2005. Distinct roles of glycinergic and GABAergic inhibition in coordinating locomotor-like rhythms in the neonatal mouse spinal cord. *Neuroscience* **131:** 745–758.

8. Gallarda, B.W. *et al.* 2008. Segregation of axial motor and sensory pathways via heterotypic trans-axonal signaling. *Science* **320:** 233–236.

9. Zhang, Y. *et al.* 2008. V3 spinal neurons establish a robust and balanced locomotor rhythm during walking. *Neuron* **60:** 84–96.

10. Mor, Y. & A. Lev-Tov. 2007. Analysis of rhythmic patterns produced by spinal neural networks. *J. Neurophysiol.* **98:** 2807–2817.

11. Torrence, C. & G.P. Compo. 1998. A practical guide to wavelet analysis. *Bull. Am. Meteorol. Soc.* **79:** 61–78.

12. Arenkiel, B.R. *et al.* 2007. *In vivo* light-induced activation of neural circuitry in transgenic mice expressing channelrhodopsin-2. *Neuron* **54:** 205–218.

13. Maraun, D. & J. Kurths. 2004. Cross wavelet analysis: significance testing and pitfalls. *Nonlinear Process. Geophys.* **11:** 505–514.

14. Maraun, D., J. Kurths & M. Holschneider. 2007. Nonstationary Gaussian processes in wavelet domain: synthesis, estimation, and significance testing. *Phys. Rev. E* **75:** 16707, DOI: 10.1103/PhysRevE.75.016707.

15. Tresch, M.C. & O. Kiehn. 2000. Motor coordination without action potentials in the mammalian spinal cord. *Nat. Neurosci.* **3:** 593–599.

16. Briggman, K., H. Abarbanel & W. Kristan, Jr. 2006. From crawling to cognition: analyzing the dynamical interactions among populations of neurons. *Curr. Opin. Neurobiol.* **16:** 135–144.

Ann. N.Y. Acad. Sci. ISSN 0077-8923

ANNALS OF THE NEW YORK ACADEMY OF SCIENCES
Issue: *Neurons and Networks in the Spinal Cord*

Presynaptic inhibition of primary afferents by depolarization: observations supporting nontraditional mechanisms

Shawn Hochman,[1] Jacob Shreckengost,[1] Hiroshi Kimura,[2] and Jorge Quevedo[3]

[1]Department of Physiology, Emory University, Atlanta, Georgia. [2]Molecular Neuroscience Research Center, Shiga University of Medical Science, Ōtsu, Japan. [3]Cinvestav del IPN, Mexico City, Mexico

Addresses for correspondence: Shawn Hochman, Ph.D., Whitehead Biomedical Research Building, Room 644, Emory University School of Medicine, 615 Michael St., Atlanta, GA 30322. shawn.hochman@emory.edu. Jorge N. Quevedo, Depto. de Fisiología, Biofísica y Neurociencias, CINVESTAV del IPN, Av. IPN, 2508. Col. Zacatenco, México, D.F., C.P. 07300, Mexico. jquevedo@fisio.cinvestav.mx

Primary afferent neurotransmission is the fundamental first step in the central processing of sensory stimuli and is controlled by pre- and postsynaptic inhibitory mechanisms. Presynaptic inhibition (PSI) is probably the more powerful form of inhibitory control in all primary afferent fibers. A major mechanism producing afferent PSI is via a channel-mediated depolarization of their intraspinal terminals, which can be recorded extracellularly as a dorsal root potential (DRP). Based on measures of DRP latency it has been inferred that this primary afferent depolarization (PAD) of low-threshold afferents is mediated by minimally trisynaptic pathways with pharmacologically identified GABAergic interneurons forming last-order axo-axonic synapses onto afferent terminals. There is still no "squeaky clean" evidence of this organization. This paper describes recent and historical work that supports the existence of PAD occurring by more direct pathways and with a complex pharmacology that questions the proprietary role of GABA and $GABA_A$ receptors in this process. Cholinergic transmission in particular may contribute significantly to PAD, including via direct release from primary afferents.

Keywords: presynaptic inhibition; dorsal horn; sensory; PAD; DRP

Presynaptic inhibition of primary afferents

The spinal cord is the neural interface between body and brain, receiving a continuous barrage of sensory information via primary afferents that requires central mechanisms to limit and channel their signaling. The intraspinal terminals of primary afferents, located predominantly in the dorsal horn (laminae I–VI) represent the first central nervous system (CNS) site for this control, and here it appears to be regulated by frighteningly complex processes.[1] A principal mechanism for reduction of afferent neurotransmission is via prior depolarization of their terminals, termed primary afferent depolarization (PAD), which paradoxically reduces transmitter release. GABAergic inhibitory interneurons are thought to mediate PAD via a trisynaptic circuit (Fig. 1A). Using pumps, sensory neurons maintain the chloride gradient to be depolarizing so that activation of intraspinal $GABA_A$ receptors results in the observed PAD (Fig. 2). PAD can be measured experimentally following its antidromic electrotonic spread to dorsal roots as a dorsal root potential (DRP).

Sensory afferents arising from skin or muscle can be broadly separated into two categories: low and high thresholds. Large-diameter/fast-conducting myelinated fibers require lower electrical stimulus intensities (low threshold) for recruitment than smaller-diameter un- or thinly myelinated fibers (high threshold). Low-threshold afferents are non-pain encoding cutaneous Aβ and muscle groups Ia, Ib, and II mechanoceptors, and the presynaptic inhibitory control of these fibers is the focus of this paper.

As alluded to earlier, the classical electrophysiological studies obtained indirect experimental evidence that afferent-evoked presynaptic inhibition of

doi: 10.1111/j.1749-6632.2010.05436.x

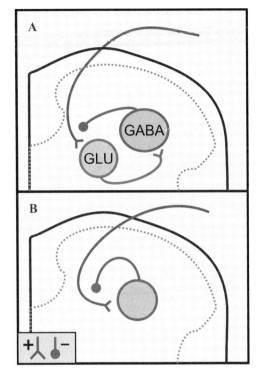

Figure 1. (A) Classical minimally trisynaptic network for presynaptic inhibition of low-threshold muscle and cutaneous afferents. (B) Recent evidence also supports more direct disynaptic pathways.

low-threshold afferents is produced via a minimally trisynaptic pathway involving last-order GABAergic inhibitory interneurons. This paper will underscore limitations in this model of afferent-evoked PAD, and then provide evidence to suggest (1) that more direct feedback mechanisms are found, (2) that GABA may not be the only transmitter involved, and (3) that the classical GABA$_A$ receptor may also not be the only receptor involved. If true, the results further expand the mechanisms by which somatosensory information processing is controlled.

Some limitations with the current model of afferent-evoked PAD

Although it is assumed that anatomically identified GABAergic axo-axonic synapses onto identified afferents arise from the GABAergic interneurons-mediating afferent activity-evoked PAD, direct electrophysiological evidence is still lacking.[1–3] Putative PAD interneurons have historically been identified based on their extracellular spike being temporally

coincident with the DRP using the technique of spike-triggered averaging.[4,5] However, as recently stated by Rudomin[6] on their earlier work, "One of the problems with the interpretation of these findings was that the spontaneous interneuronal activity of the interneurons assumed to mediate PAD of muscle afferents appeared in synchrony with a negative CDP [cord dorsum potential] which started *25–50 ms before the interneuronal activity used to trigger the DRP and VRP recordings*."[6] We concur with Wall who argued in 1998 that "we should remain cautious in the identification of those nerve cells which lead *singly* or in a chain to the generation of PAD."[7]

If PAD occurred via a trisynaptic pathway, it is worth questioning why PAD is not reduced by anesthetics such as pentobarbital, which decrease excitatory synaptic activity in all neurons.[8] Several of the studies of PAD by Rudomin *et al.* used pentobarbital as the anesthetic.[9–11] As stated by Eccles *et al.*,[3] "*The cutaneous volleys produce DRPs at such deep anaesthesia that their occurrence in the absence of all interneuronal activity has been suggested (Wall, 1958).*[12] *If this were established it would falsify the hypothesis that presynaptic inhibition is due to . . . activation of specific interneuronal pathways.*" Although it can be countered that barbiturates would also strengthen PAD by directly potentiating GABA$_A$ receptor activity,[8] in order for afferents to evoke PAD tri-synaptically, they must go through interneurons, and we now know that pentobarbital potently inhibits glutamatergic transmission (AMPA receptor IC$_{50}$ ∼50 μM ≈ 1 mg/kg).[13,14]

If the classical minimally trisynaptic interneuronal circuit does not contribute much to the observed PAD, how else might PAD be produced? The simplest answer is disynaptically. This would explain the circuit in the dorsal horn, where the location of all putative interposed interneurons is always where primary afferents terminate and never elsewhere[4,10] (see Ref. [15] for ventral horn). Disynaptic circuits mediating PAD of low-threshold afferents appear highly likely. Lamina III cholinergic interneurons receive input from myelinated and unmyelinated cutaneous afferents and appear to be interposed in negative feedback disynaptic circuits back onto the same primary afferents.[16] Moreover recent intracellular recordings from two intermediate zone interneurons monosynaptically excited

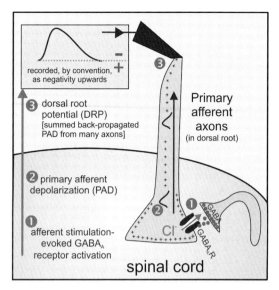

recorded, by convention,
as negativity upwards

❸ dorsal root
potential (DRP)
[summed back-propagated
PAD from many axons]

**Primary
afferent
axons**
(in dorsal root)

❷ primary afferent
depolarization (PAD)

❶ afferent stimulation-
evoked $GABA_A$
receptor activation

Cl⁻

GABA

$GABA_A$R

spinal cord

Figure 2. Measurement of primary afferent depolarization as dorsal root potential and underlying mechanisms. $GABA_A$R-mediated PSI. Unlike most synapses, Cl-gradient favors outward flow and so depolarizes afferents. Depolarizing wave can be recorded antidromically as a dorsal root potential from sensory nerve roots. Sequence of events is numbered 1–3.

by groups I and II muscle afferents were intracellularly labeled and shown to project axons directly apposed to primary afferent terminals (i.e., disynaptic circuit).[17] "These *two* interneurons are therefore likely to be the first two examples of PAD interneurons in higher vertebrates to be characterized electrophysiologically as well as labeled intracellularly,"[17] although it was not shown that they were directly linked to PAD. Importantly, based on latency measures this circuit was considered trisynaptic.[10,18]

Another possibility for PAD generation is disynaptically via a nonspiking dendroaxonic microcircuitry, which has been suggested but not demonstrated by Hounsgaard based on the observation of a TTX-insensitive PAD evoked by stimulation of high-threshold afferents in the turtle[19] (Fig. 3A). Alternatively, the actions could be direct via homosynaptic or heterosynaptic negative feedback of transmitter released from primary afferents including via spillover mechanisms[20] (Fig. 3B). Presynaptic autoreceptors represent a dominant form of PSI in CNS neuron terminals,[21] and this much simpler mechanism may explain the presence of PAD

onto their own and related terminals[1] as well as why PAD is comparatively long lasting. However, direct feedback would be inconsistent with a GABAergic mechanism because primary afferents would need to release GABA and labeling studies have failed to support GABA as a transmitter localized in primary afferents.[22] Another transmitter would need to be released from primary afferents and be capable of activation of a $GABA_A$-like receptor for such direct actions. Possibilities include acetylcholine, taurine, and β-alanine as in the elaborated section "Could another transmitter be released to produce PAD?"

Further peculiarities of PAD

Is GABA really the transmitter producing afferent-evoked PAD?

The existence of GABAergic synapses onto primary afferents clearly demonstrates that at least some GABAergic projections must exist that produce presynaptic inhibition of primary afferents.[15,23] However, they may not be associated with *all* forms of evoked PAD. One possible organization is that GABAergic interneurons are predominantly responsible for the PAD generated by descending systems but not by several afferent systems. Early work from two groups demonstrated that the evoked efflux of neuronal [3H]-GABA in amphibian spinal cord arose from Ca^{2+}-dependent release following stimulation of descending spinal tracts but not following stimulation of primary afferents.[24,25] The marginal release of [3H]-glutamate following primary afferent stimulation suggests that afferent activation may simply have been insufficient to evoke GABA release.[25] The evidence for GABA as the transmitter responsible for afferent evoked PAD is (1) the existence of GABAergic axo-axonic synapses on primary afferents[23]; (ii) afferent-evoked PAD is blocked by $GABA_A$ receptor antagonists[1,26]; and (iii) drugs blocking GABA synthesis and degradation depress or facilitate afferent-evoked PAD, respectively.[26,27] This latter point is highly suspect. The hydrazines used as blockers of synthesis are very nonspecific, and the inhibitors of GABA degradation are also nonspecific and demonstrated a facilitatory effect in only one of four studies (see references in Ref. 26). Potential weaknesses in the evidence of the first two more critical points are described later.

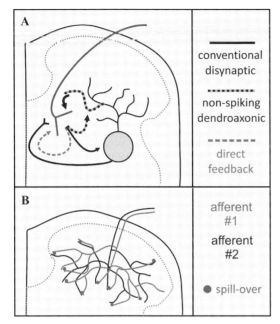

Figure 3. Putative circuits for low-threshold afferent-evoked PAD not requiring trisynaptic pathways. (**A**) As mephenesin blocks part of the DRP, a conventional disynaptic pathway may serve PAD of some primary afferents. The remaining DRP may arise from direct monosynaptic actions of transmitter onto afferent terminals or via a disynaptic nonspiking dendroaxonic microcircuit. (**B**) Heterosynaptic actions that remain after greatly restricting synaptic transmission with mephenesin may also be due to spillover effects on adjacent axons.

Is the GABA$_A$ receptor really the receptor activated to produce afferent-evoked PAD?

Regarding GABAergic terminals onto primary afferents, "little can be said to link the presynaptic terminals visualized with electron microscopy with particular spinal cord neurons or axonal arborizations."[23] In addition, although a high proportion of terminals onto primary afferents are immunopositive for GABA or its synthesis enzyme glutamic acid decarboxylase (GAD), this does not necessarily equate to a presence of postsynaptic GABA$_A$ receptors. For example, no changes were observed in autoradiographic mapping of spinal GABA$_A$ receptor ligands after degeneration of dorsal root fibers[28] with no evidence of β2/β3 labeling in primary afferent terminals using both EM and light microscopy.[23] Based on the earlier description, it is instead possible that postsynaptic

receptors to GABA$^+$ presynaptic terminals contain bicuculline/picrotoxin sensitive glycine (α1, α2, β), nicotinic (α9, α10), GABA$_A$-rho, or 5HT$_{3A}$ receptor subunits. GABA$_A$, glycine, ACh nicotinic, and 5-HT$_3$ receptors all comprise the Cys-loop family of transmitter-gated ion channels with common molecular architecture,[29] so overlapping pharmacological actions are unsurprising.

Could another Cys-loop family receptor produce PAD?

The pharmacology of low-threshold PAD has been studied in detail,[3,26,27] but not for a long time. Past interpretations of results were based on the assumption that the drugs used had rather specific actions. As described later, there are nicotinic, 5HT$_3$, and glycine receptor subunits with sensitivity to traditional GABA$_A$ antagonists.

Nicotinic receptor. The nicotinic receptor (nAChR) is a nonselective cation channel. Primary afferents contain numerous nAChR subtypes.[30,31] Bicuculline (IC$_{50}$ = 0.8 μM) and strychnine (IC$_{50}$ = 0.02 μM) potently inhibit the α9 nicotinic ACh receptor subunits[32] and nAChR α10 subunits also have sensitivity to strychnine and bicuculline. This raises the possibility that part of PAD is nicotinic receptor mediated. However, PAD is barely affected by strychnine in the *in vitro* preparation described later (Fig. 6), and does not appear to affect PAD in the cat.[33] Critically, only larger diameter (i.e., low threshold) DRG neurons contain α-bungarotoxin binding sites (examined in rat, cat, monkey, and human).[34] These neurons represent at least 12% of large-diameter afferents, and appear to selectively project to lamina III, which is the projection site of Aβ cutaneous afferents[35] and the presumed location of interneurons interposed in the PAD pathway of cutaneous afferents.[10] Dorsal horn cholinergic interneurons[36] are also located there, making them well positioned to produce PAD.[23,37]

5HT$_{3A}$ receptors. The serotonin 5HT$_3$ receptor is a nonselective cation channel. Bicuculline (IC$_{50}$ 20 μM) and picrotoxin (IC$_{50}$ 30 μM) antagonize 5HT$_{3A}$ receptors at pharmacologically relevant doses.[38] 5HT$_{3A}$ receptors are strongly expressed in myelinated primary afferents.[39]

Glycine receptors. The inhibitory glycine receptor is principally permeable to chloride. In retinal ganglion cells, glycine receptors are potently blocked by traditional GABA$_A$ receptor antagonists (bicuculline, gabazine, and picrotoxin) as were their $\alpha 1$ and $\alpha 2$ glycine receptor subunits expressed in HEK cells[40] with $\alpha 2$ subunits showing relative strychnine insensitivity.[41] Beta subunits coassembled with α subunits lead to greater bicuculline and gabazine sensitivity but reduced picrotoxin sensitivity.[42]

Unusual receptor subunit assemblies. There is also evidence of promiscuous subunit assembly between different members of the Cys-loop family. For example, GABA$_A$ $\gamma 2$s can coassemble with glycine α subunits to form functional glycine receptors.[42] There is also evidence of colocalization of $\alpha 1$ glycine receptor subunit with the GABA$_A$ $\gamma 2$ and GABA$_A$ ρ receptor subunits in spinal cord but not retina.[43] Also, glycine β and GABA$_A$ γ subunit mRNA may be coexpressed in large DRG neurons.[44]

In total, earlier conclusions stating that classical GABA$_A$ receptors are essential for PAD based on pharmacological observations can no longer be viewed as definitive.

Could another transmitter be released to produce PAD?

Acetylcholine. Lamina III is a projection site of Aβ and Aδ cutaneous afferents[35] and is the likely location of interneurons interposed in PAD of cutaneous afferents.[10] Intriguingly, it is also the predominant location of dorsal horn cholinergic interneurons[36]—well positioned to contribute to PAD.[23,37] Acetylcholine (ACh) and GABA coexist in a population of dorsal horn interneurons[37] and are found in ∼*25% of presynaptic afferent axons*.[23] Thus, there is ample anatomic evidence to support ACh as a transmitter contributing to PAD.

Intriguingly, although the early literature did not identify acetylcholine (ACh) as a neurotransmitter in primary afferents,[35] recent work strongly challenges these studies. First, an alternative splice variant of the ACh synthesis enzyme choline acetyltransferase (ChAT) has been identified. Peripheral ChAT (pChAT) is preferentially localized in peripheral neurons including in dorsal root ganglia (DRG),[45] and has sufficient enzyme activity in the adult rat DRG to produce physiological concentrations of ACh.[46] PChAT is expressed in both small and large-

diameter primary afferents[46] and immunolabeling studies identify pChAT in myelinated primary afferents that project via dorsal columns to brainstem dorsal column nuclei.[47] DRG neurons have also been shown to express the vesicular ACh transporter (VAChT) preferentially in large-diameter DRG neurons[48] as well as the ACh degradative enzyme acetylcholinesterase (AChE).[35,46] Widespread ChAT labeling in DRG was also observed in mice, including ChAT-GFP BAC transgenic mice,[49] and treatment with antisense oligonucleotides reduced labeling.[50]

Taurine and β-alanine. Taurine is released from neurons and glia upon hypo-osmotic swelling and is believed to behave chiefly as an osmoregulator. However, in spinal cord, microdialysis experiments reveal that taurine and β-alanine are released following sciatic nerve stimulation in concentrations comparable to glutamate.[51] Taurine and β-alanine are weak agonists at GABA$_A$ receptors,[26] although taurine may also be a potent activator of extrasynaptic GABA$_A$ receptors.[52] Taurine and β-alanine also directly depolarize primary afferents in the *in vitro* rat spinal cord.[53] As in frog, responses are blocked by picrotoxin (50 μM) and bicuculline (5 μM). Like GABA and glycine, taurine, and β-alanine are transported via Na$^+$-dependent high-affinity uptake systems with significant sequence homology to the GABA and glycine transporters systems.[54,55] More recently, taurine labeling has been demonstrated in spinal cord with greatest density in superficial dorsal horn, but also associated with myelinated axon terminals.[56] In addition, cysteine dioxygenase and sulfinoalanine decarboxylase, two critical enzymes in the taurine synthesis, are expressed in primary afferents[57] and synaptic vesicles contained within synaptosomes are enriched in taurine.[58]

In total, primary afferents may corelease substances that act on receptors having GABA$_A$-like pharmacology.

Experimental support for the existence of nontraditional mechanisms serving afferent-evoked PAD

The hemisected spinal cord maintained *in vitro*

Jorge Quevedo has developed a preparation to show that afferent-evoked PAD in the isolated *in vitro* spinal cord of young mouse and rat evoked by stimulation of intact peripheral nerves has many characteristics similar to those observed in the adult cat.[59] The *in vitro* model has afforded us the ability to examine the mechanisms serving PAD with greater pharmacological precision. For example, *in vivo* studies on PAD mechanisms undertaken in the presence of anesthetics (e.g., α-chloralose and barbiturates) are expected to alter the mechanisms generating PAD.[8,60] Moreover, *in vivo* studies are often necessarily undertaken in the presence of paralytic agents such as gallamine that act on nicotinic receptors and also alter the DRP.[61]

The results from experiments herein described were undertaken both in mouse and rat (P6–15). The results obtained were the same in both species but only experiments in rat are shown. The experimental setup is shown in Figure 4. The L5 dorsal root is stimulated, and DRPs are recorded from the same (homonymous) or adjacent dorsal root (L4; heteronymous). For ease of viewing, only one DRP is shown in the figures displayed. All actions were studied from putative low-threshold afferents, typically at four times the stimulus intensity that just elicits an afferent volley (threshold; 4T) or at 100 μA, 100 μs. The afferent volley was monitored to observe recruitment of low-threshold afferents and

to ensure afferent volley amplitude is unaffected by drug applications so that observed actions are due to events in the spinal cord. Also, whenever tested all recruited afferents and the DRP were completely blocked with low-dose TTX (100 nM), excluding a contribution from high-threshold TTX insensitive afferents.[19]

Low-threshold DRPs require GABA$_A$-like receptor activation

PAD generated by low-threshold afferent stimulation is blocked by GABA$_A$ receptor antagonists, as shown previously in cat,[33] rat,[53,62] and frog.[26] Here, we also demonstrate that the DRP in this preparation is blocked with bicuculline (Fig. 5A).

Bicuculline-sensitive DRPs remain after greatly restricting synaptic transmission

It is widely believed that PAD of low-threshold afferents is generated by minimally trisynaptic pathways.[1] We explored whether PAD can be generated via more direct actions of primary afferent transmitter release using mephenesin. Several labs have used mephenesin[63,64] to isolate monosynaptic components. We observed that low-threshold DRPs remain after curtailing di- and polysynaptic transmission with 1 mM mephenesin (Fig. 5A). This is consistent with an earlier *in vivo* report on the actions of mephenesin,[65] never cited in reviews on PAD. Concomitant recordings from the ventral root showed that the monosynaptic reflex amplitude was unaffected (Fig. 5B). Thus, trisynaptic and probably even disynaptic pathways were not required to generate the early component of the DRP. Overall, these results demonstrate that PAD of low-threshold primary afferents can occur by more direct synaptic mechanisms, including the possibility of direct negative feedback or nonspiking dendroaxonic pathways (Fig 3A).

DRPs can remain even after the block of glutamatergic transmission

Contrary to the dogma that primary afferent transmission is glutamatergic, much of the DRP remains after blockade of excitatory synaptic transmission with the ionotropic glutamate receptor antagonist kynurenate at a dose thought to fully block ionotropic glutamate receptors[66] (Fig. 5C). This is consistent with an earlier report in the isolated sacrococcygeal cord of adult rat.[67] To confirm

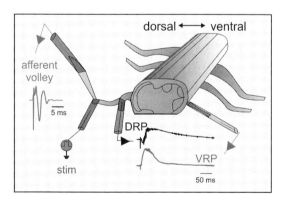

Figure 4. Methods for studying PAD-related mechanisms. Midsagittally hemisected spinal cords were isolated from mice or rats aged from postnatal days 7–14 and were prepared for *in vitro* experiments as described previously.[75] Stimulation is via the L5 dorsal root at 100 μA, 100 μs, or at 4T. A single stimulus produces a DRP that is almost entirely blocked by bicuculline. Low-threshold activation is confirmed by measuring the afferent volley produced by this stimulation and its TTX sensitivity.

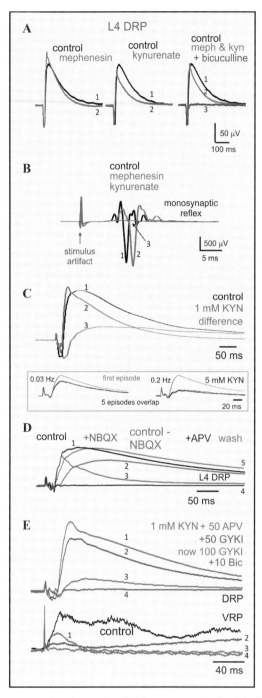

kynurenate block of glutamatergic transmission, we also showed that kynurenate always completely blocked the monosynaptic reflex (Fig. 5B) and almost blocked all of the subthreshold ventral root potential (VRP; Fig. 5E). On several occasions, kynurenate DRP block could be more substantial (e.g., at 5 mM). This is at least also partly explained by a sensitivity of the kynurenate-resistant DRP to stimulus frequency (we stimulated at a range between 0.033 and 0.2 Hz) (Fig. 5C, inset), but may also relate to recruitment of different afferents depending on the axons selected with the suction electrode. We also tested the actions of the non-NMDA receptor antagonists NBQX and GYKI52466. In the *presence* of the NMDA receptor antagonist APV, NBQX (Fig. 5D) but not GYKI (Fig. 5E) completely blocked the DRP. Note GYKI almost completely blocked the VRP at 50 μM whereas the DRP was only partially affected (5E, bottom). The differential sensitivity of glutamate receptors antagonists to afferent-evoked DRPs versus reflex actions has been observed previously *in vivo*.[68] Kynurenate insensitive afferent-evoked synaptic responses have also been reported in some dorsal horn neurons.[69] These variable results with the glutamate receptor antagonists

Figure 5. (A,B) Low-threshold DRPs remain after block both of polysynaptic transmission and ionotropic glutamate receptors. (A) Although mephenesin (1 mM) only slightly modifies the DRP, kynurenate (1 mM) reduced amplitude and more preferentially the duration of the DRP. Subsequent addition of bicuculline (10 μM) fully blocked the DRP. (B) Note that mephenesin

(1 mM) slowed onset of monosynaptic reflex but did not alter reflex amplitude. Kynurenate (1 mM), the broad spectrum glutamate ionotropic receptor antagonist completely blocked the reflex (*green trace*). (C–E) Differential sensitivity of DRPs to glutamate receptor antagonists. (C) Kynurenate blocks the longer latency component of the DRP (*difference trace*). Inset: Kynurenate actions are frequency sensitive. The DRP remaining after 5 mM kynurenate is greatly depressed by an afferent stimulation frequency of 0.2 Hz. (D) The selective AMPA receptor antagonist NBQX (10 μM) blocks the short latency component (see control—NBQX trace). Subsequent application of APV (50 μM) reversibly blocks the DRP. (E) APV has no effect subsequent to kynurenate application showing that kynurenate adequately blocked NMDA receptors. Like NBQX, GYKI52466 is a selective AMPA receptor antagonist but cannot fully block the DRP (after kynurenate and APV have already been added) even at a dose of 100 μM. Note the VRP is nearly completely blocked by 50 μM GYKI demonstrating a differential sensitivity of GYKI to VRP versus DRP. Numbers adjacent to traces reflect order of application.

suggest that a component of PAD may not require glutamatergic synaptic transmission. Moreover, some glutamate receptor antagonists could instead have direct actions at GABA$_A$-like receptors. For example, the quinoxalines (CNQX, DNQX, and NBQX) can act as antagonists of homooligomeric $\alpha 1$ and $\alpha 2$ glycine receptor subunits (NBQX IC$_{50}$ $5\,\mu M > DNQX > CNQX$)[70] and CNQX has a significant noncompetitive blocking effect on the GABA$_A$ receptor channel complex between 20 and $50\,\mu M$.[71]

Typical and atypical pharmacology of the DRP

We explored the sensitivity of the DRP to multiple ligands. Low doses of the glycine receptor antagonist strychnine (200 nM) partly blocked the DRP (Fig. 6A). Surprisingly, the nicotinic receptor antagonist tubocurarine selectively blocked the early component of the DRP in a dose-dependent manner (Fig. 6B). Moreover, the highly selective nicotinic receptor antagonist α-bungarotoxin also depressed the DRP (Fig. 6C). Sensitivity of the DRP to tubocurarine and α-bungarotoxin is consistent with actions on $\alpha 9\alpha 10$ nicotinic receptor subunits.[29,32] Remarkably, after pharmacologic isolation of the DRP with mephenesin and kynurenate, 5HT could also completely and reversibly block the DRP (Fig. 6D). Although 5-HT may be directly depressing the afferents generating the DRP, it may also be acting directly by blocking $\alpha 9\alpha 10$ nicotinic receptors.[72] Overall, these results suggest that the receptor(s) responsible for PAD have a hitherto unrecognized complex pharmacology. The common thread of these antagonists is their demonstrated actions on the Cys-loop family of transmitter-gated ion channels with common molecular architecture[29] (GABA$_A$, glycine, nicotinic, and 5-HT$_3$).

Many primary afferents are probably cholinergic

If afferent-evoked PAD occurs in part by direct negative feedback, primary afferents must release transmitters that can directly activate GABA$_A$-like receptors. One possibility is ACh acting on "GABA$_A$-like" nicotinic receptors. As stated earlier, a growing body of evidence suggests that many primary afferents have a cholinergic phenotype.[45–47,73] One of us (Kimura) has shown that pChAT, AchE, and the vesicular ACh transporter are immunodetected in DRG neurons (Fig. 7A). Importantly, Kimura and

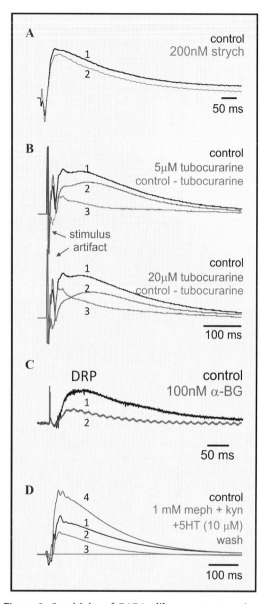

Figure 6. Sensitivity of GABA$_A$-like receptor to various ligands. (**A**) Strychnine blocks part of the early DRP. (**B**) Tubocurarine blocks the DRP in a dose-dependent manner. Subtraction from control demonstrates that the early DRP is preferentially inhibited. (**C**) α-Bungarotoxin reduces the DRP. (**D**) After synaptic isolation, 5HT reversibly blocks the DRP. 5-HT may be a competitive antagonist at the transmitter binding site that generates the DRP. Numbers adjacent to traces reflect order of application.

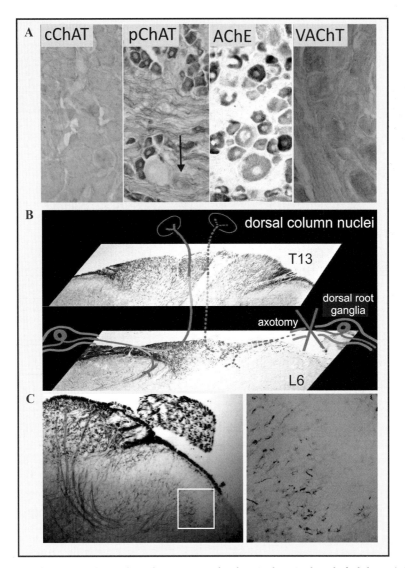

Figure 7. Expression of pChAT, AChE, and VAChT in DRG and pChAT in the spinal cord of adult rat. (A) Conventional antibody for ChAT (cChAT) does not label DRG neurons, but pChAT, AChE, and the vesicular ACh transporter (weakly) are immunodetected. Weaker staining in some larger DRG neurons (*arrow*) is consistent with lower expression detected with RT-PCR.[46] (B) pChAT immunolabeling in the dorsal columns. Note that after axotomy of the right L6 DRG, there is a complete loss of pChAT labeling in an associated band within the T13 dorsal column, verifying that all labeling arose from L6 primary afferents. (C) pChAT+ afferents project to deeper spinal laminae. Afferent entry and termination pattern is consistent with non-pain encoding cutaneous afferents.

colleagues have demonstrated that primary afferent axons that project via the dorsal columns have extensive pChAT labeling (Fig. 7B). Moreover, these afferents also project to deeper dorsal horn spinal laminae at sites consistent with termination of non-pain encoding low-threshold cutaneous afferents (Fig. 7C).

Primary afferents express taurine and β-alanine

Another possible mechanism for direct negative feedback of some afferents is the direct activation of GABA$_A$ receptors by the GABA$_A$R agonists taurine or β-alanine released from primary afferents. Although a single study inferred this for taurine,[56]

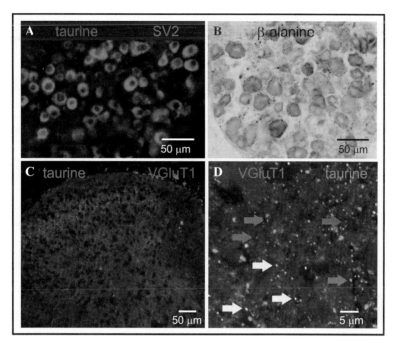

Figure 8. (A,B) Taurine/β-alanine labeling in DRG. (A) Taurine labels a population of synaptic vesicle 2 (SV2)-labeled neurons. (B) β-Alanine labeling in DRG appears more widespread. (C,D) Taurine has a distinctive labeling pattern in spinal cord. (C) Taurine punctate labeling does not appear to overlap with vGluT1+ synapses at low power. (D) In another animal, higher power confocal imaging shows that taurine colocalizes with several vGluT1+ putative primary afferent terminals in deep dorsal horn (laminae IV–V).

here we provide immunolabeling evidence for both amino acids. We have so far tested taurine in both rat and mouse and on both occasions numerous large DRG neurons were labeled (Fig. 8A). Similarly, β-alanine was tested in mouse and labeling was also in large-diameter cell bodies (Fig. 8B). Afferents with large-diameter cell bodies equate to low-threshold actions.[35]

Taurine labeling is in a subpopulation of primary afferent glutamatergic synapses

As observed previously,[56] taurine labeling is dominant in the superficial dorsal horn and largely punctate (Fig. 8C). Primary afferents are glutamatergic, so colabeling for taurine and the vesicular glutamate transporter 1 (vGluT1) would support cotransmission.[74] Preliminary observations demonstrate that taurine punctate labeling partly colocalized to a subpopulation of vGluT1 primary afferent putative glutamatergic synapses in deeper dorsal horn (Fig. 8D). These observations support the hypothesis that taurine is released from

vGluT1+ primary afferents via conventional synaptic mechanisms.

Conclusion

It is widely appreciated that presynaptic inhibition is "more powerful than postsynaptic inhibition in depressing the central excitatory actions of almost all primary afferent fibers."[9] It has been assumed, although never directly demonstrated, that this primary afferent depolarization (PAD) of low-threshold afferents is mediated by a trisynaptic pathway, and that GABAergic interneurons are essential.[1] We describe published and present further experimental evidence that PAD can also be generated by more direct synaptic pathways and may be at least partly independent of GABA and classical GABA$_A$ receptors. These findings suggest PAD mechanisms may be much more diverse than previously imagined, conceivably separated into distinct mechanisms for each genetically distinct afferent fiber population. If true, the current model of afferent-evoked PAD requires substantial updating.

Acknowledgments

SH was supported by the Christopher and Dana Reeve Foundation and the Craig Neilsen Foundation. JQ was supported by Conacyt 59873, Mexico. HK was supported by grant-in-aid for Scientific Research (JSPS), No. 20390051 (2008–2010).

Conflicts of interest

The authors declare no conflicts of interest.

References

1. Rudomin, P. & R.F. Schmidt. 1999. Presynaptic inhibition in the vertebrate spinal cord revisited. *Exp. Brain Res.* **129:** 1–37.

2. Barker, J.L. & R.A. Nicoll. 1973. The pharmacology and ionic dependency of amino acid responses in the frog spinal cord. *J. Physiol.* **228:** 259–277.

3. Eccles, J.C., R. Schmidt & W.D. Willis. 1963. Pharmacological studies on presynaptic inhibition. *J. Physiol.* 168, 500–530.

4. Jankowska, E. & J.S. Riddell. 1995. Interneurones mediating presynaptic inhibition of group II muscle afferents in the cat spinal cord. *J. Physiol. (Lond.)* **483:** 461–472.

5. Rudomin, P., M. Solodkin & I. Jimenez. 1987. Synaptic potentials of primary afferent fibers and motoneurons evoked by single intermediate nucleus interneurons in the cat spinal cord. *J. Neurophysiol.* **57:** 1288–1313.

6. Rudomin, P. 2009. In search of lost presynaptic inhibition. *Exp. Brain Res.* **196:** 139–151.

7. Wall, P.D. 1998. Some unanswered questions about the mechanisms and function of presynaptic inhibition. In *Presynaptic Inhibition and Neural Control.* P. Rudomin, R. Romo & L.M. Mendell, Eds.: 228–241. Oxford University Press. New York.

8. Franks, N.P. & W.R. Lieb. 1994 Molecular and cellular mechanisms of general anaesthesia. *Nature* **367:** 607–614.

9. Eccles, J.C. 1964. Presynaptic inhibition in the spinal cord. *Prog. Brain Res.* **12:** 65–91.

10. Jankowska, E., D. McCrea, P. Rudomin & E. Sykova. 1981. Observations on neuronal pathways subserving primary afferent depolarization. *J Neurophysiol.* **46:** 506–516.

11. Jimenez, I., P. Rudomin, M. Solodkin & L. Vyklicky.

1984. Specific and nonspecific mechanisms involved in generation of PAD of group Ia afferents in cat spinal cord. *J. Neurophysiol.* **52:** 921–940.

12. Wall, P.D. 1958. Excitability changes in afferent fibre terminations and their relation to slow potentials. *J. Physiol.* **142:** 1–21.

13. Jackson, M.F., D.T. Joo, A.A. Al Mahrouki, *et al.* 2003. Desensitization of alpha-amino-3-hydroxy-5-methyl-4-isoxazolepropionic acid (AMPA) receptors facilitates use-dependent inhibition by pentobarbital. *Mol. Pharmacol.* **64:** 395–406.

14. Marszalec, W. & T. Narahashi. 1993. Use-dependent pentobarbital block of kainate and quisqualate currents. *Brain Res.* **608:** 7–15.

15. Hughes, D.I., M. Mackie, G.G. Nagy, *et al.* 2005. P boutons in lamina IX of the rodent spinal cord express high levels of glutamic acid decarboxylase-65 and originate from cells in deep medial dorsal horn. *Proc. Natl. Acad. Sci. USA* **102:** 9038–9043.

16. Olave, M.J., N. Puri, R. Kerr & D.J. Maxwell. 2002. Myelinated and unmyelinated primary afferent axons form contacts with cholinergic interneurons in the spinal dorsal horn. *Exp. Brain Res.* **145:** 448–456.

17. Bannatyne, B.A., T.T. Liu, I. Hammar, *et al.* 2009. Excitatory and inhibitory intermediate zone interneurons in pathways from feline group I and II afferents: differences in axonal projections and input. *J. Physiol.* **587:** 379–399.

18. Eccles, J.C., F. Magni & W.D. Willis. 1962. Depolarization of central terminals of Group I afferent fibres from muscle. *J. Physiol.* **160:** 62–93.

19. Russo, R.E., R. Delgado-Lezama & J. Hounsgaard. 2000. Dorsal root potential produced by a TTX-insensitive micro-circuitry in the turtle spinal cord. *J. Physiol.* **528**(Pt 1): 115–122.

20. Kullmann, D.M., A. Ruiz, D.M. Rusakov, *et al.* 2005. Presynaptic, extrasynaptic and axonal GABAA receptors in the CNS: where and why? *Prog. Biophys. Mol. Biol.* **87:** 33–46.

21. Engelman, H.S. & A.B. MacDermott. 2004. Presynaptic ionotropic receptors and control of transmitter release. *Nat. Rev. Neurosci.* **5:** 135–145.

22. Todd, A.J. & R.C. Spike. 1993. The localization of classical transmitters and neuropeptides within neurons in laminae I-III of the mammalian spinal dorsal horn. *Prog. Neurobiol.* **41:** 609–638.

23. Alvarez, F.J. 1998. Anatomical basis for presynaptic inhibition of primary sensory fibers. In *Presynaptic Inhibition and Neural Control.* P. Rudomin, R. Romo & L. Mendell, Eds.: 13–49. Oxford University Press. New York.

24. Collins, G.G.S. 1974. The spontaneous and electrically evoked release of (3H)-GABA from the isolated hemisected frog spinal cord. *Brain Res.* **66:** 121–137.

25. Roberts, P.J. & J.F. Mitchell. 1972. The release of amino acids from the hemisected spinal cord during stimulation. *J. Neurochem.* **19:** 2473–2481.

26. Nicoll, R.A. & B.E. Alger. 1979. Presynaptic inhibition: transmitter and ionic mechanisms. In *International Review of Neurobiology* (ed. International Review of Neurobiology): 217–258. Academic Press. San Francisco.

27. Levy, R.A. 1977. The role of GABA in primary afferent depolarization. *Prog. Neurobiol.* **9:** 211–267.

28. Castro-Lopes, J.M., M. Malcangio, B.H. Pan & N.G. Bowery. 1995. Complex changes of GABA$_A$ and GABA$_B$ receptor binding in the spinal cord dorsal horn following peripheral inflammation or neurectomy. *Brain Res.* **679:** 289–297.

29. Alexander, S.P., A. Mathie & J.A. Peters. 2007. Transmitter-gated channels. *Br. J. Pharmacol.* **150**(Suppl 1): S82–S95.

30. Genzen, J.R., W. Van Cleve & D.S. McGehee. 2001. Dorsal root ganglion neurons express multiple nicotinic acetylcholine receptor subtypes. *J. Neurophysiol.* **86:** 1773–1782.

31. Lips, K.S., U. Pfeil & W. Kummer. 2002. Coexpression of alpha 9 and alpha 10 nicotinic acetylcholine receptors in rat dorsal root ganglion neurons. *Neuroscience* **115:** 1–5.

32. Rothlin, C.V., E. Katz, M. Verbitsky & A.B. Elgoyhen. 1999. The alpha9 nicotinic acetylcholine receptor shares pharmacological properties with type A gamma-aminobutyric acid, glycine, and type 3 serotonin receptors. *Mol. Pharmacol.* **55:** 248–254.

33. Jimenez, I., P. Rudomin & M. Solodkin. 1987 Mechanisms involved in the depolarization of cutaneous afferents produced by segmental and descending inputs in the cat spinal cord. *Exp. Brain Res.* **69:** 195–207.

34. Ninkovic, M. & S.P. Hunt. 1983. Alpha-bungarotoxin binding sites on sensory neurones and their axonal transport in sensory afferents. *Brain Res.* **272:** 57–69.

35. Willis, W.D., Jr. & R.E. Coggeshall. 1991. *Sensory Mechanisms of the Spinal Cord*. Plenum Press. New York.

36. Barber, R.P., P.E. Phelps, C.R. Houser, *et al.* 1984. The morphology and distribution of neurons containing choline acetyltransferase in the adult rat spinal cord: an immunocytochemical study. *J. Comp. Neurol.* **229:** 329–346.

37. Todd, A.J. 1991. Immunohistochemical evidence that acetylcholine and glycine exist in different populations of GABAergic neurons in lamina III of rat spinal dorsal horn. *Neuroscience* **44:** 741–746.

38. Das, P., C.L. Bell-Horner, T.K. Machu & G.H. Dillon. 2003. The GABA(A) receptor antagonist picrotoxin inhibits 5-hydroxytryptamine type 3A receptors. *Neuropharmacology* **44:** 431–438.

39. Zeitz, K.P., N. Guy, A.B. Malmberg, *et al.* 2002. The 5-HT3 subtype of serotonin receptor contributes to nociceptive processing via a novel subset of myelinated and unmyelinated nociceptors. *J. Neurosci.* **22:** 1010–1019.

40. Wang, P. & M.M. Slaughter. 2005. Effects of GABA receptor antagonists on retinal glycine receptors and on homomeric glycine receptor alpha subunits. *J. Neurophysiol.* **93:** 3120–3126.

41. Han, Y., P. Li & M.M. Slaughter. 2004. Selective antagonism of rat inhibitory glycine receptor subunits. *J. Physiol.* **554:** 649–658.

42. Li, P. & M. Slaughter. 2007. Glycine receptor subunit composition alters the action of GABA antagonists. *Vis. Neurosci.* **24:** 513–521.

43. Frazao, R., M.I. Nogueira & H. Wassle. 2007. Colocalization of synaptic GABA(C)-receptors with GABA (A)-receptors and glycine-receptors in the rodent central nervous system. *Cell Tissue Res.* **330:** 1–15.

44. Furuyama, T., M. Sato, K. Sato, *et al.* 1992. Co-expression of glycine receptor beta subunit and GABAA receptor gamma subunit mRNA in the rat dorsal root ganglion cells. *Brain Res. Mol. Brain Res.* **12:** 335–338.

45. Tooyama, I. & H. Kimura. 2000. A protein encoded by an alternative splice variant of choline acetyltransferase mRNA is localized preferentially in peripheral nerve cells and fibers. *J. Chem. Neuroanat.* **17:** 217–226.

46. Bellier, J.P. & H. Kimura. 2007. Acetylcholine synthesis by choline acetyltransferase of a peripheral type as demonstrated in adult rat dorsal root ganglion. *J. Neurochem.* **101:** 1607–1618.

47. Yasuhara, O., Y. Aimi, A. Matsuo & H. Kimura. 2008. Distribution of a splice variant of choline acetyltransferase in the trigeminal ganglion and brainstem of the rat: comparison with calcitonin gene-related peptide and substance P. *J. Comp. Neurol.* **509:** 436–448.

48. Tata, A.M., M.E. De Stefano, T.G. Srubek, *et al.* 2004. Subpopulations of rat dorsal root ganglion neurons express active vesicular acetylcholine transporter. *J. Neurosci. Res.* **75:** 194–202.

49. Tallini, Y.N., B. Shui, K.S. Greene, *et al.* 2006. BAC transgenic mice express enhanced green fluorescent protein in central and peripheral cholinergic neurons. *Physiol. Genomics* **27:** 391–397.

50. Matsumoto, M., W. Xie, M. Inoue & H. Ueda. 2007. Evidence for the tonic inhibition of spinal pain by

nicotinic cholinergic transmission through primary afferents. *Mol. Pain* **3:** 41.

51. Paleckova, V., J. Palecek, D.J. McAdoo & W.D. Willis. 1992. The non-NMDA antagonist CNQX prevents release of amino acids into the rat spinal cord dorsal horn evoked by sciatic nerve stimulation. *Neurosci. Lett.* **148:** 19–22.

52. Jia, F., M. Yue, D. Chandra, *et al.* 2008. Taurine is a potent activator of extrasynaptic GABA(A) receptors in the thalamus. *J. Neurosci.* **28:** 106–115.

53. Evans, R.H. 1978. The effects of amino acids and antagonists on the isolated hemisected spinal cord of the immature rat. *Br. J. Pharmacol.* **62:** 171–176.

54. Liu, Q.R., B. Lopez-Corcuera, S. Mandiyan, *et al.* 1993. Molecular characterization of four pharmacologically distinct gamma-aminobutyric acid transporters in mouse brain. *J. Biol. Chem.* **268:** 2106–2112.

55. Smith, K.E., L.A. Borden, C.H. Wang, *et al.* 1992. Cloning and expression of a high affinity taurine transporter from rat brain. *Mol. Pharmacol.* **42:** 563–569.

56. Lee, I.S., W.M. Renno & A.J. Beitz. 1992. A quantitative light and electron microscopic analysis of taurine-like immunoreactivity in the dorsal horn of the rat spinal cord. *J. Comp. Neurol.* **321:** 65–82.

57. Ledoux, M.S., L. Xu, J. Xiao, *et al.* 2006. Murine central and peripheral nervous system transcriptomes: comparative gene expression. *Brain Res.* **1107:** 24–41.

58. Bonhaus, D.W., S.E. Lippincott & R.J. Huxtable. 1984. Subcellular distribution of neuroactive amino acids in brains of genetically epileptic rats. *Epilepsia* **25:** 564–568.

59. Garcia, A. & J.N. Quevedo. 2001. PAD-evoked by selective stimulation of sensory afferents in neonatal rats and juvenile mice: an *in vitro* study. *Soc. Neurosci.* Abstracts 27.

60. Krasowski, M.D. & N.L. Harrison. 2000. The actions of ether, alcohol and alkane general anaesthetics on GABAA and glycine receptors and the effects of TM2 and TM3 mutations. *Br. J. Pharmacol.* **129:** 731–743.

61. Grinnell, A.D. 1970. Electrical interaction between antidromically stimulated frog motoneurones and dorsal root afferents: enhancement by gallamine and TEA. *J. Physiol.* **210:** 17–43.

62. Vinay, L., F. Brocard, S. Fellippa-Marques & F. Clarac. 1999. Antidromic discharges of dorsal root afferents in the neonatal rat. *J. Physiol. Paris* **93:** 359–367.

63. Lev-Tov, A. & M. Pinco. 1992. *In vitro* studies of prolonged synaptic depression in the neonatal rat spinal cord. *J. Physiol.* **447:** 149–169.

64. Quinlan, K.A. & O. Kiehn. 2007. Segmental, synaptic actions of commissural interneurons in the mouse spinal cord. *J. Neurosci.* **27:** 6521–6530.

65. Farkas, S., I. Tarnawa & P. Berzsenyi. 1989. Effects of some centrally acting muscle relaxants on spinal root potentials: a comparative study. *Neuropharmacology* **28:** 161–173.

66. Jahr, C.E. & K. Yoshioka. 1986. Ia afferent excitation of motoneurones in the *in vitro* new-born rat spinal cord is selectively antagonized by kynurenate. *J. Physiol. (Lond.)* **370:** 515–530.

67. Evans, R.H. & S.K. Long. 1989. Primary afferent depolarization in the rat spinal cord is mediated by pathways utilising NMDA and non-NMDA receptors. *Neurosci. Lett.* **100:** 231–236.

68. Farkas, S. & H. Ono. 1995. Participation of NMDA and non-NMDA excitatory amino acid receptors in the mediation of spinal reflex potentials in rats: an *in vivo* study. *Br. J. Pharmacol.* **114:** 1193–1205.

69. Schneider, S.P. & E.R. Perl. 1988. Comparison of primary afferent and glutamate excitation of neurons in the mammalian spinal dorsal horn. *J. Neurosci.* **8:** 2062–2073.

70. Meier, J. & V. Schmieden. 2003. Inhibition of alpha-subunit glycine receptors by quinoxalines. *Neuroreport* **14:** 1507–1510.

71. Jarolimek, W. & U. Misgeld. 1991. Reduction of GABA$_A$ receptor-mediated inhibition by the non-NMDA receptor antagonist 6-cyano-7-nitroquinoxaline- 2,3-dione in cultured neurons of rat brain. *Neurosci. Lett.* **121:** 227–230.

72. Rothlin, C.V., M.I. Lioudyno, A.F. Silbering, *et al.* 2003. Direct interaction of serotonin type 3 receptor ligands with recombinant and native alpha 9 alpha 10-containing nicotinic cholinergic receptors. *Mol. Pharmacol.* **63:** 1067–1074.

73. Matsuo, A., J.P. Bellier, T. Hisano, *et al.* 2005. Rat choline acetyltransferase of the peripheral type differs from that of the common type in intracellular translocation. *Neurochem. Int.* **46:** 423–433.

74. Alvarez, F.J., R.M. Villalba, R. Zerda & S.P. Schneider. 2004. Vesicular glutamate transporters in the spinal cord, with special reference to sensory primary afferent synapses. *J. Comp. Neurol.* **472:** 257–280.

75. Shay, B.L., M. Sawchuk, D.W. Machacek & S. Hochman. 2005. Serotonin 5HT2 receptors induce a long-lasting facilitation of spinal reflexes independent of ionotropic receptor activity. *J. Neurophysiol.* **94:** 2867–2877.

Ann. N.Y. Acad. Sci. ISSN 0077-8923

ANNALS OF THE NEW YORK ACADEMY OF SCIENCES

Issue: *Neurons and Networks in the Spinal Cord*

Synaptic pathways and inhibitory gates in the spinal cord dorsal horn

Tomonori Takazawa[1] and Amy B. MacDermott[1,2]

[1]Department of Physiology and Cellular Biophysics, and [2]Department of Neuroscience, Columbia University, New York, New York

Address for correspondence: Amy B. MacDermott, Department of Physiology and Cellular Biophysics, Columbia University, 630 West, 168th Street, New York, NY 10032. abm1@columbia.edu

Disinhibition in the dorsal horn accompanies peripheral nerve injury and causes the development of hypersensitivity to mild stimuli. This demonstrates the critical importance of inhibition in the dorsal horn for maintaining normal sensory signaling. Here we show that disinhibition induces a novel polysynaptic low-threshold input onto lamina I output neurons, suggesting that inhibition normally suppresses a preexisting pathway that probably contributes to abnormal pain sensations such as allodynia. In addition, we show that a significant proportion of superficial dorsal horn inhibitory neurons are activated by low-threshold input. These neurons are well situated to contribute to suppressing low-threshold activation of pain output neurons in lamina I. We further discuss several aspects of inhibition in the dorsal horn that might contribute to suppressing pathological signaling.

Keywords: inhibition; pain; tonic inhibition; dorsal horn

Introduction

The spinal cord dorsal horn is a key region in the central nervous system (CNS) in which sensory information is received, integrated, and relayed to higher brain structures. In fact, the dorsal horn receives inputs from a wide variety of primary afferent fibers including nociceptors, chemoreceptors, and thermoreceptors that respond to stimuli from the skin, muscles, joints, and viscera. The patterns of termination of primary afferents within the spinal cord are related to axonal diameter, receptive field, and sensory modality. Most nociceptive primary afferents are small-diameter thinly myelinated Aδ or unmyelinated C fibers. These terminate primarily in the superficial part of the dorsal horn, specifically in lamina I and II. Dorsal horn neurons in lamina III/IV receive low-threshold inputs from large-diameter, more heavily myelinated Aβ fibers of mechanoreceptors. Thus roughly speaking, touch sensitive fibers terminate deeper and nociceptive fibers terminate more superficially within the dorsal horn.

The dorsal horn neurons themselves are a mixture of neuron types. Nociceptive projection neurons are found in lamina I. Excitatory and inhibitory interneurons are found throughout lamina I, II, and III/IV. Some indications are beginning to emerge that there are detectable activity patterns in the dorsal horn indicating a dorsally directed flow of information. For example, a recent study used laser-scanning photostimulation to uncage glutamate to activate individual presynaptic dorsal horn neurons while recording postsynaptic responses. Excitatory synaptic drive was observed to move ventral to dorsal across lamina II toward lamina I through neurons with long ventral dendrites called vertical neurons.[1] This pattern suggested the idea that there are polysynaptic circuits that drive up toward the output neurons in lamina I.[1] The presence of such polysynaptic, ventral to dorsal circuits has been demonstrated under conditions of disinhibition[2–4] and is believed to be associated with behavioral allodynia.[3,5] Details of actual circuitries within lamina I and II, however, mostly remain obscure. Similarly, the general issue of how sensory modalities are processed properly within dorsal horn is still unclear. In this paper, we discuss the role of inhibition in dorsal horn for maintaining separation of sensory modalities such as touch and pain.

doi: 10.1111/j.1749-6632.2010.05501.x

Results and discussion

Disinhibition unmasks low-threshold input to pain output neurons

Chronic neuropathic pain often develops following peripheral nerve injury. One manifestation of that pain is allodynia, a painful response to a normally nonpainful stimulus. Behavioral studies have demonstrated that pharmacological disruption of dorsal horn inhibition *in vivo* using intrathecal antagonists for GABA$_A$ or glycine receptors transiently causes allodynia.[6–8] This suggests that inhibition is a critical element in maintaining separation between touch sensitive afferent input and projection neurons in lamina I that normally transmits information about noxious stimuli to higher centers in the CNS. Evidence that peripheral nerve injury causes a disruption of inhibition was subsequently demonstrated and shown to be, at least in part, due to a loss of Cl$^-$ gradient in lamina I neurons associated with accumulation of activated microglia.[9,10] Effective inhibition mediated by both GABA$_A$ and glycine receptors depends on a strong Cl$^-$ gradient and thus loss of the gradient diminishes inhibition.

Similarly, *in vitro* experiments have shown a strong impact of dorsal horn inhibition on excitatory synaptic drive from low-threshold peripheral fibers onto neurons in lamina I and II, a region where high-threshold fibers normally dominate. Disinhibition *in vitro* strongly enhances low-threshold activation of lamina II neurons,[11] demonstrating the importance of local inhibition for suppressing low-threshold drive. More recently, we have specifically tested whether pharmacological disinhibition is able to allow strong, low-threshold drive of lamina I output neurons.[4]

We took advantage of the fact that many projection neurons in lamina I express receptors for substance P, NK1 receptors.[12] Spinal cord slices were incubated with tetramethylrhodamine-conjugated substance P (TMR-SP) to label NK1 receptor positive (NK1R$^+$) neurons before recording dorsal-root evoked excitatory postsynaptic currents (EPSCs). Under control conditions, lamina I NK1R$^+$ neurons were shown to receive predominantly high-threshold (Aδ/C fiber) monosynaptic input. In the example shown in Figure 1A (left column), the NK1R$^+$ neuron received polysynaptic Aδ fiber and monosynaptic C fiber input.[4] However, blockade of local GABAergic and glycinergic inhibition with

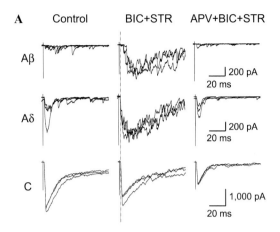

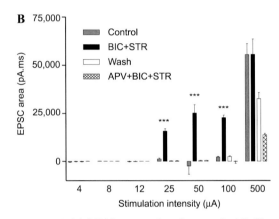

Figure 1. Disinhibition reveals polysynaptic Aβ fiber input to lamina I NK1R$^+$ neurons.[4] (A, B) Show data from a neuron with C fiber monosynaptic input that has polysynaptic Aβ fiber input revealed during disinhibition. (A, left column) Example of EPSCs evoked by stimulation (0.1 ms) using Aβ (25 μA), Aδ (100 μA), and C fiber (500 μA) stimulation intensities at low frequency under control conditions. Each trace comprises three superimposed traces evoked at 0.05 Hz. (Middle column) EPSCs evoked by the same stimulation protocol but in the presence of bicuculline (BIC; 10 μM) and strychnine (STR; 300 nM). (Right column) In the presence of APV (30 μM), BIC, and STR. B, the synaptic response stimulus-intensity profile generated by calculating the total EPSC area under the curve from the artifact to the end of the recording (900 ms) for each of the three EPSCs at each intensity tested and for all conditions.

bicuculline (10 μM) and strychnine (300 nM) revealed significant A fiber input to the lamina I NK1R$^+$ neuron that was predominantly Aβ fiber mediated (Fig. 1A, middle column). The total integrated current of EPSCs evoked using Aβ (25 μA) and Aδ (100 μA), but not C fiber (500 μA) stimulation intensities were significantly increased after disinhibition (Fig. 1B). This novel Aβ fiber input was identified as polysynaptic in nature because the input showed both failures and substantial variability of latency when recorded at high-stimulation frequencies (not shown). These results suggest the presence of an excitatory, polysynaptic pathway between low-threshold afferents and nociceptive NK1R$^+$ projection neurons that is normally suppressed by inhibition.

The polysynaptic excitatory pathway revealed by disinhibition was critically dependent upon NMDA receptor activation as shown in Figure 1A (right column). All of the novel polysynaptic activity that was activated in the presence of bicuculline and strychnine was inhibited by the NMDA selective receptor antagonist, APV (30 μM). In the presence of APV, the synaptic activity observed in the absence of bicuculline and strychnine are still apparent even though the newly revealed polysynaptic activity is blocked. These data indicate that disinhibition enhances the contribution of NMDA receptor activation to the polysynaptic low-threshold drive.

Subset of inhibitory neurons in dorsal horn receive low-threshold input

Pharmacological disinhibition, mimicking disinhibition associated with nerve injury, allowed us to observe an underlying polysynaptic excitatory pathway in the dorsal horn between low-threshold afferents and lamina I output neurons. This raises the question of how inhibition suppresses this pathway under normal, nonpathological, or nonpharmacologically altered conditions. It is known that about 30% of the neurons in the superficial dorsal horn are immunoreactive for GABA, and glycine coexists in a subpopulation of these neurons, supporting the idea that inhibitory neurons have an important role in local network activity.[13] Normal inhibition of the polysynaptic excitatory pathway acts as a gate, preventing the painful consequences. One way to control such a gate would be to simultaneously have low-threshold synaptic drive of inhibitory neurons that could suppress the existing polysynaptic excitatory pathway between low-threshold afferents and NK1R$^+$ projection neurons.

To test for low-threshold synaptic excitation of lamina I and II inhibitory neurons, we used ho-

mozygotic transgenic mice that express EGFP under control of the *gad1* gene promoter to identify glutamic acid decarboxylase 67 (GAD67) GABAergic neurons. This results in fluorescent labeling of 30–70% of the GABAergic neurons in the dorsal horn.[14–16] Recording from these neurons and stimulating the dorsal root to activate low- and high-threshold sensory afferent fibers allowed us to investigate the excitatory synaptic inputs onto GABAergic inhibitory neurons.[17] A subclass of EGFP positive GABAergic neurons had low threshold, Aβ fiber input as well as input from high-threshold fibers (Aδ and/or C). For example, the data shown in Figure 2A were recorded from a neuron that received Aβ fiber input identified as polysynaptic due to synaptic failures seen at high-frequency (20 Hz) stimulation (arrows). In addition, this neuron received both monosynaptic (arrowheads) and polysynaptic (open arrowheads) C fiber input.[17] Indeed, Aβ fibers activate a significant proportion (∼20%) of lamina I and II GABAergic neurons (Fig. 2B). This occurs with similar excitatory synaptic drive throughout postnatal maturation, but with a greater prevalence at younger ages.[17]

These GABAergic neurons receiving low-threshold, primary afferent, synaptic drive are well suited to contribute to suppressing low-threshold activation of output projection neurons. Low-threshold activation of inhibitory neurons is also consistent with the classical idea that nociceptive projection neurons are activated mainly by noxious afferent input that "opens" the gate while low-threshold, non-noxious fibers inhibit this signal and "close" the gate.[18] However, nearly all of the inhibitory neurons tested in our studies that received low threshold input also received high-threshold excitatory drive (Fig. 2B), a combination that is not predicted by the gate theory of pain. It may be that more extensive information about local circuitry considered together with sensory modality will be required to understand the impact these inhibitory neurons have on pain detection.

Mechanical allodynia

Recent evidence has been accumulating regarding a similar but different polysynaptic pathway that subserves a specific type of allodynia, dynamic mechanical allodynia. This pathway begins in inner lamina II (lamina IIi). In this region of the dorsal horn, there is a population of excitatory interneurons

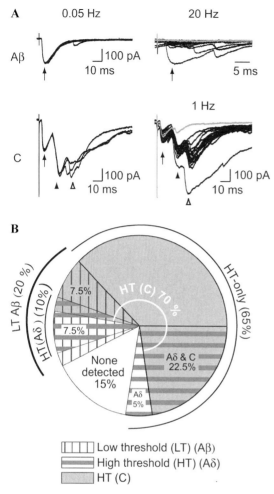

Figure 2. Low-threshold (Aβ) fiber input as well as input from high-threshold fibers (Aδ and/or C) to GABAergic neurons.[17] (A) Example recordings from a P35 GABAergic neuron with input from Aβ and C fibers. (Upper panel) Three consecutive traces show responses to low-frequency Aβ fiber stimulation (left, 0.05 Hz, 25 μA, *arrow*). Twenty consecutive Aβ fiber responses to high-frequency stimulation (right, 20 Hz, *arrow*, expanded timescale). (Lower panel) C fiber input was observed when the stimulation intensities were increased (left, 0.05 Hz, 500 μA, *arrowheads*). The C fiber response had a monosynaptic component with no failures (but note the small amplitude in the gray trace) when tested at high frequency (right, 1 Hz, *filled arrowhead*). There was also a later, polysynaptic C fiber component with failures (*open arrowhead*, illustrated by the gray trace). (B) The proportion of GABAergic neurons with input from different afferent fiber classes is summarized. For simplicity, this representation does not distinguish

that express the enzyme, PKCγ and that receive low-threshold afferent input.[19] These PKCγ+ positive (PKCγ+) neurons are a key element for activated circuits after disinhibition by intrathecal application of glycine receptor antagonist, unmasking normally blocked local excitatory circuits onto nociceptive output neurons.[2,3] However, this circuit does not involve lamina I NK1R+ neurons.[3] This evidence suggests that dynamic mechanical allodynia is transmitted through a specific pathway that involves non-nociceptive myelinated primary afferents, PKCγ+ neurons as a gateway, and NK1R negative (NK1R−) lamina I projection neurons, as shown in Figure 3. Thus, glycinergic inhibition appears to be a key player to prevent dynamic mechanical allodynia.

What is the source of this glycinergic inhibition? A significant proportion of superficial dorsal horn neurons have immunoreactivity for glycine. In addition, a recent study reported that presynaptic inhibitory neurons, which send inhibitory output onto postsynaptic lamina I–III neurons, are located relatively close to postsynaptic neurons along the dorso-ventral axis, suggesting local inhibitory synaptic connections are mostly made within the same lamina.[1] Therefore, we predict that glycinergic inhibitory neurons located near the lamina II/III border may directly inhibit PKCγ+ neurons to close the gate by blocking the pathway activated for dynamic mechanical allodynia. Figure 3 shows a schematic diagram for putative neuron networks causing mechanical allodynia and suppressing it under normal conditions.

Region- and cell type-specific inhibitory control of superficial dorsal horn neurons

Given that the distinct physiological roles of different dorsal horn neurons depend on their location and their neurochemical properties, it is important to determine whether, in fact, dorsal horn neurons receive synaptic inhibition in a region- and/or cell type-specific manner. It has been shown that adult lamina I neurons receive only glycinergic synaptic

between monosynaptic and polysynaptic responses. There is considerable overlap between the subsets of GABAergic neurons receiving input from each class of afferent fiber type.

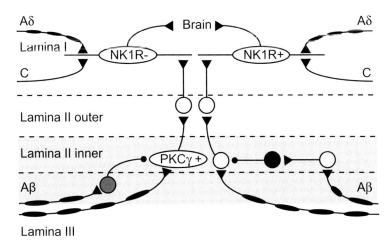

Figure 3. Schematic diagram illustrating two putative dorsal horn neural networks involved in mechanical allodynia. The schematic diagram was drawn based on evidence reported by several groups.[1–4,17,19] NK1R$^+$ neurons that receive innocuous input through polysynaptic pathways seem to be part of a local excitatory circuit that mediates mechanical allodynia after loss of GABAergic and glycinergic inhibitory control.[4] Inhibitory interneurons in lamina II (*black*) receiving polysynaptic Aβ fiber input may inhibit neurons that relay non-nociceptive information to NK1R$^+$ neurons.[17] Moreover, PKC γ$^+$ neurons that receive innocuous input via Aβ fibers at the lamina II/III border (*shaded*) are part of a local excitatory circuit that mediates dynamic mechanical allodynia after loss of glycinergic inhibitory control.[2] We tentatively put a glycinergic inhibitory interneuron (*gray*) at the lamina II/III border. Given local inhibitory synaptic connection within same lamina,[1] glycinergic inhibitory interneurons may be at lamina II/III border, although their exact location is still unknown. The target of the PKC γ$^+$ neuron appears to be lamina I neurons lacking NK1 receptors.[3]

inhibition, whereas about a half of lamina II neurons received pure GABAergic and the rest received mixed GABAergic and glycinergic inhibition.[20] In addition, other studies have focused on cell type-specific inhibition in the dorsal horn. For example, central cells, which are commonly situated in the mid-zone of the lamina II, receive GABAergic inhibition from islet cells.[21] Moreover, inhibitory synaptic connections have been demonstrated between lamina II inhibitory interneurons identified by endogenous EGFP under the control of the GAD65 promoter.[22] However, what drives the activity of identified neurons with specific physiological roles in the dorsal horn has still not been well studied. We expect that genetic and/or neurochemical approaches to neuron identification will facilitate investigations of cell type-specific inhibitory control of dorsal horn neurons. This in turn would provide insight into sensory information processing within spinal cord dorsal horn. Interestingly, some lamina II neurons receive tonic GABAergic and glycinergic inhibition, suggesting that superficial dorsal horn neurons are inhibited through two different modes, phasic, and tonic, similar to other CNS regions.[23–25]

We predict that tonic inhibition may be important in regulating the inhibitory tone in the dorsal horn.

Conclusions

There are several polysynaptic excitatory circuits in the dorsal horn that carry low-threshold signals to lamina I output neurons. The inhibition of these pathways is critically important to avoid pathological pain. This focuses attention on the mechanisms by which inhibition functions within the dorsal horn.

Acknowledgment

This study was supported by NIH NS 029797.

Conflicts of interest

The authors declare no conflicts of interest.

References

1. Kato, G. *et al.* 2009. Organization of intralaminar and translaminar neuronal connectivity in the superficial spinal dorsal horn. *J. Neurosci.* **29:** 5088–5099.

2. Miraucourt, L.S., R. Dallel & D.L. Voisin. 2007. Glycine inhibitory dysfunction turns touch into pain through PKCgamma interneurons. *PLoS ONE.* **2:** e1116.

3. Miraucourt, L.S. *et al.* 2009. Glycine inhibitory dysfunction induces a selectively dynamic, morphine-resistant, and neurokinin 1 receptor- independent mechanical allodynia. *J. Neurosci.* **29:** 2519–2527.

4. Torsney, C. & A.B. MacDermott. 2006. Disinhibition opens the gate to pathological pain signaling in superficial neurokinin 1 receptor-expressing neurons in rat spinal cord. *J. Neurosci.* **26:** 1833–1843.

5. Keller, A.F. *et al.* 2007. Transformation of the output of spinal lamina I neurons after nerve injury and microglia stimulation underlying neuropathic pain. *Mol. Pain* **3:** 27.

6. Beyer, C., L.A. Roberts & B.R. Komisaruk. 1985. Hyperalgesia induced by altered glycinergic activity at the spinal cord. *Life Sci.* **37:** 875–882.

7. Roberts, L.A., C. Beyer & B.R. Komisaruk. 1986. Nociceptive responses to altered GABAergic activity at the spinal cord. *Life Sci.* **39:** 1667–1674.

8. Yaksh, T.L. 1989. Behavioral and autonomic correlates of the tactile evoked allodynia produced by spinal glycine inhibition: effects of modulatory receptor systems and excitatory amino acid antagonists. *Pain.* **37:** 111–123.

9. Coull, J.A. *et al.* 2005. BDNF from microglia causes the shift in neuronal anion gradient underlying neuropathic pain. *Nature* **438:** 1017–1021.

10. Coull, J.A. *et al.* 2003. Trans-synaptic shift in anion gradient in spinal lamina I neurons as a mechanism of neuropathic pain. *Nature* **424:** 938–942.

11. Baba, H. *et al.* 2003. Removal of GABAergic inhibition facilitates polysynaptic A fiber-mediated excitatory transmission to the superficial spinal dorsal horn. *Mol. Cell. Neurosci.* **24:** 818–830.

12. Todd, A.J., M.M. McGill & S.A. Shehab. 2000. Neurokinin 1 receptor expression by neurons in laminae I, III and IV of the rat spinal dorsal horn that project to the brainstem. *Eur. J. Neurosci.* **12:** 689–700.

13. Todd, A.J. & A.C. Sullivan. 1990. Light microscope study of the coexistence of GABA-like and glycine-like immunoreactivities in the spinal cord of the rat. *J. Comp. Neurol.* **296:** 496–505.

14. Dougherty, K.J., M.A. Sawchuk & S. Hochman. 2005. Properties of mouse spinal lamina I GABAergic interneurons. *J. Neurophysiol.* **94:** 3221–3227.

15. Dougherty, K.J., M.A. Sawchuk & S. Hochman. 2009. Phenotypic diversity and expression of GABAergic inhibitory interneurons during postnatal development in lumbar spinal cord of glutamic acid decarboxylase 67-green fluorescent protein mice. *Neuroscience* **163:** 909–919.

16. Heinke, B. *et al.* 2004. Physiological, neurochemical and morphological properties of a subgroup of GABAergic spinal lamina II neurones identified by expression of green fluorescent protein in mice. *J. Physiol.* **560:** 249–266.

17. Daniele, C.A. & A.B. MacDermott. 2009. Low-threshold primary afferent drive onto GABAergic interneurons in the superficial dorsal horn of the mouse. *J. Neurosci.* **29:** 686–695.

18. Melzack, R. & P.D. Wall. 1965. Pain mechanisms: a new theory. *Science (New York, N.Y.)* **150:** 971–979.

19. Neumann, S. *et al.* 2008. Innocuous, not noxious, input activates PKCgamma interneurons of the spinal dorsal horn via myelinated afferent fibers. *J. Neurosci.* **28:** 7936–7944.

20. Keller, A.F. *et al.* 2001. Region-specific developmental specialization of GABA-glycine cosynapses in laminas I-II of the rat spinal dorsal horn. *J. Neurosci.* **21:** 7871–7880.

21. Lu, Y. & E.R. Perl. 2003. A specific inhibitory pathway between substantia gelatinosa neurons receiving direct C-fiber input. *J. Neurosci.* **23:** 8752–8758.

22. Labrakakis, C. *et al.* 2009. Inhibitory coupling between inhibitory interneurons in the spinal cord dorsal horn. *Mol. Pain* **5:** 24.

23. Ataka, T. & J.G. Gu. 2006. Relationship between tonic inhibitory currents and phasic inhibitory activity in the spinal cord lamina II region of adult mice. *Mol. Pain.* **2:** 36.

24. Takahashi, A., T. Mashimo & I. Uchida. 2006. GABAergic tonic inhibition of substantia gelatinosa neurons in mouse spinal cord. *Neuroreport* **17:** 1331–1335.

25. Takazawa, T. & A.B. MacDermott. 2008. Disinhibition mediated by tonic activation of GABAergic and glycinergic receptors on inhibitory interneurons in mouse superficial dorsal horn. SFN Abstracts771.778.

Ann. N.Y. Acad. Sci. ISSN 0077-8923

ANNALS OF THE NEW YORK ACADEMY OF SCIENCES
Issue: *Neurons and Networks in the Spinal Cord*

Modulation of developing dorsal horn synapses by tissue injury

Mark L. Baccei

Pain Research Center, Department of Anesthesiology, University of Cincinnati Medical Center, Cincinnati, Ohio

Address for correspondence: Dr. Mark L. Baccei, Pain Research Center, Department of Anesthesiology, University of Cincinnati Medical Center, 231 Albert Sabin Way, Cincinnati, OH 45267. mark.baccei@uc.edu

Although tissue injury can evoke significant hyperalgesia in infants from the first days of life, little is known about how injury affects emergent central pain networks at the synaptic level. Recent studies have investigated whether tissue damage at different ages has distinct consequences for synaptic function in the rat superficial dorsal horn (SDH) using *in vitro* patch clamp recordings from spinal cord slices prepared at different times after an injury. The results demonstrate that tissue damage during the first postnatal week transiently increases the frequency (but not amplitude) of miniature excitatory postsynaptic currents (mEPSCs), while no changes are observed at inhibitory synapses onto the same neurons. Prolonged blockade of sciatic nerve activity *in vivo* with bupivacaine hydroxide or tetrodotoxin prevented the elevation in mEPSC frequency following early injury. In contrast, tissue damage during the third postnatal week failed to significantly alter spontaneous excitatory or inhibitory synaptic transmission in the SDH. These data show that afferent activity arising from injured peripheral tissue selectively regulates glutamatergic synaptic signaling in the developing SDH in a highly age-dependent manner.

Keywords: inflammation; glutamate; neonatal; spinal cord; patch clamp; nerve block

Introduction

Infants and children can experience considerable pain as the result of disease, surgery, or intensive care therapy. A recent study found that neonates in the intensive care unit (NICU) underwent >10 tissue-damaging procedures each day during the first days of life.[1] However, the clinical management of pain in this population remains inadequate.[2,3] Efforts to design improved analgesic strategies that are more developmentally appropriate have been hampered by a lack of information regarding how immature pain circuits in the central nervous system (CNS) respond to tissue damage at a cellular and molecular level.

It is now well known that neonatal pain networks are not simply less mature forms of those found in adults, but are rather organized in a fundamentally different manner. Nociceptive withdrawal reflexes are exaggerated in the neonate compared to the adult, as evidenced by lower thresholds, larger receptive fields, and prolonged muscle contractions,[4] which suggests an altered balance between synaptic excitation and inhibition exists within the neonatal spinal cord. In support of this, recent work has demonstrated that synaptic function within the superficial dorsal horn (SDH), which receives dense projections from nociceptive (Aδ and C-fiber) sensory neurons in the dorsal root ganglion and thus represents a critical relay station in the pain pathway, changes significantly during the early postnatal period. For example, neonatal SDH neurons are distinguished by their relatively weak C-fiber inputs,[5,6] lack of glycinergic inhibition, and the presence of GABAergic depolarizations[7] which likely reflect an immature Cl$^-$ extrusion capacity.[8]

This distinct organization of the SDH synaptic network at early postnatal ages might predict novel effects of neonatal tissue injury on synaptic signaling within the dorsal horn. It is clear that tissue damage can enhance the overall excitability of the spinal cord (termed "central sensitization") in both neonates and adults, as behavioral hyperalgesia is

doi: 10.1111/j.1749-6632.2009.05425.x

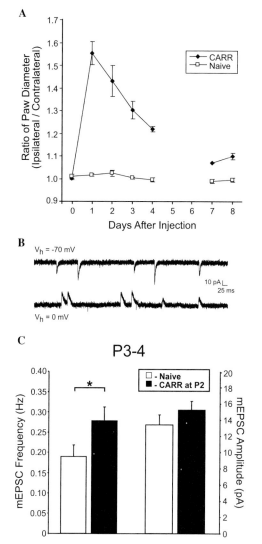

observed under pathological conditions throughout postnatal development.[9–11] However, the underlying synaptic mechanisms of this spinal hyperexcitability could depend on postnatal age. Unfortunately, little is known about how tissue injury at different ages modulates synaptic function within developing pain circuits. As a result, the aim of the current studies was to investigate whether tissue damage evokes age-dependent alterations in synaptic transmission within the SDH.

Results

Peripheral inflammation during early life selectively facilitates glutamatergic signaling in the superficial dorsal horn

To evaluate the effect of neonatal tissue damage on synaptic function within the SDH, λ-carrageenan (a polysaccharide from the cell walls of red algae) was injected into the plantar surface of the rat hindpaw at postnatal day (P)2. Carrageenans are well-known to evoke the release of inflammatory mediators such as 5-HT and bradykinin in the rodent skin, resulting in significant and persistent swelling of the ipsilateral hindpaw following subcutaneous injection (Fig. 1A). Spinal cord slices were prepared from carrageenan-treated (CARR) pups or naïve littermates 1–2 days later and miniature excitatory postsynaptic currents (mEPSCs) and inhibitory postsynaptic currents (mIPSCs) were recorded in neonatal SDH neurons using *in vitro* patch-clamp techniques (Fig. 1B). All sampled neurons were located between

(i.e., day 0 after injection) increases the ipsilateral paw diameter compared to the contralateral side ($P < 0.001$ compared to naïve; two-way ANOVA). (B) Examples of traces illustrating mEPSCs isolated at a holding potential (V_h) of -70 mV (*top*) and mIPSCs recorded in the same neuron from a V_h of 0 mV (*bottom*). (C) Carrageenan (CARR) treatment at P2 evoked a significant increase in mEPSC frequency (*left*; $^*P = 0.011$; Mann–Whitney test), but not mEPSC amplitude (*right*), in P3–4 SDH neurons compared to naïve littermate controls. (D) Neither the mIPSC frequency (*left*) nor mIPSC amplitude (*right*) at P3–4 was affected by peripheral inflammation from P2. [This figure has been reproduced with permission of the International Association for the Study of Pain® (IASP®).]

Figure 1. Peripheral inflammation during the early postnatal period facilitates excitatory signaling in the neonatal rat SDH.[13] (A) Subcutaneous injection of carrageenan (0.7 μL/g body weight at 2%) into the left hindpaw at P2

50 and 150 μm from the edge of the dorsal white matter, suggesting that the majority of these neurons resided in lamina II.[12]

Peripheral inflammation from P2 significantly increased mEPSC frequency at P3–4 compared to naïve controls (Naïve: 0.19 ± 0.03 Hz, n = 34; CARR: 0.28 ± 0.03 Hz, n = 34; $P = 0.011$; Mann–Whitney test; see Fig. 1C) without significantly changing mEPSC amplitude. In contrast, CARR treatment failed to alter mIPSC frequency or amplitude in the same neurons (Fig. 1D), suggesting a selective effect of tissue injury on glutamatergic synaptic function in the neonatal SDH.[13] Meanwhile, the naïve and CARR groups exhibited a similar mEPSC frequency by P10–11 (data not shown), suggesting that the potentiation of glutamatergic transmission did not persist beyond the duration of the original tissue damage.[13]

Does the effect of peripheral inflammation on SDH synapses depend on postnatal age? To address this question, adjusted volumes of CARR were injected at either postnatal day (P) 9 or P17 in order to evoke tissue injury of a similar degree to that observed following CARR administration at P2, and again miniature synaptic currents from lamina II neurons were analyzed at the height of the inflammatory response.[13] The results clearly demonstrate that peripheral inflammation occurring during the second or third postnatal week has different consequences for SDH synaptic function compared to an inflammation at P2, as no significant differences in mEPSC frequency or amplitude were observed between the naïve and inflamed groups at the later ages (Fig. 2).

A selective increase in mEPSC frequency after carrageenan treatment during the early postnatal period predicts changes in presynaptic function at glutamatergic terminals within the SDH under pathological conditions. To determine whether peripheral inflammation alters the probability of glutamate release at primary afferent synapses within the neonatal SDH, we measured the effect of CARR injections at P2 on the paired-pulse ratio (PPR) of monosynaptic EPSCs evoked by dorsal root stimulation at P3–4.[13] There were no significant differences in the PPR of primary afferent-evoked EPSCs between the naïve and CARR groups at any interstimulus interval examined (Naïve: n = 18; CARR: n = 23; $P = 0.836$; Two-way ANOVA; see Fig. 3B). As illustrated in Figure 3D, similar re-

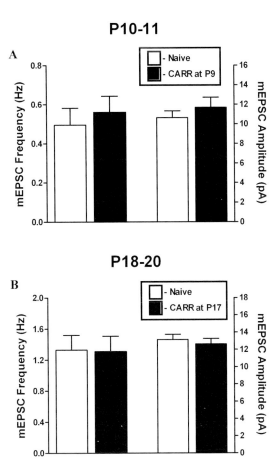

Figure 2. Peripheral inflammation during the second or third postnatal week fails to modulate glutamatergic synaptic transmission in the SDH.[13] (A) Hindpaw injections of carrageenan at P9 had no significant effects on spontaneous excitatory synaptic signaling in P10–11 SDH neurons. (B) Excitatory synaptic function at P18–20 was similarly unaffected by carrageenan treatment at P17, suggesting that the ability of tissue injury to facilitate glutamatergic synaptic signaling is restricted to the early postnatal period. [This figure has been reproduced with permission of the International Association for the Study of Pain® (IASP®).]

sults were observed when activating local excitatory interneurons using focal stimulation within the SDH.[13] Collectively, the results strongly suggest that the enhanced mEPSC frequency produced by peripheral inflammation during the first postnatal week is not accompanied by significant alterations in the probability of glutamate release within the dorsal horn.

A

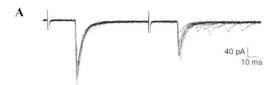

40 pA | 10 ms

B

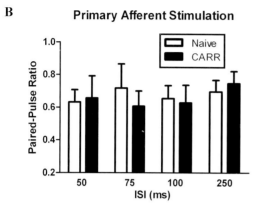

Primary Afferent Stimulation

Paired-Pulse Ratio (y-axis: 0.2 to 1.0)

Legend: Naive (white), CARR (black)

ISI (ms): 50, 75, 100, 250

C

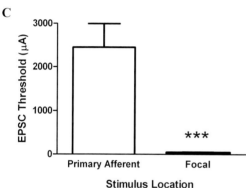

EPSC Threshold (μA) (y-axis: 0 to 3000)

Primary Afferent | Focal ***

Stimulus Location

D

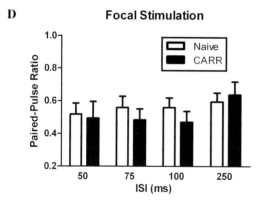

Focal Stimulation

Paired-Pulse Ratio (y-axis: 0.2 to 1.0)

Legend: Naive (white), CARR (black)

ISI (ms): 50, 75, 100, 250

Figure 3. Increased excitatory signaling after early tissue injury does not result from alterations in the probability of glutamate release within the neonatal dorsal horn.[13] (**A**) Representative traces showing monosynaptic EPSCs evoked in a P3 dorsal horn neuron following paired electrical stimulation of the attached dorsal root.

Ongoing primary afferent activity is required for the potentiation of excitatory signaling after early injury

While the aforementioned data suggest that glutamatergic transmission onto developing lamina II neurons is enhanced by aberrant input from sensory afferents following tissue damage, there is no direct evidence that the observed synaptic changes are activity-dependent. To investigate this issue, we used an incision through the skin and muscle of the mid-thigh as a model of surgical injury, which has the additional advantage of providing access to the sciatic nerve in order to manipulate the level of sensory input to the developing spinal cord *in vivo* during the post-injury period.[14] As seen with the carrageenan model, surgical injury during the first postnatal week (at P3) selectively increased the mEPSC frequency in lamina II cells compared to naïve littermates (Naïve: 0.24 ± 0.05 Hz, n = 30; Incision: 0.50 ± 0.11 Hz, n = 27; $P = 0.030$; Mann–Whitney test; see Figure 4A), while the same incision performed at P17 failed to modulate glutamatergic function in the SDH at 2–3 days postinjury (Fig. 4B). As expected, mIPSC properties at this time point were not altered by the skin/muscle incision at either age (data not shown). In addition, a third experimental group undergoing incision at P3 exhibited a significantly *lower* mEPSC

Ten pairs of stimuli were delivered (at 2X threshold) at each interstimulus interval (ISI; 50–250 ms), the traces averaged, and the paired-pulse ratio (PPR) calculated as mean EPSC2/mean EPSC1 at each ISI for a given neuron. (**B**) There were no significant differences in the mean PPR of primary afferent-evoked EPSCs between the naïve and carrageenan-treated littermates across the range of ISI examined. (**C**) Significantly lower stimulus intensities (at a duration of 100 μs) were required to evoke an EPSC in P3–4 SDH neurons using focal stimulation within the SDH compared to the use of primary afferent (i.e., dorsal root) stimulation (*** $P < 0.0001$; Mann–Whitney test), suggesting the recruitment of different populations of synaptic inputs onto SDH neurons. (**D**) Inflammation at P2 also failed to alter the PPR of focally evoked EPSCs across the range of ISI at P3–4. [This figure has been reproduced with permission of the International Association for the Study of Pain® (IASP®).]

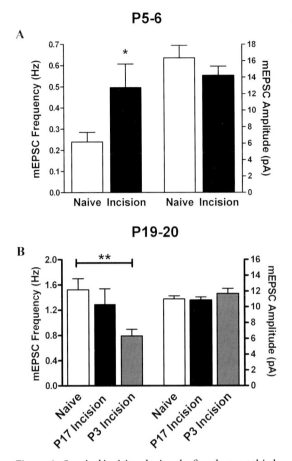

Figure 4. Surgical incision during the first, but not third, postnatal week transiently increases mEPSC frequency in SDH neurons.[14] (A) Incision at P3 causes a significant elevation in the mEPSC rate (*$P = 0.03$; Mann–Whitney test) at P5–6. (B) P3 surgical incision (*gray bars*) selectively decreased mEPSC frequency at P19–20 compared to naïve (*white*) littermates (**$P < 0.01$; Kruskal–Wallis test), while incision at P17 had no significant effect at the same time point.

frequency compared to naïve littermates at P19–20 (Naïve: 1.53 ± 0.17 Hz, n = 83; P3 Incision: 0.79 ± 0.10 Hz, n = 55; $P < 0.01$; Fig. 4B), suggesting that early tissue damage can evoke a biphasic modulation of glutamatergic transmission in the developing dorsal horn.[14]

To determine whether the transient facilitation of glutamatergic signaling requires ongoing peripheral input, we employed two different approaches to reduce primary afferent drive to the spinal cord *in vivo* during the 2–3 day post-injury period and

subsequently characterized synaptic function in the SDH as described earlier.

Immediately following the mid-thigh surgical incision at P3, bupivacaine hydroxide (BUPI) was implanted into the wound site around the sciatic nerve. Figure 5A demonstrates that BUPI evoked a significant reduction in mechanical sensitivity (i.e., lower number of hindpaw withdrawals) on the ipsilateral paw compared to the contralateral paw or littermates undergoing incision without BUPI treatment.[14] A prolonged unilateral sensory block was also confirmed by a reduction in capsaicin-evoked c-fos activation in the dorsal horn (data not shown). Importantly, blocking primary afferent input with BUPI prevented the enhancement of mEPSC frequency following the incision at P3 (Naïve: 0.18 ± 0.04 Hz, n = 18; Incision only: 0.44 ± 0.07 Hz, n = 9; Incision + BUPI: 0.11 ± 0.03 Hz, n = 8; $P < 0.01$, Kruskal–Wallis test; Fig. 5B), without significantly affecting mEPSC amplitude (Fig. 5C) or mIPSC properties (data not shown).

To confirm the role of afferent activity, we employed an additional method for prolonged sensory blockade *in vivo* in which TTX was slowly released from microcapillaries inserted under the epineurium of the sciatic nerve.[15,16] TTX application at P3 produced a significant increase in the mechanical withdrawal threshold on the ipsilateral paw compared to naïve and vehicle-treated littermate controls (Fig. 6A). To confirm that this reflected a spatially restricted block of sciatic nerve conduction by TTX, *in vitro* compound action potentials (CAPs) were recorded from sensory fibers in the L4/L5 dorsal roots 3 days after the microcapillaries were inserted. Average stimulus-response curves for dorsal root CAPs from the naïve, vehicle and TTX-treated groups demonstrate that TTX application causes a significant decrease in the excitability of sciatic nerve fibers when stimulation occurs below (i.e., more distal to) the location of the TTX microcapillary (n = 5), yet when the electrical stimulation is delivered above (i.e., more proximal to) the site of the microcapillary the stimulus-response relationship for the TTX-treated nerves is similar to naïve (n = 3) and vehicle-treated (n = 4) controls (Fig. 6B). These results clearly demonstrate that TTX delivery to the immature sciatic nerve *in vivo* produces a highly localized conduction block.[14]

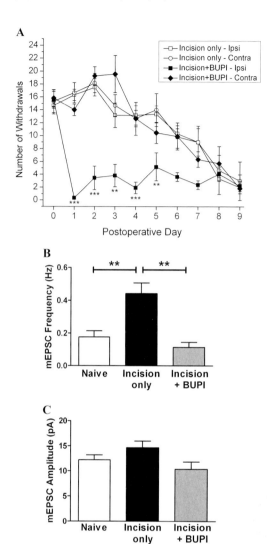

Figure 5. Reducing sensory input to the developing SDH *in vivo* with bupivacaine hydroxide prevents the increase in excitatory synaptic transmission following surgical incision.[14] (A) Plot showing the total number of hindpaw withdrawals evoked by mechanical stimulation (with von Frey hairs 6–12; each applied 5X) following incision at P3 (postoperative day 0) with or without subsequent implantation of bupivacaine hydroxide (BUPI). BUPI application to the sciatic nerve (n = 11) led to a significant decrease in mechanical sensitivity on the ipsilateral paw (**$P < 0.01$; ***$P < 0.001$; two-way ANOVA). (B) Surgical incision at P3 failed to significantly change mEPSC frequency at P5–6 when accompanied by implantation of BUPI to the sciatic nerve at the time of injury (**$P < 0.01$; Kruskal–Wallis test). (C) There were no significant differences in mean mEPSC amplitude between the three groups at this time point ($P > 0.05$; Kruskal–Wallis test).

Surgical incision at P3 was combined with the insertion of microcapillaries containing either TTX (7.5 mM) or vehicle into the sciatic nerve, and synaptic function in the SDH was subsequently examined at P5–6.[14] First, neither the presence of the microcapillary itself nor perfusion with the vehicle solution caused significant modifications at immature SDH synapses, as we observed that the properties of spontaneous transmission in the vehicle-treated group (Incision + Vehicle; see Fig. 6C) were similar to those previously documented for pups receiving incision alone (see Figs. 5B and C). More importantly, as might be predicted from the BUPI experiments, block of sciatic nerve conduction with TTX caused a significant decrease in mEPSC frequency (Incision + Vehicle: 0.41 ± 0.06 Hz, n = 34; Incision + TTX: 0.22 ± 0.03 Hz, n = 23; $P = 0.046$; Mann–Whitney test; Fig. 6C *left*) without an accompanying change in mEPSC amplitude (Fig. 6C, *right*) or significant alterations in mIPSC properties (data not shown). Meanwhile, the administration of TTX (30 mM) microcapillaries from P17 failed to influence glutamatergic signaling at P19–20 (Fig. 6D), suggesting that older SDH neurons exhibit fundamentally different responses to fluctuations in sensory input.

Collectively, the results demonstrate that excitatory, but not inhibitory, synaptic transmission onto SDH neurons strongly depends on the level of primary afferent input to the spinal cord during a limited period of early postnatal development.

Discussion

The aforementioned findings clearly show that tissue damage during a defined period of early life transiently potentiates glutamatergic synaptic function in the developing spinal dorsal horn in an activity-dependent manner. In contrast, peripheral inflammation fails to modulate spontaneous excitatory signaling in the mature SDH.[17] In addition, while the efficacy of glycinergic synaptic inhibition is compromised in the adult dorsal horn under inflammatory conditions,[18,19] we did not observe any alterations in synaptic inhibition following neonatal tissue damage, although we cannot discount potential effects on chloride homeostasis as reported in the adult after injury.[20] Overall, the available evidence suggests that a developmental

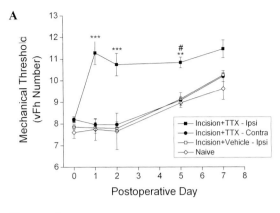

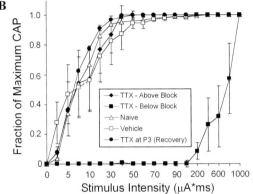

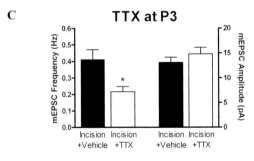

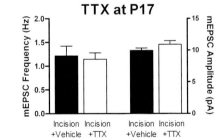

Figure 6. TTX delivery to the sciatic nerve *in vivo* during the first postnatal week decreases glutamatergic synaptic function in the SDH.[14] (**A**) Plot of mechanical withdrawal thresholds (vFh number evoking flexion withdrawal in 50% of trials) versus postoperative day after insertion of microcapillaries containing TTX or vehicle into the sciatic nerve at P3. TTX (n = 8) significantly elevated mechanical thresholds on the ipsilateral paw compared to the contralateral side, vehicle (n = 7) or naïve (n = 2) controls ($^{**}P < 0.01$, $^{***}P < 0.001$; two-way ANOVA; #$P < 0.05$ compared to naïve at this particular time point). (**B**) Summary plot of the normalized amplitude of dorsal root CAP versus stimulus strength at P20 (following microcapillary insertion at P17), showing that the thresholds of TTX-treated nerve fibers are similar to vehicle and naïve controls if stimulation occurs proximal to the TTX delivery site. Nerves which had been treated with TTX from P3 exhibited a similar stimulus-response relationship as vehicle and naïve controls by P20, arguing against any permanent alterations in the excitability of sciatic nerve fibers by the TTX application. (**C**) Reduction in primary afferent drive to the developing SDH from P3 decreased mEPSC frequency at P5–6 compared to vehicle controls ($^{*}P = 0.046$, Mann–Whitney test) without altering mEPSC amplitude. (**D**) In contrast, TTX application at P17 failed to alter mEPSC frequency ($P = 0.527$; Mann–Whitney test) or amplitude ($P = 0.153$; t-test) at P19–20 compared to vehicle controls.

shift in the synaptic mechanisms underlying central sensitization occurs during the early postnatal period.

The precise mechanisms underlying the observed increase in mEPSC frequency remain to be elucidated. An increase in the probability of glutamate release in the immature SDH under pathological conditions seems unlikely to explain the enhanced mEPSC rate, since peripheral inflammation failed to affect the PPR of evoked EPSCs (Fig. 3). This raises the possibility that early tissue damage elevates the number of glutamatergic synapses (or release sites) in the developing dorsal horn. Interestingly, an expansion in the central projections of nociceptive afferents is known to selectively occur following inflammation during the early postnatal period.[21,22] In addition, the sprouting of sensory fibers within the dorsal horn following mild tissue damage[22] and the elevation in mEPSC frequency described here were both reversible. Further experiments will determine if the increased mEPSC frequency does in fact reflect a transient expansion of C-fiber synaptic inputs within the SDH.

Although the enhanced mEPSC frequency could reflect the conversion of "silent" ("NMDAR only") synapses, which are present in the SDH during the first two postnatal weeks,[23,24] to functional connections via the insertion of AMPARs into the postsynaptic membrane,[25] it should be noted that there was no effect of neonatal incision on the AMPAR/NMDAR ratio (data not shown). In addition, while pure NMDAR-only synapses account for only ~20% of the total number of glutamatergic synapses onto immature SDH cells,[23] we observed a much greater (~100%) increase in mEPSC frequency following incision at P3. Finally, we cannot exclude the possibility that early tissue injury selectively modulates spontaneous excitatory neurotransmission in the developing SDH. Different subtypes of voltage-gated Ca^{2+} channels are known to regulate miniature versus evoked EPSCs in the adult dorsal horn[26] and spontaneous and evoked glutamate release in the CNS can originate from separate pools of synaptic vesicles.[27]

Additional work will also be necessary to explain the reduction in mEPSC frequency in P19–20 SDH neurons following surgical injury at P3 (Fig. 4B). Because a developmental decrease in the number of synaptic contacts has been reported in other regions of the CNS under normal conditions,[28] it is possible that early tissue damage enhances the rate at which this "synaptic pruning" occurs, and this may become evident only after the initial expansion of C-fiber inputs has resolved. Interestingly, stress during the neonatal period, which undoubtedly accompanies early surgical injury, is known to produce a delayed attenuation of synaptic development in the hippocampus.[29] Similar stress-evoked changes could occur in the SDH and contribute to the delayed reduction in glutamatergic signaling during the third postnatal week.

These findings raise additional questions that will be essential to address. For example, it is critical to determine which subtypes of lamina II neurons receive the increased glutamatergic input under pathological conditions, since the functional implications of the observed synaptic changes for the overall excitability of the SDH network will clearly depend on whether excitatory and/or inhibitory interneurons are affected by the tissue damage. We are currently investigating this issue using transgenic mice which express GFP in selective subpopulations of neurons within the CNS.[30,31] In addition, while a restricted developmental period exists (Figs. 1 and 2) during which tissue injury can facilitate excitatory transmission in the SDH, the cellular and molecular mechanisms which define this sensitive period remain unknown. The postnatal maturation of inhibitory synapses within the SDH[7,8] could limit any changes in glutamatergic synaptic function following tissue damage during the third postnatal week. Alternatively, the closure of the sensitive period could be initiated by myelin-derived signals in the SDH, as myelin expression begins to exhibit an adult-like pattern in the dorsal horn by P16[32] and is known to restrict the anatomical plasticity of nociceptive primary afferent fibers following injury.[33] Finally, since repetitive injury is an inevitable component of intensive care treatment, it will be important to characterize any potential cumulative effects of recurring insults on short- and long-term synaptic function within the developing dorsal horn network.

Conflicts of interest

The author declares no conflicts of interest.

References

1. Stevens, B. *et al*. 2003. Procedural pain in newborns at risk for neurologic impairment. *Pain* **105:** 27–35.
2. Alexander, J. & M. Manno. 2003. Underuse of analgesia in very young pediatric patients with isolated painful injuries. *Ann. Emerg. Med.* **41:** 617–622.
3. Schechter, N.L., D.A. Allen & K. Hanson. 1986. Status of pediatric pain control: a comparison of hospital analgesic usage in children and adults. *Pediatrics* **77:** 11–15.
4. Fitzgerald, M. 2005. The development of nociceptive circuits. *Nat. Rev. Neurosci.* **6:** 507–520.
5. Baccei, M.L., R. Bardoni & M. Fitzgerald. 2003. Development of nociceptive synaptic inputs to the neonatal rat dorsal horn: glutamate release by capsaicin and menthol. *J. Physiol.* **549:** 231–242.
6. Fitzgerald, M. & S. Gibson. 1984. The postnatal physiological and neurochemical development of peripheral sensory C fibres. *Neuroscience* **13:** 933–944.
7. Baccei, M.L. & M. Fitzgerald. 2004. Development of GABAergic and glycinergic transmission in the neonatal rat dorsal horn. *J. Neurosci.* **24:** 4749–4757.
8. Cordero-Erausquin, M. *et al*. 2005. Differential maturation of GABA action and anion reversal potential in spinal lamina I neurons: impact of chloride extrusion capacity. *J. Neurosci.* **25:** 9613–9623.

9. Marsh, D. *et al.* 1999. Epidural opioid analgesia in infant rats II: responses to carrageenan and capsaicin. *Pain* **82:** 33–38.

10. Ren, K. *et al.* 2004. Characterization of basal and re-inflammation-associated long-term alteration in pain responsivity following short-lasting neonatal local inflammatory insult. *Pain* **110:** 588–596.

11. Ririe, D.G. *et al.* 2003. Age-dependent responses to thermal hyperalgesia and mechanical allodynia in a rat model of acute postoperative pain. *Anesthesiology* **99:** 443–448.

12. Lorenzo, L.E. *et al.* 2008. Postnatal changes in the Rexed lamination and markers of nociceptive afferents in the superficial dorsal horn of the rat. *J. Comp. Neurol.* **508:** 592–604.

13. Li, J. & M.L. Baccei. 2009. Excitatory synapses in the rat superficial dorsal horn are strengthened following peripheral inflammation during early postnatal development. *Pain* **143:** 56–64.

14. Li, J. *et al.* 2009. Activity-dependent modulation of glutamatergic signaling in the developing rat dorsal horn by early tissue injury. *J. Neurophysiol.* **102:** 2208–2219.

15. Bray, J.J., J.I. Hubbard & R.G. Mills. 1979. The trophic influence of tetrodotoxin-inactive nerves on normal and reinnervated rat skeletal muscles. *J. Physiol.* **297:** 479–491.

16. Martinov, V.N. & A. Nja. 2005. A microcapsule technique for long-term conduction block of the sciatic nerve by tetrodotoxin. *J. Neurosci. Meth.* **141:** 199–205.

17. Baba, H., T.P. Doubell & C.J. Woolf. 1999. Peripheral inflammation facilitates Abeta fiber-mediated synaptic input to the substantia gelatinosa of the adult rat spinal cord. *J. Neurosci.* **19:** 859–867.

18. Harvey, R.J. *et al.* 2004. GlyR alpha3: an essential target for spinal PGE2-mediated inflammatory pain sensitization. *Science* **304:** 884–887.

19. Muller, F., B. Heinke & J. Sandkuhler. 2003. Reduction of glycine receptor-mediated miniature inhibitory postsynaptic currents in rat spinal lamina I neurons after peripheral inflammation. *Neuroscience* **122:** 799–805.

20. Zhang, W., L.Y. Liu & T.L. Xu. 2008. Reduced potassium-chloride co-transporter expression in spinal cord dorsal horn neurons contributes to inflammatory pain hypersensitivity in rats. *Neuroscience* **152:** 502–510.

21. Ruda, M.A. *et al.* 2000. Altered nociceptive neuronal circuits after neonatal peripheral inflammation. *Science* **289:** 628–631.

22. Walker, S.M. *et al.* 2003. Neonatal inflammation and primary afferent terminal plasticity in the rat dorsal horn. *Pain* **105:** 185–195.

23. Bardoni, R., P.C. Magherini & A.B. MacDermott. 1998. NMDA EPSCs at glutamatergic synapses in the spinal cord dorsal horn of the postnatal rat. *J. Neurosci.* **18:** 6558–6567.

24. Li, P. & M. Zhuo. 1998. Silent glutamatergic synapses and nociception in mammalian spinal cord. *Nature* **393:** 695–698.

25. Isaac, J.T. *et al.* 1997. Silent synapses during development of thalamocortical inputs. *Neuron* **18:** 269–280.

26. Bao, J., J.J. Li & E.R. Perl. 1998. Differences in Ca^{2+} channels governing generation of miniature and evoked excitatory synaptic currents in spinal laminae I and II. *J. Neurosci.* **18:** 8740–8750.

27. Sara, Y. *et al.* 2005. An isolated pool of vesicles recycles at rest and drives spontaneous neurotransmission. *Neuron* **45:** 563–573.

28. Bourgeois, J.P. & P. Rakic. 1993. Changes of synaptic density in the primary visual cortex of the macaque monkey from fetal to adult stage. *J. Neurosci.* **13:** 2801–2820.

29. Andersen, S.L. & M.H. Teicher. 2004. Delayed effects of early stress on hippocampal development. *Neuropsychopharmacology* **29:** 1988–1993.

30. Daniele, C.A. & A.B. MacDermott. 2009. Low-threshold primary afferent drive onto GABAergic interneurons in the superficial dorsal horn of the mouse. *J. Neurosci.* **29:** 686–695.

31. Heinke, B. *et al.* 2004. Physiological, neurochemical and morphological properties of a subgroup of GABAergic spinal lamina II neurones identified by expression of green fluorescent protein in mice. *J. Physiol.* **560:** 249–266.

32. Kapfhammer, J.P. & M.E. Schwab. 1994. Inverse patterns of myelination and GAP-43 expression in the adult CNS: neurite growth inhibitors as regulators of neuronal plasticity? *J. Comp. Neurol.* **340:** 194–206.

33. Schwegler, G., M.E. Schwab & J.P. Kapfhammer. 1995. Increased collateral sprouting of primary afferents in the myelin-free spinal cord. *J. Neurosci.* **15:** 2756–2767.

Ann. N.Y. Acad. Sci. ISSN 0077-8923

Role of NKCC1 and KCC2 in the development of chronic neuropathic pain following spinal cord injury

Tera Hasbargen,[1] Mostafa M. Ahmed,[1] Gurwattan Miranpuri,[1] Lin Li,[1] Kristopher T. Kahle,[3] Daniel Resnick,[1] and Dandan Sun[1,2]

[1]Department of Neurosurgery, University of Wisconsin School of Medicine and Public Health. [2]Waisman Center, Madison, Wisconsin. [3]Department of Neurosurgery, Massachusetts General Hospital and Harvard Medical School, Boston, Massachusetts

Address for correspondence: Dandan Sun, M.D., Ph.D., Department of Neurological Surgery, University of Wisconsin Medical School, T513 Waisman Center, 1500 Highland Ave., Madison, WI 53705. sun@neurosurg.wisc.edu

Neuropathic pain is a common problem following spinal cord injury (SCI). Effective analgesic therapy has been hampered by the lack of knowledge about the mechanisms underlying post-SCI neuropathic pain. Current evidence suggests GABAergic spinal nociceptive processing is a critical functional node in this complex phenotype, representing a potential target for therapeutic intervention. Normal GABA neurotransmission is dependent on precise regulation of the level of intracellular chloride, which is determined by the coordinated activities of two cation/chloride cotransporters (CCCs) in the *SLC12* family: the inwardly directed Na^+-K^+-Cl^- cotransporter isoform 1 (NKCC1) and outwardly directed K^+-Cl^- cotransporter isoform 2 (KCC2). Inhibition of NKCC1 with its potent antagonist bumetanide reduces pain behavior in rats following SCI. Moreover, the injured spinal cord tissues exhibit a significant transient upregulation of NKCC1 protein and a concurrent downregulation of KCC2 protein. Thus, imbalanced function of NKCC1 and KCC2 may contribute to the induction and maintenance of the chronic neuropathic pain following SCI.

Keywords: ion transport; chloride homeostasis; bumetanide

Introduction

Spinal cord injury (SCI) results in motor and sensory deficits and disabling chronic neuropathic pain.[1] Effective analgesic therapy has been hampered by the lack of knowledge about the mechanisms underlying post-SCI neuropathic pain. The GABAergic system is an essential component in spinal nociceptive processing and involved in primary afferent nociceptive attenuation.[2,3] GABA receptors are found on pre- and postsynaptic sites of primary afferent terminals, as well as on interneurons in laminae I–IV in the spinal cord dorsal horn.[4] GABAergic interneurons in the dorsal horn are important for nociceptive attenuation.[5,6] Subarachnoid implantation of GABA-producing neuronal cells in rats attenuates allodynia and hyperalgesia following excitotoxic injury.[7] Furthermore, administration of the GABA_A receptor agonist muscimol

prevents long-lasting potentiation of hyperalgesia following peripheral nerve injury.[8] Therefore, altered Cl^- homeostasis and GABAergic function are associated with nociceptive input hypersensitivity.[9]

Normal GABA_A receptor function is critically dependent on the activity of intracellular Cl^- which is determined by two major intracellular Cl^- regulatory proteins, the inwardly directed Na^+-K^+-Cl^- cotransporter isoform 1 (NKCC1) and outwardly directed K^+-Cl^- cotransporter isoform 2 (KCC2).[10–14] In the early developmental stages, GABA acts primarily as an excitatory neurotransmitter in the nervous system.[6,15] This is due, to a large extent, to early development-dependent expression of NKCC1 and delayed expression of KCC2. Therefore, immature neurons maintain the intracellular Cl^- concentration at a high level and exhibit a membrane depolarization upon activation of GABA_A receptors, resulting from a net outward

doi: 10.1111/j.1749-6632.2010.05462.x

flow of Cl^- (the Cl^- equilibrium potential $E_{Cl} >$ membrane potential E_m).[16] Elevation of intracellular Cl^- can lead to GABAergic hypersensitivity by reversing both E_{Cl} and the normal inhibitory action of GABA.[17,18] Both NKCC1 and KCC2 are expressed in spinal cords and function to regulate intracellular Cl^- concentration. Increasing evidence suggests that changes of the transporter expression play a role in inflammatory or neuropathic pain.[5,6,12,13] A recent study suggests that NKCC1 and KCC2 play a role in chronic hyperalgesia following SCI.[19] Moreover, there might be a functional link between activation of TRPV1 and NKCC1 in referred hyperalgesia.[20] This review will center on these issues. Readers shall find extensive information about the role of NKCC1 and KCC2 in hyperalgesia in other recent review articles.[3,5]

NKCC1 and KCC2 in hyperalgesia

The inhibitory action of GABA is a critical component of numerous neuronal circuits. It has been proposed that large, myelinated Aβ-fibers could antagonize nociceptive primary afferent inputs to the dorsal horn through inhibitory mechanisms mediated by interneurons. These interneurons release GABA, which activates $GABA_A$ receptors on primary afferent terminals and produces primary afferent depolarization (PAD). PAD shunts the magnitude of incoming action potentials and decreases excitatory amino release at the primary afferent central terminals.[5,6] However, under inflamed conditions, PAD may be enhanced such that it leads to excessive depolarization of Aδ- and C-fibers above their thresholds for action potential generation.

Any injury-induced modification of this inhibitory action has the potential to alter the processing of nociceptive information in the spinal dorsal horn. Therefore, the generation of Cl^--dependent $GABA_A$ receptor response is critically dependent on the activity of NKCC1 and KCC2 (Fig. 1). NKCC1 knockout mice ($NKCC1^{-/-}$) lack the $GABA_A$ receptor-mediated anion outward flux current.[12] $NKCC1^{-/-}$ mice have deficits in thermal nociceptive thresholds and display a decrease in Aβ-fiber-mediated touch-evoked allodynia following capsaicin injection.[12] Moreover, the NKCC1 antagonist bumetanide inhibits itch and flare responses to histamine in human skin, and attenuates phase I and II behavioral responses in the formalin model

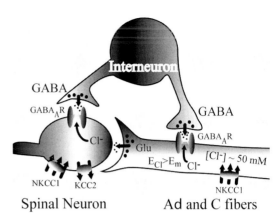

Figure 1. Outline of the current view on role of NKCC1 and KCC2 in Cl^- homeostasis and hyperalgesia. Periphery nerve inflammation, nerve injury, or spinal cord injury cause a differential change of NKCC1 and KCC2 expression and function, the latter increases intracellular Cl^- concentration and promotes GABA-mediated excitatory responses and nociceptive input hypersensitivity.

of tissue injury-induced pain.[10] After intracolonic capsaicin injection in mice, NKCC1 plasma membrane expression and phosphorylation are increased in the dorsal spinal cord, although it is unknown whether it is accompanied by KCC2 downregulation.[2] Inhibition of NKCC1 and vanilloid receptor-1 (TRPV1) attenuates capsaicin-induced allodynia.[20] These results suggest that NKCC1 plays a role in the development of hyperalgesia. On the other hand, intraplantar formalin stimulation triggers a significant decrease in KCC2 protein expression without changes in NKCC1 in the rat spinal cord.[21] Taken together, these studies suggest that alteration of Cl^- homeostasis by changes in NKCC1 and/or KCC2 function may contribute to hyperalgesia development (Fig. 1).

NKCC1 and KCC2 in neuropathic pain

A recent report suggests that changes of NKCC1 and KCC2 protein expression are involved in the development of chronic neuropathic pain following a contusion SCI. In this study, Sprague–Dawley rats underwent a contusive SCI at T9 and developed hyperalgesia between days 21 and 42 post-SCI.[19] NKCC1 protein level was elevated on day 7 post-SCI and increased by ∼60% on day 14 post-SCI.[19] In contrast, KCC2 protein was decreased on 2–7 days post-SCI and fell by ∼40% on day 14 post-SCI.

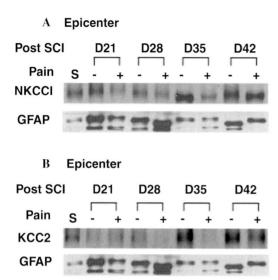

A   Epicenter

Post SCI	D21	D28	D35	D42
Pain	S - +	- +	- +	- +

NKCCl

GFAP

B   Epicenter

Post SCI	D21	D28	D35	D42
Pain	S - +	- +	- +	- +

KCC2

GFAP

Figure 2. Changes in NKCC1 and KCC2 expression in nonhyperalgesic and hyperalgesic rats. NKCC1 protein expression in the injury epicenter spinal cord tissues at 21, 28, 35, and 42 days post-SCI. Sham (S) samples were acquired from animals subject to laminectomies without subsequent spinal cord contusion. *Top panel:* the blot was probed with anti-NKCC1 antibody and anti-GFAP (glial fibrillary acidic protein) antibody. *Lower panel:* the blot was probed with anti-KCC2 antibody and anti-GFAP antibody. Hyperalgesic rats (labeled as pain) were identified with the thermal hyperalgesia withdrawal latency test as described above. (+): hyperalgesia; (−): without hyperalgesia. n = 2. (Adapted from Cramer *et al.* (Ref. 19).)

These data indicate a significant increase in the expression of NKCC1 and, conversely, a decrease in KCC2 expression at the epicenter on day 14 post-SCI (which is prior to the chronic phase of post-SCI neuropathic hyperalgesia).

The presence of chronic thermal hyperalgesia can be detected in rats on days 21–42 post-SCI. Moreover, inhibition of NKCC1 with its potent antagonist bumetanide (30 mg/kg, i.p.) significantly reduced pain behavior in these rats.[19] On days 21–35 post-SCI, a moderate reduction of NKCC1 in the contusion epicenter of spinal cord occurred. KCC2 proteins remained downregulated during days 21 and 35 post-SCI (Fig. 2). Interestingly, in rats exhibiting no thermal hyperalgesia, both NKCC1 and KCC2 proteins remained unchanged as compared to sham. In contrast, the hyperalgesic rats displayed a sustained loss of KCC2 protein, with expression

of KCC2 observed to be 34% and 40% of sham in lesion epicenter tissue at days 28 and 35 post-SCI, respectively (due to neuronal death and astrogliosis, no routine loading control markers were appropriate for a quantitative immunoblotting analysis). These data suggest that despite reduction of both NKCC1 and KCC2 proteins, the relative higher ratio of NKCC1/KCC2 in lesion epicenter may play a role in development of chronic neuropathic pain following SCI. This view is supported by the antialgesia effects of NKCC1 inhibition by bumetanide.[19]

Numerous reports illustrate that alteration of KCC2 function is involved in nociceptive input hypersensitivity following periphery nerve injury. Partial nerve injury (induced by a sciatic cuff) disrupted anion homeostasis in lamina I neurons and shifted the normally inhibitory synaptic currents to excitatory, thereby increasing lamina I neuronal excitability *in vitro*.[22] The nerve injury was associated with a decrease in KCC2 mRNA and protein levels. Moreover, inhibition of KCC2 activity *in vivo* reduces mechanical and thermal nociceptive thresholds in control and uninjured animals.[22] In addition, *in vivo* axonal injury causes a reduction of KCC2 mRNA in motor neurons and results in an increased intracellular Cl^- concentration and, consequently, $GABA_A$ receptor-mediated excitatory responses.[23] A recent report shows that this transient downregulation of KCC2[24] and the early pain behavior depends on activation of TrkB receptor via BDNF in nerve injury.[13] Posttranslational modulation of KCC2 appears to be involved in the downregulation of KCC2 protein. A loss of tyrosine phosphorylation of KCC2 and a reduction of surface-expression of KCC2 in the plasma membrane is largely attributable to tyrosine phosphatases.[25] Moreover, it was reported recently that selective downregulation of KCC2 protein also occurs in motorneurons following spinal cord transaction in adult rats, which may play a role in the pathophysiology of spasticity following SCI.[6]

Potential interactions between TRPV1 and NKCC1

Activation of TRPV1-mediated signaling pathway plays an important role in referred allodynia and thermal hyperalgesia.[20,26] TRPV1 is activated by heat, capsaicin, and lipoxygenase products.[27] A greater than threefold increase in TRPV1 mRNA expression was detected in dorsal horn of rats

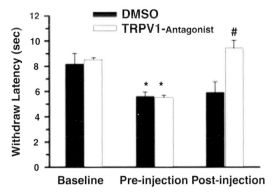

Figure 3. Antihyperalgesic effects of TRPV1 antagonist AMG9810 in hyperalgesic rats. The mean withdrawal latency time was recorded in Sham rats (baseline control), rats with SCI prior to, or post-drug administration. Group 1 received vehicle (DMSO, i.p.) as controls ($n = 4$) and group 2 received TRPV1 antagonist AMG9810 (30 mg/kg, i.p., $n = 12$). After 1 h of treatment, WLT was remeasured and the mean WLT recorded. Data are mean ± SE. $^*P < 0.05$ versus pre-SCI. $^\#P < 0.05$ versus vehicle. (Adapted from Rajpal *et al.* (Ref. 26).)

exhibiting chronic neuropathic pain following SCI.[14] Moreover, TRPV1 antagonist AMG 9810 exhibited a significant antihyperalgesic effect in rats following SCI (Fig. 3). TRPV1 upregulation may contribute to neuropathic pain development through stimulation of NKCC1 function post-SCI. Intracolonic injection of capsaicin was shown to increase dorsal spinal phosphorylated NKCC1 within 10 min of injection.[2] In addition to the change in NKCC1 phosphorylation, NKCC1 protein was translocated to the cell membrane in the dorsal spinal cord.[2] These data suggest that peripheral TRPV1 activation may increase spinal NKCC1 activity.[2] Intrathecal application of the NKCC1 antagonist bumetanide attenuated referred allodynia and hyperalgesia.[20] More importantly, activation of TRPV1 with an endogenous agonist, narachidonoyl-dopamine, induced stroking allodynia in the hindpaw, which can be blocked by the NKCC1 inhibitor bumetanide.[20] The underlying mechanisms are unknown, but likely involve activation of TRPV1 receptors and kinases-mediated phosphorylation of NKCC1.[3]

Summary

Chloride homeostasis through the function of ionotropic GABA receptors is one important mech-

anism in regulation of nociceptive processing. Two major intracellular Cl^- regulatory proteins, NKCC1 and KCC2, play a critical role in hyperalgesia and allodynia after peripheral nerve inflammation or nerve injury. The recent report illustrates that expression of NKCC1 and KCC2 proteins was differentially altered following SCI. The antihyperalgesic effect of NKCC1 inhibition suggests that normal or elevated NKCC1 function and loss of KCC2 function play a role in the development and maintenance of SCI-induced neuropathic pain.

Acknowledgments

The authors would like to thank Douglas Kintner for his assistance in manuscript preparation. Tera Hasbargen, Mostafa Ahmed, and Lin Li were supported by Shapiro Research Summer Fellowship for Medical Students at University of Wisconsin, Madison.

Conflicts of interest

References

1. Yezierski, R.P. 2005. Spinal cord injury: a model of central neuropathic pain. *Neurosignals* **14:** 182–193.
2. Galan, A. & F. Cervero. 2005. Painful stimuli induce *in vivo* phosphorylation and membrane mobilization of mouse spinal cord NKCC1 co-transporter. *Neuroscience* **133:** 245–252.
3. Price, T.J., F. Cervero, M.S. Gold, *et al.* 2009. Chloride regulation in the pain pathway. *Brain Res. Rev.* **60:** 149–170.
4. Bowery, N.G., A.L. Hudson & G.W. Price. 1987. GABAA and GABAB receptor site distribution in the rat central nervous system. *Neuroscience* **20:** 365–383.
5. Price, T.J., F. Cervero & Y. de Koninck. 2005. Role of cation-chloride-cotransporters (CCC) in pain and hyperalgesia. *Curr. Top. Med. Chem.* **5:** 547–555.
6. Vinay, L. & C. Jean-Xavier. 2008. Plasticity of spinal cord locomotor networks and contribution of cation-chloride cotransporters. *Brain Res. Rev.* **57:** 103–110.
7. Eaton, M.J., S.Q. Wolfe, M. Martinez, *et al.* 2007. Subarachnoid transplant of a human neuronal cell line attenuates chronic allodynia and hyperalgesia after excitotoxic spinal cord injury in the rat. *J. Pain.* **8:** 33–50.
8. Miletic, G., P. Draganic, M.T. Pankratz, *et al.* 2003. Muscimol prevents long-lasting potentiation of dorsal horn

field potentials in rats with chronic constriction injury exhibiting decreased levels of the GABA transporter GAT-1. *Pain* **105**: 347–353.

9. Ahn, S.H., H.W. Park, B.S. Lee, *et al.* 2003. Gabapentin effect on neuropathic pain compared among patients with spinal cord injury and different durations of symptoms. *Spine* **28**: 341–346.

10. Granados-Soto, V., C.F. Arguelles & F.J. Alvarez-Leefmans. 2005. Peripheral and central antinociceptive action of Na$^+$-K$^+$-2Cl$^-$ cotransporter blockers on formalin-induced nociception in rats. *Pain* **114**: 231–238.

11. Misgeld, U., R.A. Deisz, H.U. Dodt, *et al.* 1986. The role of chloride transport in postsynaptic inhibition of hippocampal neurons. *Science* **232**: 1413–1415.

12. Sung, K.W., M. Kirby, M.P. McDonald, *et al.* 2000. Abnormal GABAA receptor-mediated currents in dorsal root ganglion neurons isolated from Na-K-2Cl cotransporter null mice. *J. Neurosci.* **20**: 7531–7538.

13. Miletic, G. & V. Miletic. 2008. Loose ligation of the sciatic nerve is associated with TrkB receptor-dependent decreases in KCC2 protein levels in the ipsilateral spinal dorsal horn. *Pain* **137**: 532–539.

14. DomBourian, M.G., N.A. Turner, T.A. Gerovac, *et al.* 2006. B1 and TRPV-1 receptor genes and their relationship to hyperalgesia following spinal cord injury. *Spine* **31**: 2778–2782.

15. Ben Ari, Y. 2002. Excitatory actions of GABA during development: the nature of the nurture. *Nat. Rev. Neurosci.* **3**: 728–739.

16. Ge, S., E.L. Goh, K.A. Sailor, *et al.* 2006. GABA regulates synaptic integration of newly generated neurons in the adult brain. *Nature* **439**: 589–593.

17. Blaesse, P., M.S. Airaksinen, C. Rivera, *et al.* 2009. Cation-chloride cotransporters and neuronal function. *Neuron* **61**: 820–838.

18. Kahle, K.T., K.J. Staley, B.V. Nahed, *et al.* 2008. Roles of the cation-chloride cotransporters in neurological disease. *Nat. Clin. Pract. Neurol.* **4**: 490–503.

19. Cramer, S.W., C. Baggott, J. Cain, *et al.* 2008. The role of cation-dependent chloride transporters in neuropathic pain following spinal cord injury. *Mol. Pain.* **4**: 36–44.

20. Pitcher, M.H., T.J. Price, J.M. Entrena, *et al.* 2007. Spinal NKCC1 blockade inhibits TRPV1-dependent referred allodynia. *Mol. Pain.* **3**: 17–25.

21. Nomura, H., A. Sakai, M. Nagano, *et al.* 2006. Expression changes of cation chloride cotransporters in the rat spinal cord following intraplantar formalin. *Neurosci. Res.* **56**: 435–440.

22. Coull, J.A., D. Boudreau, K. Bachand, *et al.* 2003. Trans-synaptic shift in anion gradient in spinal lamina I neurons as a mechanism of neuropathic pain. *Nature* **424**: 938–942.

23. Nabekura, J., T. Ueno, A. Okabe, *et al.* 2002. Reduction of KCC2 expression and GABAA receptor-mediated excitation after *in vivo* axonal injury. *J. Neurosci.* **22**: 4412–4417.

24. Rivera, C., H. Li, J. Thomas-Crusells, *et al.* 2002. BDNF-induced TrkB activation down-regulates the K+-Cl- cotransporter KCC2 and impairs neuronal Cl- extrusion. *J. Cell Biol.* **159**: 747–752.

25. Wake, H., M. Watanabe, A.J. Moorhouse, *et al.* 2007. Early changes in KCC2 phosphorylation in response to neuronal stress result in functional downregulation. *J. Neurosci.* **27**: 1642–1650.

26. Rajpal, S., T.A. Gerovac, N.A. Turner, *et al.* 2007. Anti-hyperalgesic effects of vanilloid-1 and bradykinin-1 receptor antagonists following spinal cord injury in rats. *J. Neurosurg. Spine.* **6**: 420–424.

27. Hagenacker, T., J.C. Czeschik, M. Schafers, *et al.* 2010. Sensitization of voltage activated calcium channel currents for capsaicin in nociceptive neurons by tumor-necrosis-factor-alpha. *Brain Res. Bull.* **81**: 157–163.

Ann. N.Y. Acad. Sci. ISSN 0077-8923

ANNALS OF THE NEW YORK ACADEMY OF SCIENCES
Issue: *Neurons and Networks in the Spinal Cord*

Bone cancer pain

Juan Miguel Jimenez-Andrade,[1] William G. Mantyh,[1] Aaron P. Bloom,[1] Alice S. Ferng,[2] Christopher P. Geffre,[2] and Patrick W. Mantyh[1,3,4]

[1]Department of Pharmacology, University of Arizona, Tucson, Arizona. [2]Department of Physiological Sciences, College of Medicine University of Arizona, Tucson, Arizona. [3]Arizona Cancer Center, University of Arizona, Tucson, Arizona. [4]Research Service, VA Medical Center, Minneapolis, Minnesota

Address for correspondence: Patrick W. Mantyh, Ph.D., Department of Pharmacology, College of Medicine, University of Arizona, 1656 E. Mabel, Rm. #119, PO Box 245215, Tucson, AZ 85724. Voice: 520-626-0742; fax: 520-626-4182. pmantyh@email.arizona.edu

In the United States, cancer is the second most common cause of death and it is expected that about 562,340 Americans will have died of cancer in 2009. Bone cancer pain is common in patients with advanced breast, prostate, and lung cancer as these tumors have a remarkable affinity to metastasize to bone. Once tumors metastasize to bone, they are a major cause of morbidity and mortality as the tumor induces significant skeletal remodeling, fractures, pain, and anemia. Currently, the factors that drive cancer pain are poorly understood. However, several recently introduced models of bone cancer pain, which closely mirror the human condition, are providing insight into the mechanisms that drive bone cancer pain and guide the development of mechanism-based therapies to treat the cancer pain. Several of these mechanism-based therapies have now entered human clinical trials. If successful, these therapies have the potential to significantly enlarge the repertoire of modalities that can be used to treat bone cancer pain and improve the quality of life, functional status, and survival of patients with bone cancer.

Keywords: osteosarcoma; prostate; therapies

Bone cancer pain in humans

The majority of patients with metastatic bone disease experience moderate to severe pain and bone pain is one of the most common types of chronic pain in these patients.[1] Although bone is not a vital organ, many common tumors (breast, prostate, thyroid, kidney, and lung) have a strong predilection to simultaneously metastasize to multiple bones.[1,2] It has been reported that tumor mestastases to the skeleton affect over 400,000 individuals in the United States annually. Tumor growth in bone results in pain, hypercalcemia, anemia, increased susceptibility to infection, skeletal fractures, compression of the spinal cord, spinal instability, and decreased mobility, all of which compromise the patient's functional status, quality of life, and survival.[1,3] Once tumor cells have metastasized to the skeleton, tumor-induced bone pain is usually described as dull in character, constant in presentation, and gradually increasing in intensity with time.[3] Adherence to the World Health Organization

analgesic ladder, along with adjuvant therapies such as bisphosphonates, corticosteroids, radiotherapy, and radionuclides, can frequently control ongoing bone cancer pain. However, both opiates and nonsteroidal anti-inflammatory drugs may have significant dose-limiting side effects.

As tumor growth and tumor-induced bone remodeling progress, severe "incident pain" frequently occurs.[3] Incident pain is also known as "breakthrough pain" as the pain breaks through the analgesic regime that is controlling the ongoing pain. This pain is defined as an intermittent episode of extreme pain which occurs spontaneously, during non-noxious movement,[4] or mechanical loading of the tumor-bearing bone(s). A major problem with incident pain in bone cancer is that it is usually more severe than ongoing pain, it appears suddenly (within seconds to minutes) and it can occur multiple times each day.[4] Given the therapies that are currently available, as well as the rapid onset and severity of incident pain, this pain remains one of the most challenging of cancer pains to fully

doi: 10.1111/j.1749-6632.2009.05429.x
Ann. N.Y. Acad. Sci. 1198 (2010) 173–181 © 2010 New York Academy of Sciences.

control.[4] When present, incident pain can be highly debilitating to the patient's functional status and quality of life.[2–4]

Preclinical models of bone cancer pain

Previously, there were two commonly used *in vivo* mouse models to study tumor-induced bone destruction. In the first model, tumor cells are injected into the left ventricle of the heart and then spread to multiple sites including the bone marrow where they grow and induce remodeling of the surrounding bone.[5,6] While this model replicates the observation that most tumor cells metastasize to multiple sites including bone, a major problem with this model is the animal-to-animal variability in the sites, size, and extent of the metastasis. Because the tumors frequently metastasize to vital organs such as the lung or liver, the general health of the animal is also variable, making behavioral assessment of bone pain difficult. Given these problems, intracardiac injection of cancer cells as a model for bone cancer pain has proven difficult.

The second major model used to study tumor-induced bone destruction involves the direct injection of osteolytic sarcoma cells into the intramedullary space of the mouse tibia or femur (Fig. 1A). A major advance leading to the currently used model was to plug the injection hole with a dental amalgam or bone cement (Fig. 1B), which by tightly binding and sealing the injection hole, confining tumor cells to the marrow space of the bone and prevents tumor invasion into surrounding soft tissue (Fig. 1C).[7]

Mouse osteosarcoma tumor cells were the first cell type that was extensively used in this model (Fig. 1C). These cells were injected and confined to the intramedullary space of the mouse femur (Fig. 1C).[8] The tumor cells grow in a highly reproducible fashion (Fig. 2E) and, as they proliferate, replace the hemapoetic cells that normally populate the bone marrow (Fig. 2D).[7,8] Eventually, the entire marrow space is filled with tumor cells and tumor-associated inflammatory/immune cells (Fig. 2E).[7,8] In terms of bone remodeling, injection of osteosarcoma cells into the femur induces a dramatic proliferation and hypertrophy of osteoclasts at the tumor–bone interface, as well as significant bone destruction in both the proximal and distal heads of the femur (Figs. 2B and E).[7] In

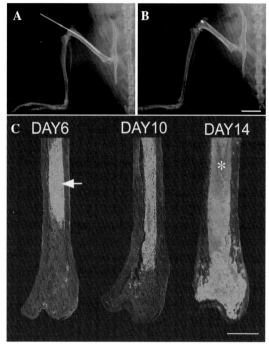

Figure 1. Development of a mouse model of bone cancer pain and disease progression. Low-power anterior–posterior radiograph of a mouse femur showing the unilateral injection of sarcoma cells into the femur (**A**) and confinement of the tumor cells in marrow space with an amalgam plug (**B**). The present model allows a simultaneous visualization and quantitative evaluation of the tumor burden by using 2472 sarcoma cancer cells genetically manipulated to express enhanced green fluorescent protein (GFP). (**C**) GFP-transfected tumor cells (*green*) injected into the ipsilateral femurs at day 6 (*arrow*), day 10, and day 14 postinjection. Scale bar: 6 mm in (**A, B**) and 1.5 mm in (**C**).

this model, ongoing and movement-evoked pain behaviors increase in severity with time and are correlated with the tumor growth and progressive tumor-induced bone destruction,[7,8] which mirrors what occurs in patients with primary or metastatic bone cancer. Although osteosarcoma cells were the first cells used in this model, other animal and human tumor cells, including prostate, breast, melanoma, colon, and lung tumors, have now been used in the closed femur model of bone cancer pain.[9]

Prostate cancer is unique in that bone is often the only clinically detectable site of metastasis. Prostate

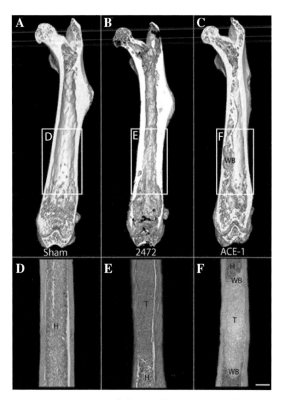

Figure 2. Bone remodeling and tumor growth in the 2472 sarcoma and ACE-1 prostate carcinoma-injected femurs have different characteristics depending on the osteolytic or osteoblastic component of the tumor cells as assessed by μCT imaging and hematoxilin and eosin (H&E) staining. Sham-injected femurs present relative absence of bone formation or bone destruction (**A**, **D**). The 2472 sarcoma-injected femurs display a primarily osteolytic appearance visible as regions absent of trabecular bone at the proximal and distal heads (**B**) as well as replacement of normal hematopoietic cells by tumor cells (**E**). The ACE-1 prostate carcinoma-injected femurs mainly present an osteoblastic appearance which is characterized by pathologic bone formation in the intramedullary space (**C**) surrounding pockets of tumor cells which generate diaphyseal bridging structures (**F**). (**A–F**) Scale bar: 0.5 mm. T, tumor; H, normal hematopoietic cells; WB, ACE-1-induced woven bone formation.

tumors that have metastasized to bone frequently induce bone pain, which can be difficult to fully control as it seems to be driven simultaneously by inflammatory, neuropathic, and tumorigenic mechanisms. In an effort to develop mechanism-based therapies that attenuate bone cancer pain due to other metastatic tumors, such as those from the prostate, we recently characterized another bone cancer pain model[10] (Figs. 2C and F). This model utilizes canine prostate tumor cells (ACE-1) that are injected and confined to the intramedullary space in the femur of nude mice.[10] Using this model it was shown that significant tumor-induced, pain-related behaviors were first observed at 9 days following injection of prostate tumor cells and continued to increase until 19 days postinjection at which time the mice were euthanized.[10] Prostate tumor cells induce significant formation of new woven bone at the proximal head, distal end, and the diaphysis of the bone (Figs. 2C and F). The marked bone formation induced by prostate cancer cells is also accompanied by bone destruction, giving the tumor-bearing femur a unique scalloped appearance when assessed by micro-computed tomography (μCT) (Fig. 2C) or with traditional histological methodology (Fig. 2F). This appearance is consistent with what is observed in human patients with prostate tumor metastases.

Tumor and osteoclast-induced acidosis and bone cancer pain

Studies in both humans and animals have suggested that osteoclasts (the cells that break down bone) play a significant role in cancer-induced bone loss[11] and that osteoclasts contribute to the etiology of bone cancer pain.[12,13] Osteoclasts are terminally differentiated, multinucleated, monocyte lineage cells that resorb bone by maintaining an extracellular microenvironment of acidic pH (4.0–5.0) at the osteoclast–mineralized bone interface (Fig. 3).[14] Both osteolytic (bone destroying) and osteoblastic (bone forming) cancers are characterized by osteoclast proliferation and hypertrophy.[7,15,16] Thus, osteoclast-mediated bone remodeling results in robust production of extracellular protons,[17] which are known to be potent activators of nociceptors (Fig. 3B).[18] This raises the possibility that the acidic microenvironment produced by osteoclasts contributes significantly to bone cancer-associated pain through activation of acid-sensitive nociceptors that innervate the marrow, mineralized bone, and periosteum.[19]

The finding that sensory neurons can be directly excited by protons originating from cells, such as osteoclasts in bone, has generated clinical interest in targeting acid sensing channels expressed by

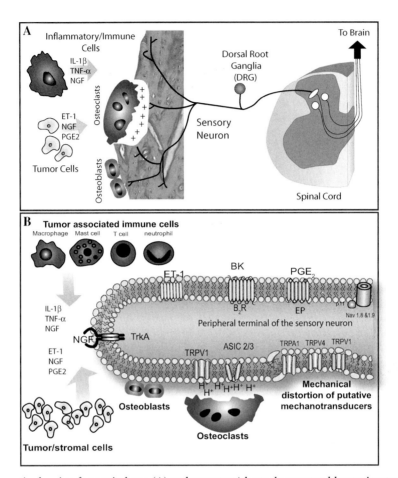

Figure 3. Schematic showing factors in bone (**A**) and receptors/channels expressed by nociceptors that innervate the skeleton (**B**) that drive bone cancer pain. A variety of cells (tumor cells and stromal cells including inflammatory/immune cells, osteoclasts, and osteoblasts) drive bone cancer pain (**A**). Nociceptors that innervate the bone use several different types of receptors to detect and transmit noxious stimuli that are produced by cancer cells (*yellow*), tumor-associated immune cells (*blue*), or other aspects of the tumor microenvironment. There are multiple factors that may contribute to the pain associated with cancer (**B**). The transient receptor potential vanilloid receptor-1 (TRPV1) and acid sensing ion channels (ASICs) detect extracellular protons produced by tumor induced tissue damage or abnormal osteoclast-mediated bone resorption. Tumor cells and associated inflammatory (immune) cells produce a variety of chemical mediators including prostaglandins (PGE2), nerve growth factor (NGF), endothelins (ET-1) and bradykinin (BK). Several of these proinflammatory mediators have receptors on peripheral terminals and can directly activate or sensitize nociceptors. It is suggested that movement-evoked breakthrough pain in cancer patients is partially due to the tumor-induced loss of the mechanical strength and stability of the tumor-bearing bone so that normally innocuous mechanical stress can now produce distortion of the putative mechanotransducers (TRPV1, TRPV4, and TRPA1) that innervate the bone.

nociceptors. Studies have shown that subsets of sensory neurons express different acid-sensing ion channels.[18] Two acid-sensing ion channels expressed by nociceptors are transient receptor potential vanilloid 1 (TRPV1) and acid-sensing ion channel-3 (ASIC-3) (Fig. 3B).[18] Both of these channels are sensitized and excited by a decrease in pH in the range of 4.0–5.0, which is generated by osteoclasts (Fig. 3B).[18] In addition to osteoclast-induced acidosis, the tumor stroma[20] and areas of the tumor which are necrotic typically exhibit lower extracellular pH than surrounding normal tissues. As inflammatory and immune cells invade the tumor stroma, these cells also release protons that generate a local acidosis.[12,19]

Animal and clinical studies of bone cancer have reported that the antiresorptive effects of bisphosphonate therapies simultaneously reduce bone cancer pain, tumor-induced bone destruction, and tumor growth within the bone.[12,13,21] Bisphosphonates are a class of antiresorptive compounds that are pyrophosphate analogues which display high affinity for calcium ions, causing them to rapidly and avidly bind to the mineralized matrix of bone.[15] As osteoclasts resorb bone they use endocytosis and transcytosis to clear the bone breakdown products from the osteoclast–bone interface (including the bisphosphonate, which is bound to the mineralized bone). Bisphosphonates, once taken up by the osteoclasts, induce loss of function and ultimately apoptosis of the osteoclasts.[15]

It should be stressed that while bisphosphonates are approved and are frequently used to reduce tumor-induced bone destruction and bone cancer pain, bisphosphonates do have unwanted side effects (including induction of arthralgias and osteonecrosis of the jaw),[15] and it has yet to be definitively shown that bisphosphonates increase the survival of patients with bone cancer. For this reason, other therapies targeting osteoclasts are already in mid- to late-stage clinical trials and hold significant promise for alleviating bone cancer pain and tumor-induced bone remodeling. One line of therapies attempts to block the binding of receptor activator for nuclear factor κB ligand (RANKL), which is an essential regulator of osteoclasts.[11] Studies in mice have shown that sequestration of RANKL with OPG attenuates sarcoma-induced bone pain, bone remodeling, and tumor growth within the bone (Figs. 4B–E).[7] Recent small clinical studies have shown that in humans with multiple myeloma or breast cancer metastasis to bone, Denosumab (a fully humanized monoclonal antibody that inhibits RANKL) markedly reduces tumor-induced bone resorption and skeletal-related events (which include fracture and pain).[22] Currently, phase III clinical trials are underway for assessing Denosumab's effects on attenuating cancer-induced bone loss in breast and prostate cancers,[23] skeletal related events (pain, fracture) due to the spread of cancer to the bone in

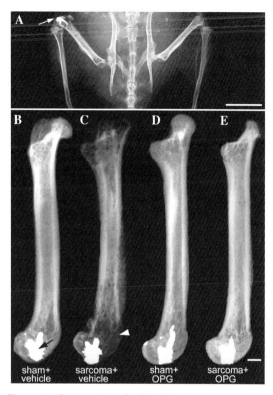

Figure 4. Osteoprotegerin (OPG) attenuates sarcoma-induced bone destruction in a mouse model of bone cancer pain. (**A**) Low-power frontal radiograph of mouse pelvis and hind limbs following unilateral injection of 2472 murine osteosarcoma cells into the distal end of the femur and closure of the injection with a dental amalgam plug (*arrow*). The amalgam plug was used to prevent tumor cells from growing outside the bone. High-resolution radiographs of sham-injected (**B** and **D**) and sarcoma-injected (**C** and **E**) femurs from mice that received vehicle (**B** and **C**) or OPG (**D** and **E**). Note that at day 17 after the injection of the osteosarcoma cells, there is significant bone destruction in the distal femur without OPG (**C**; *white arrowhead*), whereas tumor induced bone destruction is not evident in sarcoma-injected mouse that received OPG (**E**). Scale bars represent 10 mm (a) and 0.5 mm (b−e; *bottom panel*). (With permission from Honore, P. *et al.*[7])

multiple myeloma and multiple solid tumors, as well as the potential to delay bone metastases in prostate cancer.[24]

The mechanisms by which inhibition of osteoclast activity (either by bisphosphonates or OPGL/RANKL binding molecules) attenuates bone cancer pain may involve, at least in part, the reduction of osteoclast-induced acidosis. Tissue acidosis may activate nociceptors that innervate the bone through multiple mechanisms,[12,18] but TRPV1 has been proposed to play a major role in acid-induced activation of nociceptors (Fig. 3B). Recent pharmacological studies showed that selective TRPV1 antagonists significantly decreased ongoing (JNJ-17203212, ABT-102, and SB366791) and movement-evoked (JNJ-17203212 and ABT-102) pain-related behaviors in the mouse model of bone cancer pain, without any observable behavioral side effects, such as ataxia or hypoactivity.[19,25]

Although the above discussion has focused on osteoclast-mediated acidosis as a mechanism that drives bone cancer pain, both osteolytic and osteoblastic tumors induce a loss of the mechanical strength and stability of the tumor-bearing bone so that normally innocuous mechanical stress can now produce distortion of the mechanosensitive sensory nerve fibers that innervate the bone (Fig. 3B). Previous results have shown that the pain associated with fracture is significantly attenuated if the bone is stabilized and returned to its normal orientation.[26] Preservation of the mechanical strength of bone should reduce movement-induced incident pain, as this pain is probably driven by activation of normally silent mechanosensitive nociceptors that innervate the bone.

Tumor-derived products in generation of bone cancer pain

In most cancers, the tumor mass is composed of tumor and tumor stromal cells, the latter of which includes macrophages, neutrophils, T-lymphocytes, fibroblasts, and endothelial cells. Tumor and/or tumor stromal cells have been shown to secrete a variety of factors that sensitize or directly excite primary afferent neurons (Fig. 3). These factors include prostaglandins, bradykinin, tumor necrosis factor-alpha, endothelins, interleukins-1 and -6, epidermal growth factor, transforming growth factor-alpha, platelet-derived growth factor, and nerve growth factor (NGF) (Fig. 3).[12,27]

One tumor/stromal cell product that is of significant interest in the etiology of bone cancer pain is NGF. Previous studies have shown that NGF may directly activate sensory neurons that express the TrkA receptor and/or modulate the expression of proteins of sensory neurons expressing TrkA or p75 receptor (Fig. 3).[28] Anti-NGF antibody therapy may be particularly effective in blocking bone cancer pain as NGF appears to be integrally involved in the up-regulation, sensitization, and disinhibition of multiple neurotransmitters, ion channels and receptors in the primary afferent nerve fibers that synergistically increase nociceptive signals originating from the tumor-bearing bone.

To test the hypothesis that blocking NGF from binding to its cognate receptor TrkA is efficacious in reducing bone cancer pain, the analgesic efficacy of a murine anti-NGF monoclonal antibody was evaluated in two animal models of bone cancer.[10,29] These models included the primarily osteolytic mouse osteosarcoma line that expresses high levels of NGF,[29] and the primarily osteoblastic canine ACE-1 prostate, where NGF expression is undetectable (Fig. 5).[10] In both of these models it was demonstrated that administration of an anti-NGF antibody was efficacious in reducing both early- and late-stage bone cancer pain-related behaviors (Fig. 5) and that this reduction in pain-related behaviors was greater than that achieved with acute administration of 10 mg/kg of morphine sulfate.[10,29] This data suggests that therapeutic targeting of NGF, or its cognate receptor TrkA, may be useful in blocking bone cancer pain whether or not the tumor that has metastasized to bone expresses NGF. Presumably, in the case where the tumor cells themselves do not express NGF, it is the tumor stromal cells that are expressing and secreting NGF, as tumor stromal cells comprise 2–60% of the total tumor mass. Currently, a fully humanized monoclonal antibody to NGF (Tanezumab) has been tested in human patients with osteoarthritis (OA) and this therapy was effective at reducing OA pain.[30] Human clinical trials evaluating Tanezumab's effects at reducing bone cancer pain in patients with advanced breast or prostate cancer were scheduled to commence mid-2009.[31]

Neuropathic component of bone cancer pain

Because sensory and sympathetic neurons are present within the bone marrow, mineralized bone, and periosteum, and all these compartments are ultimately impacted by fractures, ischemia, or the presence of tumor cells, sensory fibers in any of

A

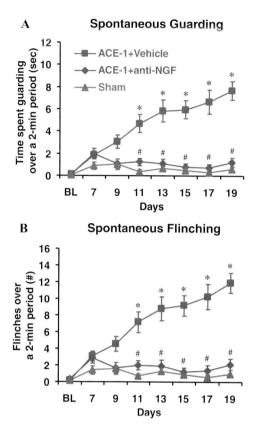

Spontaneous Guarding

B

Spontaneous Flinching

Figure 5. Anti-NGF attenuates spontaneous bone cancer pain in a model where the tumor cells (canine prostate cells) do not express NGF. Anti-NGF treatment (10 mg/kg, i.p., given on days 7, 12, and 17 posttumor injection) attenuated ongoing bone cancer pain behavior on days 7–19 posttumor injection. In these experiments, canine prostate carcinoma (ACE-1) cells were injected into the femur of adult male mice. The time spent guarding (**A**) and number of spontaneous flinches (**B**) of the afflicted limb over a 2-minute observation period were used as measures of ongoing pain. Anti-NGF significantly reduced ongoing pain behaviors in tumor-injected mice as compared with ACE-1 + vehicle. Note that ACE-1 cells *in vitro* express undetectable levels of NGF mRNA or protein, suggesting that NGF could be released mainly from tumor-associated macrophage and immune cells. Bars represent mean ± S.E.M. *$P < 0.05$ versus sham + vehicle; #$P < 0.05$ versus ACE-1 + vehicle. (With permission from Halvorson, K.G. *et al.*[10])

these tissues may play a role in the generation and maintenance of bone cancer pain.

In examining the changes in the sensory innervation of bone that are induced by the primarily oste-

olytic sarcoma cells, sensory fibers were observed at and within the leading edge of the tumor in the deep stromal regions of the tumor.[32] These sensory nerve fibers displayed a discontinuous and fragmented appearance, suggesting that following initial activation by the osteolytic tumor cells, the distal processes of the sensory nerve fibers were injured by the invading tumor cells.[32]

The tumor-induced injury and/or remodeling of sensory nerve fibers in these bone cancer pain models was also accompanied by an increase in ongoing and movement-evoked pain behaviors, an upregulation of galanin by sensory neurons that innervate the tumor-bearing femur, an upregulation of glial fibrillary acidic protein, hypertrophy of satellite cells surrounding sensory neuron cell bodies within the ipsilateral DRG, and macrophage infiltration of the DRG ipsilateral to the tumor-bearing femur.[12] Similar neurochemical changes have been described following peripheral nerve injury in other noncancerous neuropathic pain states.[33] In addition, chronic treatment with Gabapentin in the sarcoma model attenuated both ongoing and movement-evoked bone cancer-related pain behaviors, but did not influence tumor growth or tumor-induced bone destruction.[32] In light of these findings, we can suggest that bone cancer pain is driven by a neuropathic pain component. Currently, clinical trials are underway for assessing the effects of pregabalin (structurally related to gabapentin) on attenuating chronic bone pain related to metastases.[34]

Conclusions

Over the last decade, progress has been made in laying the foundation for a mechanism-based understanding of the factors that drive bone cancer pain. Interestingly, several therapies that attenuate bone cancer pain may also reduce tumor growth and tumor-induced bone remodeling. Thus, bisphosphonates are commonly used to treat bone cancer pain and other therapies including Denosumab (anti-RANKL; Amgen Inc., Thousand Oaks, CA), Tanezumab (anti-NGF; Pfizer Inc., New York, NY), and Pregabalin (Pfizer) are in mid- to late-stage clinical trials. We are beginning to understand the mechanisms that drive bone cancer. If this progress can be sustained and expanded, these advances have the potential to enlarge the repertoire of therapies available to treat bone cancer pain and significantly improve the quality of life, functional status, and survival of affected patients.

Conflicts of interest

The authors declare no conflicts of interest.

References

1. Coleman, R.E. 2006. Clinical features of metastatic bone disease and risk of skeletal morbidity. *Clin. Cancer Res.* **12:** 6243s–6249s.

2. Coleman, R.E. 1997. Skeletal complications of malignancy. *Cancer* **80:** 1588–1594.

3. Mercadante, S. 1997. Malignant bone pain: pathophysiology and treatment. *Pain* **69:** 1–18.

4. Zeppetella, G. 2009. Impact and management of breakthrough pain in cancer. *Curr. Opin. Support Palliat. Care* **3:** 1–6.

5. Arguello, F., R.B. Baggs & C.N. Frantz. 1988. A murine model of experimental metastasis to bone and bone marrow. *Cancer Res.* **48:** 6876–6881.

6. Yoneda, T., A. Sasaki & G.R. Mundy. 1994. Osteolytic bone metastasis in breast cancer. *Breast Cancer Res. Treatment* **32:** 73–84.

7. Honore, P. *et al.* 2000. Osteoprotegerin blocks bone cancer-induced skeletal destruction, skeletal pain and pain-related neurochemical reorganization of the spinal cord. *Nat. Med.* **6:** 521–528.

8. Schwei, M.J. *et al.* 1999. Neurochemical and cellular reorganization of the spinal cord in a murine model of bone cancer pain. *J. Neurosci.* **19:** 10886–10897.

9. Sabino, M.A. *et al.* 2003. Different tumors in bone each give rise to a distinct pattern of skeletal destruction, bone cancer-related pain behaviors and neurochemical changes in the central nervous system. *Int. J. Cancer* **104:** 550–558.

10. Halvorson, K.G. *et al.* 2005. A blocking antibody to nerve growth factor attenuates skeletal pain induced by prostate tumor cells growing in bone. *Cancer Res.* **65:** 9426–9435.

11. Lipton, A. 2006. Future treatment of bone metastases. *Clin. Cancer Res.* **12:** 6305s–6308s.

12. Mantyh, P.W. 2006. Cancer pain and its impact on diagnosis, survival and quality of life. *Nat. Rev. Neurosci.* **7:** 797–809.

13. von Moos, R. *et al.* 2008. Metastatic bone pain: treatment options with an emphasis on bisphosphonates. *Support Care Cancer* **16:** 1105–1115.

14. Delaisse, J.M. & G. Vaes. 1992. Mechanism of mineral solubilization and matrix degradation in osteoclastic bone resorption. In *Biology and Physiology of the Osteoclast.* B.R. Rifkin & C.V. Gay, Eds.: 289–314. CRC. Ann Arbor.

15. Drake, M.T., B.L. Clarke & S. Khosla. 2008. Bisphosphonates: mechanism of action and role in clinical practice. *Mayo Clin. Proc.* **83:** 1032–1045.

16. Halvorson, K.G. *et al.* 2006. Similarities and differences in tumor growth, skeletal remodeling and pain in an osteolytic and osteoblastic model of bone cancer. *Clin. J. Pain* **22:** 587–600.

17. Teitelbaum, S.L. 2007. Osteoclasts: what do they do and how do they do it? *Am. J. Pathol.* **170:** 427–435.

18. Julius, D. & A.I. Basbaum. 2001. Molecular mechanisms of nociception. *Nature* **413:** 203–210.

19. Ghilardi, J.R. *et al.* 2005. Selective blockade of the capsaicin receptor TRPV1 attenuates bone cancer pain. *J. Neurosci.* **25:** 3126–3131.

20. Griffiths, J.R. 1991. Are cancer cells acidic? *Br. J. Cancer* **64:** 425–427.

21. Lipton, A. 2008. Emerging role of bisphosphonates in the clinic—antitumor activity and prevention of metastasis to bone. *Cancer Treat Rev.* **34**(Suppl 1): S25–S30.

22. Body, J.J. *et al.* 2006. A study of the biological receptor activator of nuclear factor-kappaB ligand inhibitor, denosumab, in patients with multiple myeloma or bone metastases from breast cancer. *Clin. Cancer Res.* **12:** 1221–1228.

23. http://clinicaltrials.gov. Accessed April 2009. NCT00556374, NCT00321620.

24. Lipton, A. & S. Jun. 2008. RANKL inhibition in the treatment of bone metastases. *Curr. Opin. Support Palliat. Care* **2:** 197–203.

25. Niiyama, Y. *et al.* 2009. SB366791, a TRPV1 antagonist, potentiates analgesic effects of systemic morphine in a murine model of bone cancer pain. *Br. J. Anaesth.* **102:** 251–258.

26. Rubert Cynthia, H.R. & M. Martin. 2000. Orthopedic management of skeletal metastases. In *Tumor Bone Disease and Osteoporsis in Cancer Patients.* J.-J. Body, Ed.: 305–356. Marcel Dekker. New York City.

27. Joyce, J.A. & J.W. Pollard. 2009. Microenvironmental regulation of metastasis. *Nat. Rev. Cancer* **9:** 239–252.

28. Pezet, S. & S.B. McMahon. 2006. Neurotrophins: mediators and modulators of pain. *Annu. Rev. Neurosci.* **29:** 507–538.

29. Sevcik, M.A. *et al.* 2005. Anti-NGF therapy profoundly reduces bone cancer pain and the accompanying increase in markers of peripheral and central sensitization. *Pain* **115:** 128–141.

30. Schnitzer, T.J. *et al.* 2008. Efficacy and safety of Tanezumab (PF04383119), an anti-nerve growth factor (NGF) antibody, for moderate to severe pain due to osteoarthritis (OA) of the knee: a randomized trial. In *12th World Congress of Pain: PT 214*. Glasgow. Scotland, UK.

31. http://clinicaltrials.gov. Accessed April 2009. NCT00545129, NCT00830180.

32. Peters, C.M. *et al.* 2005. Tumor-induced injury of primary afferent sensory nerve fibers in bone cancer pain. *Exp. Neurol.* **193:** 85–100.

33. Obata, K. *et al.* 2003. Contribution of injured and uninjured dorsal root ganglion neurons to pain behavior and the changes in gene expression following chronic constriction injury of the sciatic nerve in rats. *Pain* **101:** 65–77.

34. http://clinicaltrials.gov. Accessed April 2009. NCT00381095.

Ann. N.Y. Acad. Sci. ISSN 0077-8923

Timing and mechanism of a window of spontaneous activity in embryonic mouse hindbrain development

Martha M. Bosma

Department of Biology, University of Washington, Seattle, Washington

Address for correspondence: Martha M. Bosma, Department of Biology, University of Washington, Seattle, WA 98195-1800. Voice: (206) 616-9031; fax: (206) 616-2011. martibee@u.washington.edu

Spontaneous activity (SA) in the developing vertebrate brain is required for correct wiring of circuits and networks. In almost every brain region studied to date, SA is recorded during a period of synaptogenesis, and may deploy ionic mechanism(s) that are not expressed in the adult structure. Eventually the conditions in the immature neurons that allow SA are replaced with ion channels found in the mature neuron; this replacement may itself require SA. In the embryonic (E) 11.5 mouse hindbrain, SA is initiated by a subgroup of serotonergic neurons derived from former rhombomeres 2 and 3; SA events propagate rostrally and caudally along the midline, and into the lateral hindbrain. In this review, I describe the properties of mouse hindbrain SA and the developmental window during which it is expressed, summarize the known mechanisms by which SA arises, and describe other brain regions where this SA is similar (chick hindbrain) or influential (mouse midbrain).

Keywords: motor patterns; hindbrain; spontaneous activity; serotonin

Introduction

The mature brain is wired to respond to signals, either from sensory inputs or other neurons, which cause an electrical response; with the exception of a few neuron types, few CNS neurons participate in electrical signaling by large synchronous groups, except under unusual conditions. The situation is quite different in the developing brain, in which large regions of the brain synchronously express spontaneous activity. Such spontaneous activity (SA) has been shown to be required for a variety of developmental processes in network formation, including neuronal proliferation, cell body migration, neurite extension and pathfinding, and synaptic formation and maintenance.[1] SA has been recorded in a number of CNS structures, sometimes during a discrete window that corresponds to a period of specific network formation; such structures include the cortex, hippocampus, retina, cochlea, and spinal cord.

One example of network formation control by SA is found in the connections between the retina and its major target, the lateral geniculate nucleus of the thalamus. The retina undergoes waves of SA which are able to initiate in any region, but which may be elicited by a specific group of retinal neurons, the starburst amacrine cells.[2,3] Alterations in the frequency or spread of SA waves alter the specificity and coarseness of the retinal map on the LGN, demonstrating that the mechanisms that elicit and propagate SA are crucial in correct network formation.[4,5]

Our work concentrates on the development of the hindbrain, which in the adult becomes the pons, medulla and, very rostrally, the cerebellum. These structures receive sensory input and deliver motor output to the face and head, coordinate sensory input in the cerebellum, contain many axon tracts between the spinal cord and higher CNS, and are home to many neurons of the reticular formation, including serotonergic neurons. The hindbrain, in early development, is organized in the rostral-caudal axis by segmentation into rhombomeres, cell-specification segments setting up transversely arranged bands of gene expression. As development proceeds, longitudinal tracts are formed that course between vestibular networks, the spinal cord, and higher CNS structures.

doi: 10.1111/j.1749-6632.2009.05423.x

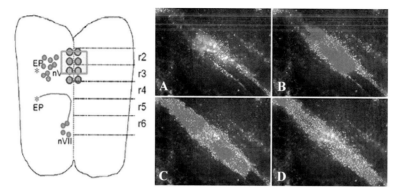

Figure 1. Spontaneous activity propagates from an initiation zone (InZ). Inset (*left*) shows main features of hindbrain, in open book preparation. On the right are the borders of the former rhombomeres, designated by numbers (r). *Red circles* show the cell bodies of motoneurons from the trigeminal (V) and facial (VII) nerves, with exit points shown as *red asterisks* (EP). *Blue circles* near midline indicate location of serotonin-positive cell bodies (caudal group does not develop until E12.5.); *green box* is initiation zone (InZ). (**A**)–(**D**) Live $[Ca^{2+}]_i$ imaging of hindbrain, with midline crossing diagonally from *upper left* (rostral) to *lower right* (caudal). Single event initiating at center of screen, propagating both rostrally and caudally. High $[Ca^{2+}]_i$ levels are shown in *red*, superimposed on bright-field image of hindbrain. Frames taken every 0.4 sec.

The serotonergic neurons originating in the rostral hindbrain later develop into the raphe nuclei of the reticular formation.[6,7] The raphe innervates many brain structures and is involved in a wide range of complex behaviors, such as sleep, circadian rhythms, and mood and is composed of several groups of 5HT-positive neurons.[8] We have previously demonstrated that the early differentiating neurons of the serotonergic raphe play a role in early hindbrain development, where they act as a driver or initiator zone (InZ) that mediates synchronous SA in the hindbrain, and in the adjoining midbrain as well.[9]

In this review, I will discuss the properties of the initiator region in driving hindbrain SA. When rhombomeric segmentation ends, synchronized SA emerges in the mouse hindbrain, driven by the InZ, which initiates over 85% of the events. This pacemaker persists in initiating events between E11.5 and E13.5, and then becomes inactive. We have observed a similar phenomenon in chick hindbrain, with differences attributable to the more mature properties of chick hindbrain. This conservation suggests that SA is important in network development in the hindbrain. We have also observed that the events initiated in the hindbrain trigger waves of SA in the more rostral midbrain, the first time that an identified initiator can control activity in a different brain structure.

Results

Description of mouse hindbrain spontaneous activity

SA was examined using the open-brain preparation, in which the dorsal midline is opened and the hindbrain placed in a $[Ca^{2+}]_i$ imaging chamber (Fig. 1, *inset*). The positions and trajectories of the branchiomeric motoneurons (trigeminal and facial) were delineated by retrograde labeling, and the serotonergic neuronal groups identified using immunocytochemistry. In the E11.5 mouse hindbrain, more than 85% of recorded events initiate from the midline in former rhombomere 2;[10] we thus term this region the initiator zone (InZ). InZ-initiated events propagate rostrally and caudally along the midline, as well as laterally (see later). Figure 1A shows an event initiating in the midline InZ (red color indicates increase in $[Ca^{2+}]_i$); this event then propagates in both the rostral and caudal directions along the midline (Figs. 1B–D). Interestingly, events moving in the rostral direction propagate at a more rapid velocity (359 ± 5 μm/s) than the same event propagating caudally (168 ± 35 μm/s) ($n = 23$)[10], suggesting that differential mechanisms mediate propagation in the two directions. Other rostral midline regions can initiate events (approximately 15%), but we have never observed initiation of events by lateral regions.

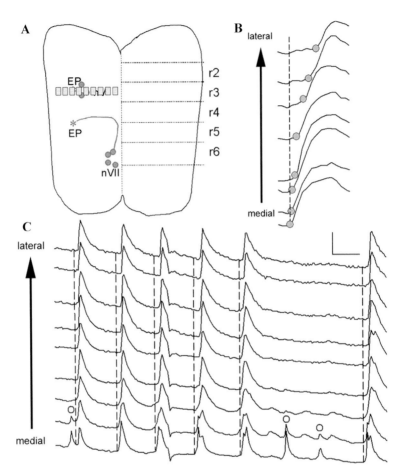

Figure 2. Single SA events propagate from medial to lateral. (**A**) Drawing of hindbrain showing recording sites arrayed from midline to lateral regions (*rectangles*). (**B**) Recordings from sites plotted from medial (*bottom trace*) to lateral (*top trace*), showing single event propagating from medial to lateral. (**C**) Events shown on slower time scale, in different hindbrain, demonstrating medial-to-lateral propagation; some events do not propagate outside of the InZ (*open circles*). The propagation rate was approximately 240 μm/sec. Time scale is 0.4 sec for B, 2 sec for C.

InZ-triggered events also propagate laterally from the midline. Figure 2A shows the placement of multiple $[Ca^{2+}]_i$ imaging sites on the hindbrain, starting from the midline InZ and covering the entire medio-lateral extent of the hindbrain. Changes in fluorescence at each site are plotted from bottom to top in Figures 2B and C, demonstrating that events initiate medially and propagate laterally. When a longitudinal cut is made between the InZ and a lateral position, the activity in the midline is not affected, while the lateral activity is smaller, significantly lower in frequency, and not coordinated with the midline, after the cut. [9]

We used pharmacological manipulation to elucidate interactions that elicit hindbrain SA. Block-

ers of glutamatergic, GABA$_A$ and GABA$_B$, nicotinic, glycinergic, dopaminergic, tachykinin, purinergic, and histaminergic receptors did not abolish activity.[11] The only transmitter system that appears to be required for expression of hindbrain SA is serotonin (5HT), acting through 5HT2$_A$ and 5HT2$_C$ receptors. In addition, gap junctional coupling appears to be crucial to SA, as block by the relatively nonspecific agents octanol, carbenoxolone, and mefloquine all abolish SA, while the addition of ammonium transiently augments SA.

Transverse cryosections of the E11.5 hindbrain labeled with an antibody against serotonin showed that serotonin-positive neurons were located with 125 μm of the midline of the hindbrain, and send

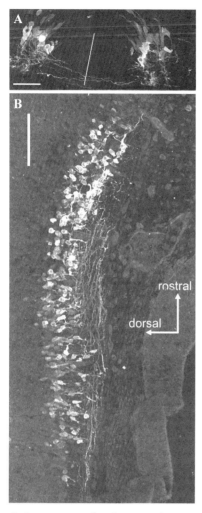

Figure 3. Immunocytochemistry against serotonin (5HT) demonstrates newly postmitotic neurons at E11.5. (**A**) Transverse section showing serotonin-positive neurons leaving the ventricular zone, and clustering in the marginal zone very close to the midline (*white line*). Axons cross the floor plate ventral to the ventricular zone. Scale bar is 50 μm. (**B**) Parasagittal section 30 μm from midline showing rostral cluster of serotonin-positive neurons stretching from isthmus (at rostral end) to the rostral edge of former r4 (as measured in dextran-identified animals; not shown). Scale bar is 100 μm.

their axons both contralaterally across the floor plate and into the marginal zone (Fig. 3A). In sagittal sections, the serotonin-positive neurons were clustered in a group that extended from the isthmus (hindbrain–midbrain organizer) to the rostral end of former rhombomere 4 (Fig. 3B), encompassing

the identified InZ. These neurons send axons across the isthmus into the midbrain, which becomes highly innervated by E13.5, and into more rostral regions of the brain. (A second serotonergic group, located caudal to former rhombomere 4, develops at E12.5 and innervates the spinal cord.[8]) Counting serial transverse sections showed that within the midline InZ region, 85% of the postmitotic neurons were serotonin-positive, suggesting that the InZ is composed almost exclusively of serotonergic neurons.[9] This combined evidence of initiation site, proportion of serotonergic neurons within the InZ, and pharmacological dependence of SA on 5HT receptors, implies that the developing neurons of the rostral raphe are the drivers of SA in the hindbrain.

Developmental window of SA

SA in mouse hindbrain is a transient phenomenon, recorded only in the interval of E9.5–E13.5. Early experiments examining the development of SA utilized recordings from identified trigeminal and facial motor neurons, retrogradely labeled by Texas Red-conjugated dextrans injected into the target branchial arches (Fig. 4A).[12] At E9.5, individual neurons have spontaneous events which are long in duration, and neurons undergo events independently (Fig. 4B). Twenty-four hours later, at E10.5, events are significantly shorter in duration, suggesting that some mechanism for more rapid termination of events has developed; events are still independently expressed in individual neurons (Fig. 4C). After an additional 24 h of development, at E11.5, events between individual motor neurons become highly synchronized, and almost no independent events are observed (Fig. 4D).

The synchronized SA, initially observed in identified motoneurons lateral to the midline, was determined to be driven by the midline InZ, as shown by the medio-lateral mapping experiments described above. Thus, at E11.5, the InZ becomes active, and synchronizes SA across the entire hindbrain (green area, Fig. 5A), driving neurons that are already close to threshold in propagating waves of activity. The relative frequency of midline activity is slightly higher near the pontine flexure (PF) (right histogram, Fig. 5A), which includes the InZ. The InZ remains active until E13.5, but the area of the hindbrain that is able to be synchronized by InZ input diminishes over time.[10] Thus, the midline remains

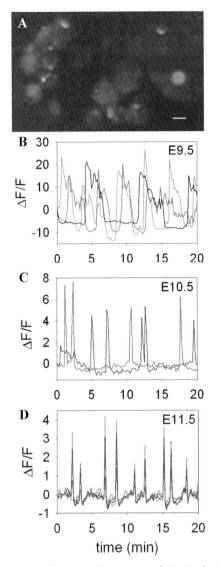

Figure 4. Developmental sequence of SA in dextran-identified motoneurons. (A) Living motoneurons retrogradely filled with dextran (*red*) by injection into target tissue, and loaded with fluo4-AM (*green*). Single identified neurons were recorded for fluctuations in $[Ca^{2+}]_i$. Scale bar is 15 µm. In B–D, each color trace represents recording from an individual neuron. (B) At E9.5, events in individual neurons are long duration, and independent. (C) At E10.5, events are significantly shorter in duration, and events in individual neurons are still independent. (D) At E11.5, events are short-duration, and highly synchronized between neurons.

driven by the InZ at E12.5, although the most rostral and caudal extremes have a reduced frequency of activity (green area and histogram, Fig. 5B); lateral regions of the hindbrain no longer respond to the InZ signal. By E13.5, the rostral and caudal regions of the midline respond to InZ activity at only very low frequency (green area and histogram, Fig. 5C), and by E14.5, no SA is recorded in the hindbrain. The area that responds to the InZ at E13.5 is only 14% of that at E11.5. The absolute frequency of InZ-initiated events decreases by approximately twofold between E11.5 and E12.5, remains constant to E13.5 (*inset*, Fig. 5), and is disappears at E14.5.

These experiments show that SA in the hindbrain is expressed over the interval of E9.5–E13.5, but each day of that period has a unique and characteristic form of SA. Independent spontaneous events at E9.5 have long durations, and shorten significantly at E10.5; events in all neurons are then synchronized by InZ input at E11.5. After this 24-h period of whole-hindbrain response to the InZ driver, the lateral areas begin to become refractory at E12.5, followed by the midline outside of the InZ at E13.5. Thus, the unique aspects of SA on each developmental day overlie other developmental events in the hindbrain.

Mechanisms of SA initiation

The ability to observe the relationship between several cells or groups of cells was integral to the discovery of the propagation of SA in the hindbrain. We then examined the electrophysiological properties of individual neurons in medial versus lateral positions within the hindbrain.[13] Neurobiotin was included in the pipette in order to measure the coupling of the recorded neuron to neighboring neurons. Within the delineated InZ (up to 100 µm from the midline), in current clamp recording, neurons had spontaneous events comprised of two components: the first was a large amplitude, spike-like event; the second was a slower plateau (Fig. 6(A)1). Outside of the midline area comprising the InZ, neurons had spontaneous events that were small in amplitude, and consisted of only the plateau component (Fig. 6(A)2). In several tens of recordings, the components were measured and compared to the position in the hindbrain. These data showed that the spike was recorded only in medial neurons, and the plateau was significantly larger in medial neurons.

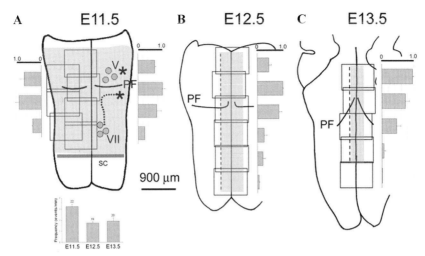

Figure 5. Between E11.5 and E13.5, SA retracts from lateral, then medial tissue. Hindbrains from each stage were laid in open-book configuration, and drawings to scale made of each stage. Boxed frames in each figure correspond to camera frames during each recording, which were positioned over each hindbrain in random order; a multiple array of sites within each frame were then recorded. Scale bar applies to A–C. (A) At E11.5, SA is recorded in the entire hindbrain (*green area*). At the midline, the relative frequency of activity was highest in the most rostral frame (graph on right of figure); in lateral region, frequency was highest in more caudal region, suggesting that propagation is more efficacious at that level of the tissue. (B) At E12.5, SA is largely retracted from the lateral regions, and is found only in midline tissue; frequency of activity is highest just above the pontine flexure (PF). *Dashed line* indicates most extreme lateral extent of SA. (C) At E13.5, SA is even more restricted within the midline, with frequency highest at the most rostral end of the hindbrain near the isthmus. Events are able to propagate to PF, and then stop well before the end of the hindbrain. Inset shows absolute frequency of SA at each stage, which is significantly higher at E11.5.

We sought to identify the underlying currents that engendered the differential expression of event properties between medial and lateral neurons. When the tissue containing the recorded cells was reacted for the neurobiotin from the pipette, medial neurons had a small cluster size, while lateral neurons were coupled to significantly more neighboring neurons (Figs. 6(B)1 and 2). The neurobiotin-permeable connections are likely to be gap junctions, as octanol and mefloquine block SA, while ammonium transiently augments SA. Thus, midline neurons have small, but significant, cluster sizes that may be important in initiating activity, while lateral neurons have connections to more neighboring neurons, most likely to aid in propagation of events.

We then asked whether the differential expression of neuron coupling was reflected in the resting conductance of the neurons. Using voltage clamp recording, we applied ramp potentials from -110 to $+30$ mV. Resultant currents in lateral cells showed a much larger resting conductance compared to those in medial cells, likely a consequence of the increased coupling between neurons (Fig. 6C).

In addition, the resultant currents in medial neurons showed a small inflection near -40 mV, raising the possibility that an inward current was expressed in medial cells, but not evident in lateral cells. We used Cs^+-based pipette solutions to ask whether hindbrain neurons expressed inward currents. We found that medial, but not lateral neurons, expressed an inward current that was sensitive to Ni^{2+}, peaked at about -45 mV, and had kinetics similar to T-type Ca^{2+} channels (*inset*, Fig. 6C). Thus, medial neurons have inward currents that are available near the resting potential of the neuron, and have relatively little resting conductance, both properties that would allow them to act as initiators of activity. Lateral neurons, in contrast, have no inward currents and have high resting conductance, consigning them to a follower behavior in the hindbrain.

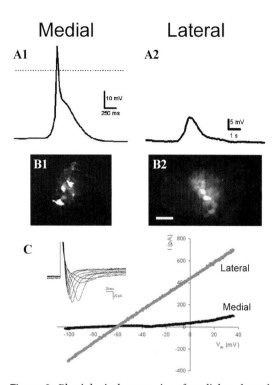

Medial   Lateral

Figure 6. Physiological properties of medial *vs.* lateral neurons. (**A1 and 2**) Representative traces in current clamp mode from a medial neuron (**A1**) and a lateral neuron (**A2**), showing the two-component spontaneous events (spike plus plateau) in medial neurons, and events with only plateaus in lateral neurons. *Dotted line* in A1 indicates 0 mV for both figures. (**B1 and 2**) Representative neurobiotin-reacted fills from medial (*left*) and lateral (*right*) neurons, showing that lateral neurons are coupled to significantly more neurons via gap junctions. (**C**) Main graph shows resultant currents in voltage clamp from a voltage ramp from −110 to +30 mV, showing that lateral neurons (*gray trace*) have high resting leak conductance, while medial neurons (*black trace*) have significantly less. Inset shows inward current responses in a medial neuron to depolarizations from a holding potential of −80 mV in voltage clamp; 5 mV steps to −40 to 0 mV elicit inward currents resembling T-type Ca^{2+} currents. Only medial neurons express measurable inward currents.

SA in chick hindbrain

To characterize the relevance of hindbrain SA across species, we examined the expression of SA in developing chick hindbrain.[14] In chick hindbrain, SA was recorded at E5, but only under conditions of increased $[K^+]_o$ (5 mM, in contrast to our standard 2.5 mM). During the developmental period between E6 and E9, intervals between events were very regular, and increased from approximately 4 min at E6 to 18 min at E9 (Fig. 6). In contrast to mouse hindbrain SA, which has a single initiation point near the former r2, chick SA was initiated from two sites, one near the former r2, and the other more caudally located, at the former r4 (Fig. 7). Another striking difference between chick and mouse was the involvement of spinal cord in chick SA; when the preparation included the spinal cord, lateral waves of spinal cord activity could be seen that appeared to be synchronized with hindbrain SA; however, the presence of the spinal cord was not required for independent hindbrain SA. Spinal cord involvement in mouse hindbrain SA was never observed, irregardless of the length of spinal cord that was present.

Pharmacologically, SA in chick was not exclusively dependent on 5HT receptors, as blockers of nAChR, $GABA_A$, and glycine receptors all blocked activity.[14] As chick develops more rapidly than mouse, it may not be surprising that other neurotransmitter systems are involved in chick SA, as many more axon tracts and networks are in place at these developmental stages in chick.[15]

We examined the serotonergic system in E6 chick hindbrain, and found that both the rostral and caudal serotonergic groups were in place, with extensive axon extension and cell body migration to more mature positions. Interestingly, the gap in serotonin-positive cells between the rostral and caudal group was situated more rostrally in chick than in mouse, at approximately former rhombomere 2; thus, both initiation points are located in the caudal serotonergic group. The anatomical differences between chick and mouse are summarized in Figure 7, which shows the initiation points (asterisks) and serotonergic midline groups (both rostral and caudal in chick, and the rostral and future caudal in mouse). These comparative experiments show that hindbrain SA is strongly conserved within vertebrate species suggesting a role for hindbrain SA in network formation.

Hindbrain SA drives activity in the midbrain

Events from the hindbrain InZ propagate rostrally and caudally along the midline; those that

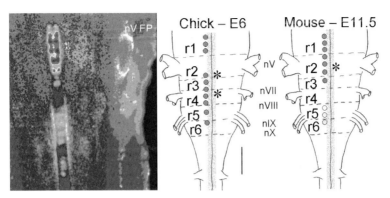

Figure 7. SA in chick hindbrain. (*Left*) Frame from video showing two midline initiation regions in chick hindbrain, the first just caudal to the nV exit point, the other closer to the nVII exit point. *Red* indicates relatively high $[Ca^{2+}]_i$ levels; fluorescence trace is superimposed on bright-field image of the hindbrain. (*Right*) Comparison drawings of chick and mouse hindbrain. In each, the cranial nerves and former rhombomeres are indicated; the gray dots represent the positions of serotonin-positive neurons (white dots in the mouse hindbrain are the caudal group that does not appear until E12.5); asterisks show the initiation regions for each species. Note the differential position of the gap in serotonergic neurons: in former rhombomere 2 in chick, and in former rhombomere 4 in mouse. Scale bar is 1 mm for chick, 0.5 mm for mouse hindbrain. (Figure modified from Figure 9 of Hughes *et al.*, 2009.)

propagate caudally dissipate well before they encounter the spinal cord. Events that propagate in the rostral direction can cross the isthmus (also known as the hindbrain–midbrain organizer), and sweep across the tegmentum of the midbrain.[16] Events initiated in the hindbrain InZ travel along the midline towards the isthmus, where they pause before propagating into the midbrain (Fig. 8). The ability to cross the isthmus is dependent on developmental stage, as hindbrain events at E12.5 have a higher probability of crossing into the midbrain than those at either E11.5, even though the frequency of activity in the hindbrain decreases slightly during that interval. This is likely due to the increased length of serotonin-positive projections towards the midbrain and crossing the isthmus over this developmental period; since the hindbrain events travel rostrally along these projections, their increasing length may facilitate crossing the isthmus. Events cross into the midbrain along the midline through the isthmus; they then propagate rostrally and laterally to fan across the entire tegmentum of the midbrain. Groups of nicotinic and GABAergic neurons, located laterally to the midline, are likely crucial in the lateral propagation,

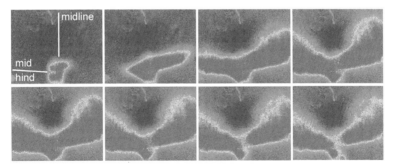

Figure 8. Hindbrain SA initiates activity in the mouse midbrain. Successive frames show propagation of a midline (*vertical white line*) event moving across the isthmus (*horizontal white line*) to fan laterally and rostrally across the midbrain tegmentum. Each frame is 1 mm wide. Frames taken every 0.68 sec. (Figure modified from figure 2 and cover of Rockhill *et al.*, 2009.)

as it is abolished by blockers of those receptors. Strikingly, although each wave of midbrain activity crosses the developing dopaminergic neurons, those neurons are not themselves required for SA, as blockers of either D1 or D2 receptors do not affect midbrain SA. However, the dopaminergic neurons may themselves contribute to, or be influenced by, the waves of midbrain activity.

In the chick midbrain, it has been shown that concentric torii of gene expression are located within the tegmentum; each torus opens facing caudally, and each underlies a specific mature neuron population.[17] The most caudal and medial group is the anlage of the dopaminergic neurons of the substantial nigra, while more lateral torii underlie GABergic and cholinergic neurons. The propagation of midbrain SA events occurs in a fan which moves orthogonally to the established torii of gene expression. We have observed hindbrain-to-midbrain propagation in chick (unpublished) as well as in mouse, implying that along with conservation of hindbrain SA between species, hindbrain-driven midbrain events are also conserved.

Discussion

SA in mouse hindbrain is first recorded as individual neurons engaged in spontaneous events that are not coordinated. Synchronized waves of InZ-driven SA are expressed exactly at E11.5, when the transient borders between rhomobomeres disappear.[18] Segmented gene expression is the conserved mechanism for establishment of anterior–posterior identity in vertebrates and invertebrates; this segmentation determines insect segmental identity as well as hindbrain neuronal fates (for example, the differential determination of trigeminal versus facial motoneurons). We postulate that as the role of the anterior–posterior fate determination by rhombomeric segregation decreases, waves of SA that repeatedly emanate from one site become the mechanism by which neurons localize their spatial relationship. A single point source of propagating excitation allows developing neurons in a longitudinal or horizontal group to discriminate neighbor relationships; those that are close neighbors may then reinforce their developing synapses in a Hebbian manner.

This hindbrain InZ is the first example where an identified driver causes SA in a neighboring brain structure, the midbrain.[16] The frequency of midbrain events is determined by the ability of serotonergic axons to carry the event through the isthmus into the midbrain; as these axons are longer at E12.5 than E11.5, midbrain activity is higher in frequency at that stage. The frequency decreases at E13.5, as the midline of the hindbrain becomes refractory to the InZ signal. The phenomenon of the hindbrain driving the midbrain may be a mechanism by which connections between the two structures are guided: for example, axons of the medial and lateral longitudinal funiculi derive from neurons in the rostral hindbrain and midbrain,[19] and may require SA in order to pathfind appropriately. In addition, the rostrally directed axons of the serotonergic neurons are themselves elongating extensively, and the robust midline SA may be an important guidance mechanism by which they find and traverse the isthmus.

Interestingly, the strongest and longest-lasting axis of SA propagation is rostro-caudal, which places SA propagation orthogonal to the former transverse bands of gene expression which were initially established by rhombomere segmentation. As these waves of activity enter the midbrain, they fan rostro-laterally from the isthmus across the tegmentum, again moving orthogonally across bands of gene expression. It is possible that in each of these cases, spontaneous electrical activity is replacing gene patterning mechanisms in neuron specification or differentiation.

At E11.5, both the frequency of events and the total area that is able to be driven by each event is significantly higher than later stages. We have yet to determine the mechanism by which first the lateral (at E12.5), then the midline neurons (at E13.5), lose their ability to be driven by the InZ. Possibilities include the down-regulation of connexin expression such that the signal cannot propagate between cells or the up-regulation of K^+ channels that oppose depolarizing influences.

When the InZ is cut into successively smaller pieces the probability of SA decreases as the pieces get smaller. This phenomenon suggests that the InZ is composed of a network of serotonergic neurons interacting to initiate events which then propagate into other hindbrain regions. Although individual cells undergo spontaneous electrical events without obvious evidence of synaptic input from other neurons, and ionotropic receptors are not involved in hindbrain SA, the events may be a consequence of electrical coupling and G-protein-coupled receptor input.

A further area of study is the ionic mechanism(s) which turn off the expression of SA within the InZ. One mechanism may be the developmental down-regulation of T-type Ca^{2+} channels, which have a window current near the resting potential which might allow SA; without such a depolarizing drive, cells may not undergo spontaneous events.

The changing pattern of SA in the hindbrain, from independent long-duration events (at E9.5), to all-over synchronized waves (at E11.5), to retraction back to the InZ (at E13.5), is unique to the hindbrain. The mechanisms that cause each step— independent SA, synchronization, and retraction— are not yet understood, nor is the mechanism of differential ion channel expression between medial and lateral neurons. However, this robust phenomenon is maintained between relatively distant vertebrates (mouse and chicken), and thus has been conserved strongly. It is possible that alterations resulting from brain insult, fever, or fetal seizures may disrupt the balance of this pattern over the developmental window of SA, resulting in abnormal network properties not just in hindbrain, but midbrain as well. An additional point to consider is that maternal use of serotonergic modulators may influence the synchronization, frequency or propagation of hindbrain SA, possibly altering developing circuits.

Conflicts of interest

The author declares no conflicts of interest.

References

1. Moody, W.J. & M.M. Bosma. 2005. Ion channel development, spontaneous activity, and activity-dependent development in nerve and muscle cells. *Physiol. Rev.* **85:** 883–941.

2. Zheng, J., S. Lee & Z.J. Zhou. 2006. A transient network of intrinsically bursting starburst cells underlies the generation of retinal waves. *Nat. Neurosci.* **9:** 363–371.

3. Feller, M. 2009. Retinal waves are likely to instruct the formation of eye-specific retinogeniculate projections. *Neural Dev.* **4:** 24.

4. Shatz, C.J. 1996. Emergence of order in visual system development. *Proc. Natl. Acad. Sci. USA* 93: 602–608.

5. Wong, R.O. 1999. Retinal waves and visual system development. *Ann. Rev. Neurosci.* **22:** 29–47.

6. Wallace, J.A. & J.M. Lauder. 1983. Development of the serotonergic system in the rat embryo: an immunocytochemical study. *Brain Res. Bull.* **10:** 459–479.

7. Hornung, J.P. 2003. The human raphe nuclei and the serotonergic system. *J. Chem. Neuroanat.* **26:** 331–343.

8. Jacobs, B.L. & E.C. Azmitia. 1982. Structure and function of the brain: serotonin system. *Physiol. Rev.* **72:** 165–229.

9. Hunt, P.N., A.K. McCabe & M.M. Bosma. 2005. Midline serotonergic neurons drive widespread synchronized activity in embryonic mouse hindbrain. *J. Physiol.* **566:** 807–819.

10. Hunt, P.N., J. Gust, A.K. McCabe & M.M. Bosma. 2006. Primary role of the serotonergic midline system in synchronized spontaneous activity during development of the embryonic mouse hindbrain. *J. Neurobiol.* **66:** 1239–1252.

11. Hunt, P.N., A.K. McCabe, J. Gust & M.M. Bosma. 2006. Spatial restriction of spontaneous activity towards the rostral primary initiating zone during development of the embryonic mouse hindbrain. *J. Neurobiol.* **66:** 1225–1238.

12. Gust, J., J.J. Wright, E.B. Pratt & M.M. Bosma. 2003. Development of synchronized activity of cranial motor neurons in the segmented embryonic mouse hindbrain. *J. Physiol.* **550:** 123–133.

13. Moruzzi, A.M., N.C. Abedini, M.A. Hansen, *et al.* 2009. Differential expression of membrane conductances underlies spontaneous event initiation by rostral midline neurons in the embryonic mouse hindbrain. *J. Physiol.* **587:** 5081–5093.

14. Hughes, S.M., C.R. Easton & M.M. Bosma. 2009. Properties and mechanisms of spontaneous activity in the embryonic chick hindbrain. *Dev. Neurobiol.* **69:** 477–490.

15. Glover, J.C. & G. Petursdottir. 1991. Regional specificity of developing reticulospinal, vestibulospinal, and vestibulo-ocular projections in the chicken embryo. *J. Neurobiol.* **22:** 353–376.

16. Rockhill, W., J.L. Kirkman & M.M. Bosma. 2009. Spontaneous activity in the developing mouse midbrain driven by an external pacemaker. *Dev. Neurobiol.* **69:** 689–704.

17. Sanders, T.A., A. Lumsden & C.W. Ragsdale. 2002. Arcuate plan of chick midbrain development. *J. Neurosci.* **22:** 10742–10750.

18. Guthrie, S. 1996. Patterning the hindbrain. *Curr. Opin. Neurobiol.* **6.1:** 41–48.

19. Glover, J.C. 2000. Development of specific connectivity between premotor neurons and motoneurons in the brain stem and spinal cord. *Phys. Rev.* **80:** 615–647.

Ann. N.Y. Acad. Sci. ISSN 0077-8923

ANNALS OF THE NEW YORK ACADEMY OF SCIENCES
Issue: *Neurons and Networks in the Spinal Cord*

Human stem cells as a model of motoneuron development and diseases

Yan Liu[1,2] and Su-Chun Zhang[2]

[1]Department of Human Anatomy and Histology, Institute of Stem Cells and Regenerative Medicine, Shanghai Medical School, Fudan University, Shanghai, China. [2]Departments of Anatomy and Neurology, School of Medicine and Public Health, Waisman Center, University of Wisconsin, Madison, Wisconsin

Address for correspondence: Dr. Su-Chun Zhang, Waisman Center, University of Wisconsin, 1500 Highland Avenue, Madison, WI 53705. zhang@waisman.wisc.edu

Human embryonic stem cells (hESCs) and human induced pluripotent stem cells (hiPSCs) possess the potential to become all cell and tissue types of the human body. Under chemically defined culture systems, hESCs and hiPSCs have been efficiently directed to functional spinal motoneurons and astrocytes. The differentiation process faithfully recapitulates the developmental process predicted from studies in vertebrate animals and human specimens, suggesting the usefulness of stem cell differentiation systems in understanding human cellular development. Motoneurons and astrocytes differentiated from genetically altered hESCs or disease hiPSCs exhibit predicted phenotypes. They thus offer a simplified dynamic model for analyzing pathological processes that lead to human motoneuron degeneration, which in turn may serve as a template for pharmaceutical screening. In addition, the human stem cell-derived motoneurons and astrocytes, including those specifically derived from a patient, may become a source for cell therapy.

Keywords: embryonic stem cells; induced pluripotent stem cells; astrocytes; spinal muscular atrophy (SMA); amyotrophic lateral sclerosis (ALS)

Introduction

Motoneurons in the spinal cord innervate skeletal muscles, which is necessary for controlling movements. They originate from neuroepithelial cells in a restricted area of the developing spinal cord (neural tube) at around 4–5 weeks of human gestation. During embryonic development, motoneurons extend their processes (nerves) to the periphery to innervate skeletal muscles that are adjacent to the spinal cord. In an adult human body, however, motoneuron's axons are projected as far as 1 m away from the cell bodies in the spinal cord to reach their target muscles. In order to achieve this, motoneurons contain a high content of structural proteins, like neurofilaments. This geophysical feature of motoneurons demands a high metabolic rate compared to smaller neurons, which potentially renders motoneurons more susceptible to genetic, epigenetic, and/or environmental changes. Because motoneurons are generally nonrenewable, degeneration or loss of spinal motoneurons is often associated with debilitating or fatal neurological conditions such as pediatric spinal muscular atrophy (SMA) and adult onset amyotrophic lateral sclerosis (ALS).

Development of therapeutics for motoneuron diseases will depend upon our understanding of how human motoneurons are generated during embryogenesis, functionally maintained during adult life, degenerate under pathological conditions, and how the disease process may be halted or reversed. Human pluripotent stem cells, including human embryonic stem cells (hESCs) and human induced pluripotent stem cells (hiPSCs), can renew themselves for an extended period and be induced to generate all cell types in the body, including spinal motoneurons and their neighboring glial cells. Because of this, they provide an ideal model to study human motoneurons and glial cells directly. Over the past several years, hESCs have been successfully directed to spinal motoneurons[1,2] and astrocytes.[3] What is important to note is that the *in vitro*

doi: 10.1111/j.1749-6632.2010.05537.x

differentiation process mirrors *in vivo* development in terms of temporal time course, response to extrinsic morphogens, activation of transcriptional networks, and functional maturation.[14] Hence, stem cell differentiation offers a simplified model to understand human motoneuron and astrocyte development that is otherwise inaccessible. The *in vitro* produced human motoneurons and astrocytes could potentially become a source for cell therapy. In recent years, progress on genetically altered hESCs or disease hiPSCs, including those with ALS[4] and SMA,[5] would allow for tracing the degenerative process of human motoneurons and may be further modified for drug screening, thus leading to therapeutic development.

Stem cell model for human motoneuron and astrocyte development

Molecular interactions underlying the specification of motoneurons in vertebrate animals have been well defined. During chick embryo development, in response to a specific gradient (concentration) of sonic hedgehog (SHH) diffused from the notochord and floor plate, naïve neuroepithelial cells in the motoneuron progenitor (pMN) domain are specified to motoneuron progenitors by expressing a set of transcription factors including Olig2. During the neurogenic phase, the Olig2-expressing progenitors migrate a short distance ventrally, downregulate Olig2 expression, upregulate neurogenic transcription factors such as Ngn2 and HB9, and become post-mitotic motoneurons.[6] Based on this principle, mouse ESCs, after being neuralized by retinoic acid (RA), can be efficiently differentiated to spinal motoneurons in the presence of SHH.[7] In light of this, the molecular mechanism underlying motoneuron specification appears to be preserved *in vitro*.

To determine whether motoneuron differentiation from hESCs follows the same mechanism, we first guide the naïve hESCs to a synchronized population of neuroepithelial cells. Differentiation of neuroepithelia is achieved by plating individual hESC aggregates at a low density under a chemically defined medium.[8] This neural induction process is very efficient, yielding over 90% of the differentiated progenies being Pax6+ and Sox1+, which are markers for neuroepithelial cells.[9] Despite the absence of any exogenous neural inducers, differentiating hESCs produce molecules at multiple levels to block

transforming growth factor ß (TGF ß) signaling and to activate fibroblast growth factor signaling,[10] suggesting a conserved mechanism underlying human neural induction. It was recently suggested that addition of dual inhibitors of bone morphogenetic proteins (BMPs) can significantly increase the neural differentiation from human stem cells.[11] We did find that addition of BMP antagonists, such as Noggin, can inhibit BMP signaling in our neural differentiation system. However, such treatment does not significantly alter the neural differentiation efficiency given the already high yield.[10] We reason that the dual inhibition of BMPs during differentiation may be helpful if the starting hESCs or other stem cells have poor neural induction due to the presence of a high amount of BMPs in partially differentiated cells.

Besides the conserved molecular mechanisms described above, neural differentiation of hESCs manifests in morphological transformation that is readily identifiable. After 6–8 days of hESC differentiation, the round hESCs become columnar epithelia, which organize into neural tube-like rosettes by 14 days of culture.[8] This timeline of *in vitro* neural differentiation strikingly resembles the temporal course of neural plate and neural tube formation at the end of the third gestation week in human embryos, suggesting the preservation of an intrinsic developmental program in the hESC differentiation *in vitro*. It is in this differentiation process that we discovered a multipotent neural stem cell stage that can be readily patterned to versatile regional progenitors.[1] We refer to these precursors as primitive anterior neuroepithelia because they express anterior transcription factors including Otx2, Lhx2, and Pax6, but not the definitive neuroectoderm marker Sox1, and because they can be patterned to progenitors with various regional identities in response to morphogens.[9] Indeed, treatment with specific position-inducing morphogens of the primitive, but not the definitive, neuroepithelia results in differentiation of forebrain, midbrain, spinal cord, and dorsal-ventral progenitors.[1,12,13] This finding sets the foundation for differentiating human stem cells to specific neuronal and glial subtypes, including spinal motoneurons (Fig. 1).[14]

For motoneuron differentiation, the primitive neuroepithelia are patterned to ventral spinal progenitors by treatment with RA, a caudalizing morphogen, and SHH, a glycoprotein that induces

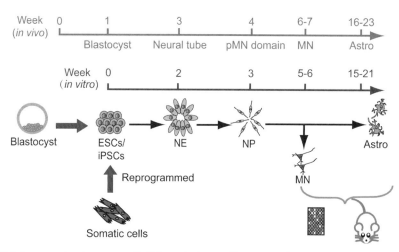

Figure 1. Parallels between *in vitro* stem cell differentiation and human embryo development. hESCs derived from a blastocyst or hiPSCs established from somatic cells are first differentiated to neuroepithelia that organize into neural tube-like rosettes in 2 weeks. This corresponds to the formation of neural plate/tube in a 3-week-old human embryo. In response to SHH and RA the neuroepithelia become ventral spinal progenitors in the next 10 days. This corresponds to the expansion of neural progenitors in a developing spinal cord. These progenitors then give rise to postmitotic motoneurons in the 4th and 5th week of culture. In the human spinal cord, motoneurons appear at the 5th–6th week. Additional 2 months of culture results in generation of astrocytes. It should be noted that hESCs are developmentally equivalent to 1-week-old embryos. Both motoneurons and astrocytes generated from transgenic hESCs or disease hiPSCs may be modified as templates for drug screening whereas those from nonmutated stem cells may be a source for cell therapy. Modified from Krencik and Zhang.[42]

ventralization. In 2 weeks, a large population of progenitors will express Olig2, a transcription factor specific for motoneuron progenitors. These progenitors then downregulate Olig2, upregulate HB9, a transcription factor specific for spinal motoneurons, exit the cell cycle, and become post-mitotic motoneurons by 4 weeks of hESC differentiation.[1] These motoneurons carry additional markers that are normally expressed in those of the spinal cord, including Islet 1/2 and Lhx3. Like mouse ESCs, treatment of hESC-derived neuroepithelia with RA results in differentiation of motoneurons of mainly the cervical and brachial spinal cord, as shown by their expression of HoxC5 and 8.[1] Furthermore, the *in vitro* differentiation of spinal motoneurons corresponds to the appearance of motoneurons in the human spinal cord at around 5 weeks of development. Again, these findings indicate that the *in vitro* differentiation process follows the same transcriptional program in response to a similar set of morphogens at a predictable time course (Fig. 1). This suggests that the *in vitro* stem cell differentiation system may be instrumental for understanding how individual subtypes of motoneurons are specified by

examining the transcriptional networks in response to specific sets of extracellular factors.

The *in vitro* generated spinal motoneurons gradually mature over the next several weeks. Shortly after the expression of HB9, the motoneurons express acetylcholine transferase, an enzyme necessary for synthesizing the neurotransmitter acetylcholine.[1] It is presently unknown what instructs the motoneurons to adopt this cholinergic fate. In addition, motoneurons express vesicular choline transferase, an enzyme required for storing and releasing the transmitter, suggesting functionality of the *in vitro* produced motoneurons. Indeed, when co-cultured with myocytes, the human motoneurons induce aggregation of acetylcholine receptors on myocytes, as indicated by bungarotoxin staining, and form neuro-muscular junctions, reminiscent of that which occurs *in vivo*. They further induce muscular contraction *in vitro*.[1] These findings confirm that the human motoneurons are functional. The stem cell differentiation system will likely provide an ideal platform to address this fundamental question about how to obtain a cholinergic identity.

Along with the cellular and molecular changes, motoneurons become electrophysiologically active after about 7–8 weeks of hESC differentiation. Synaptic currents are more readily detected with additional weeks of cultures. This is likely due to the enhanced synaptogenesis by the presence of differentiating astrocytes.[12] Astrocytes have been shown to be critical for synaptogenesis and synaptic transmission in animals[15] as well as in hESC-derived neurons.[12] Therefore, functional development of motoneurons is critically affected by the timing of differentiation and the presence of surrounding astrocytes.

Astrocytes are involved in virtually every aspect of physiology and pathology of the CNS.[16] However, directed differentiation and functional assessment of hESC-derived astrocytes has been surprisingly unexplored. Part of the reason is the paucity of information on the molecular mechanism of astrocytic development and lack of specific markers for astrocyte progenitors.[17,18] In hESC neural differentiation cultures, astrocytes appear after the differentiation of neurons,[8,12] which mirrors the sequence of neurogenesis first and gliogenesis at a later time. Systematic analysis of astrocytic markers, including nuclear factor NF1A, CD44, S100ß, and glial fibrillary acidic protein (GFAP) revealed that astrocyte progenitors began to appear as early as 1 month of hESC differentiation, though the majority emerged at 2–4 months in culture (Fig. 1). These astroglial progenitors were then enriched by dissociation and expansion in the presence of EGF, a condition that minimizes the presence of neurogenic progenitors. By 4 months in culture, the expanded progenitors gave rise to a nearly pure population of astrocytes in the presence of ciliary neurotrophic factor (CNTF), determined by their typical stellate morphology, immunoreactivity to CD44, S-100ß, and GFAP, and their ability to take up glutamate and transmit calcium waves.[3] In human development, the earliest astrocyte generation, indicated by expression of GFAP, is around 3 months of gestation. Thus, astrocyte differentiation from hESCs *in vitro* mirrors generation of astrocytes *in vivo*.

Astrocytes in different regions of the CNS possess differential cellular and functional phenotypes, which may play important roles in the health of neighboring neurons. While it is well established that regional patterning of neuroepithelia determines the identity of neuronal subtypes, it is unknown whether astrocyte subtypes are endowed in a similar way or rather are due to adaptation to the local brain environment. Using the stem cell differentiation model that allows tracing of lineage development (Fig. 1), we discovered that the regional identity of astrocyte subtypes is determined when the neuroepithelia are patterned to regional progenitors, which produce different types of astrocytes during the gliogenic phase. Furthermore, the *in vitro* generated human astrocyte subtypes exhibit differential functional properties.[3] Therefore, early patterning of neuroepithelia not only defines the neuronal subclasses but also determines astrocyte subtypes and at least some of the astrocyte functions. The close relationship between motoneurons and astrocytes during development provides one explanation why the health of motoneurons is tied with astrocytes under homeostatic environment and during pathological conditions.

Modeling human motoneuron degeneration

Most disease processes involve multiple cellular and tissue types, which are best modeled using intact animals. Indeed, animal models have been instrumental to our understanding of human disease pathogenesis. However, many neurodegenerative diseases, including those affecting motoneurons, do not naturally occur in commonly used laboratory animals, though introduction of certain pathogenic aspects of human diseases into animals can often create phenotypes that resemble human diseases. In familial cases of ALS, mutations in the superoxide dismutase 1 (SOD1) gene are associated with motoneuron degeneration. Introduction of mutant SOD1 into mice induces disease phenotypes that resemble those manifested in patients. In these cases, expression of multiple copies of mutant SOD1 is required for provoking phenotypes.[19,20] In human patients, a single copy is sufficient. The most prevalent form of mutant SOD1 in ALS patients, the alanine to valine substitution (A4V), does not appear to generate phenotypes in mice.[21] Therefore, differences do exist between humans and mice in supporting the pathogenic potential of the mutant SOD1. In another motoneuron disease, SMA, a loss-of-function mutation in the survival of motoneuron SMN1 gene results in progressive motoneuron degeneration in the spinal cord.[22,23] In animals, knockout of SMN1 is lethal. This is because SMN is a housekeeping protein that is expressed in all tissues. In humans, there are two copies of SMNs, SMN1 and SMN2, and the SMN2 gene generates a small proportion of the full-length functional SMN protein. Hence, a human SMN2 gene needs to be introduced to the SMN knockout background in mice in order to create an SMA model. Additionally, astrocytes, which were found to be significantly different between rodents and humans,[24] are also critical in the pathogenesis of ALS and potentially also SMA. Therefore, model systems with a human background would supplement our current investigations on the pathogenesis of motoneuron degeneration.

There are two major routes to building disease models using human stem cells. One is to genetically alter human stem cells, whereas the other is to derive stem cells from patients with target diseases, especially those with inheritable changes. Genetic alteration of hESCs is essentially the same as the first step in building transgenic animals. Targeting specific gene loci by homologous recombination in mouse ESCs is now a routine technique for most laboratories. This in principle also works in hESCs.[25] Nevertheless, repeated cellular cloning required by traditional homologous recombination often renders the established hESC lines unstable. Random gene insertion, by lentiviruses for instance, can reduce the cloning cycles, but the transgenes that are integrated during the stem cell stage are often downregulated along differentiation.[26] We therefore first screened gene loci that are resistant to transgene silencing using a lentiviral vector with a built-in Cre-loxP cassette. While the initial selection of clones is time-consuming, the established cell lines are generally resistant to gene silencing after the hESCs are differentiated to cells of the three embryonic germ layers, including functional neurons and astrocytes.[27] Because of a built-in Cre-loxP cassette, any gene of interest, including disease-provoking genes, may be introduced through Cre-mediated recombination with high efficiency. These hESCs are therefore referred to as master cell lines. The most recent technological development in the field is the use of zinc fingers that can target specific loci with high efficiency,[28] thus potentially alleviating the burden of screening large numbers of cell clones. Nevertheless, whether the transgene expression is sustained following stem cell differentiation remains to be seen.

Human stem cells with disease traits may now be generated directly from human patients using the technology established by Yamanaka and colleagues.[29] These induced pluripotent stem cells (hiPSCs), can now be generated from somatic cells such as dermal fibroblasts by expressing pluripotent transcription factors, including Oct3/4 and Sox2 combined with either Klf4 and c-Myc, or Lin28 and nanog.[29,30] hiPSCs exhibit very similar phenotypes of hESCs. Using similar approaches, hiPSCs have also been generated from patients with motoneuron diseases including ALS[5] and SMA.[4] For hiPSCs to be useful, it is essential that the hiPSCs can differentiate to targeted functional cell types. In parallel comparison with hESCs, we found that hiPSCs, generated with various methods from diverse sources of donor cells, still differentiate to neural precursors albeit at a much lower efficiency.[31] Nevertheless, these hiPSC-derived neural precursors can be further differentiated to motoneurons and astrocytes (Fig. 2).[31] For example, hiPSCs from ALS and SMA patients can differentiate to motoneurons.[4,5] Preliminary results indicate that some of the disease phenotypes, such as death of motoneurons, appear to occur in those from SMA hiPSCs.[4] Therefore, patient hiPSCs could provide a useful model to dissect cellular and molecular mechanisms underlying motoneuron degeneration.

Whether transgenic hESCs and disease hiPSCs model more detailed pathological processes besides cell death remains largely untested. In particular, neural degeneration occurs mostly in adult life, suggesting that pathological phenotypes may not manifest in neural cells that are cultured from the transgenic hESCs or hiPSCs. Additional interventions, such as oxidative stress, may be necessary to instigate pathological traits. Alternatively, introduction of multiple copies of disease genes or induction of disease genes at a particular condition (via inducible transgene expression) may accelerate the pathogenic process, which endows transgenic hESCs an advantage. The additional advantage of culture systems is that it permits separation or mixing of different cell types, which helps dissecting cellular contributions to pathological processes. For example, co-culturing hESC-derived motoneurons with human primary astrocytes expressing mutant SOD1[32] or mouse primary glial cells carrying SOD1 mutation[33] results in loss of motoneurons but not other neuronal subtypes, indicating the specific effect of these mutant

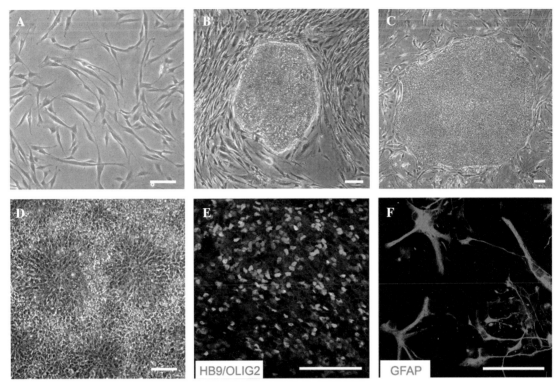

Figure 2. Differentiation of spinal motoneurons and astrocytes from hiPSCs. (**A**) Human fibroblasts were infected with retrovirus to express Oct3/4, Sox2, Klf4, and c-Myc. (**B**) Stem cell-like colonies appeared 3–4 weeks following viral infection. (**C**) The stem cell-like colonies were isolated and expanded, and hiPSC lines were subsequently established. (**D**) Under a chemically defined culture, the hiPSCs were differentiated to neuroepithelia, which form neural tube-like rosettes in 2 weeks. (**E**) The neuroepithelia further generated Olig2+ (*green*) motoneuron progenitors and HB9+ (*red*) postmitotic motoneurons in an additional 3 weeks. (**F**) GFAP+ astrocytes were generated from hiPSCs after 3 months of stem cell differentiation. Scale bar: 50 μm.

astrocytes on motoneurons. These findings are consistent with *in vivo* transgenic studies that mutant SOD1-expressing astrocytes are toxic to motoneurons and accelerate the disease progression,[34] validating the usefulness of the culture system to model certain aspects of the disease process. Of course, a simple life or death of motoneurons is far from sufficient to model the slowly progressive nature of degeneration. Furthermore, both transgenic hESCs and disease hiPSCs may be transplanted into animals to follow their pathological process *in vivo* over a long period. Once certain aspects of neurodegeneration are modeled, they could be modified as a template for screening drugs that potentially slow down or stop the degeneration process (Fig. 1).

Developing stem cell-based therapy for motoneuron diseases

Cell-based therapy has been tried in a number of neurological diseases with focal pathology, notably Parkinson's disease.[35] Replacement of diseased or lost cells in widespread areas of the brain and spinal cord, such as in the case of ALS and SMA, will likely be very difficult. However, replacement of diseased cells in critical parts of the brain and spinal cord, such as the respiratory centers of the spinal cord, could be life-saving. Progression of motoneuron diseases like ALS, and possibly also SMA, is subject to the dynamic interactions between motoneurons and their neighboring astrocytes. Therefore, replacing diseased or toxic astrocytes at an early stage could rescue motoneurons from further degeneration. By the time most motoneurons are lost, replacement of motoneurons and astrocytes becomes necessary.

Replacement of astrocytes to support the health of motoneurons has been demonstrated in a rat model of ALS in which primary astrocytes not only survive the transplant but also contribute to the increased life span of the grafted animals.[36] In this case, grafted astrocytes appear to migrate along the spinal cord a certain distance, offering a possibility of supporting motoneurons in the transplant site and neighboring areas. Of course, the human spinal cord is substantially larger and longer than that of a mouse. Nevertheless, it is surgically feasible to inject cells to multiple sites. More importantly, an enriched or pure population of human astrocytes can now be readily differentiated from hESCs and hiPSCs in a chemically defined culture system in large quantities.[3] This culture system can be readily adapted to a clean facility for production of a clinical grade of human astrocytes. In particular, astrocytes can be generated from the patient's own somatic cells through reprogramming to hiPSCs, which can be transplanted back to the patient to avoid immune rejection.

Replacement of motoneurons through transplantation is technically very challenging. First, differentiation of motoneurons from human stem cells, though the most reproducible procedure to date, does not yield a pure population. We have recently modified our original protocol and increased the differentiation efficiency to nearly 50%. Furthermore, we replaced protein growth factors with small molecules in the differentiation procedure so that the motoneuron differentiation process can now be readily adapted to production in a clean facility.[37] Second, unlike glial cell transplants, grafted human stem cells-derived postmitotic motoneurons usually have a poor survival rate. In contrast, motoneurons derived from mouse ESCs have been shown to survive well in embryonic and neonatal CNS environment, and their axons innervate muscles.[7,38] They also appear to survive in the adult mouse spinal cord. Remarkably, their axons grow to denervated muscles.[39] Nevertheless, transplantation of hESC-derived motoneurons into adult mouse brain survived poorly.[40] Strategies must be developed to promote the survival of human motoneurons, either by grafting committed motoneuron progenitors or by co-grafting with astrocytes. Perhaps what is even

more daunting is that the grafted and survived motoneurons need to travel a long distance in order to reach target muscles and make functional connection with muscles. In an SMA mouse model, HB9-GFP motoneurons transplanted into the neonatal spinal cord not only survive but also grow out nerves and innervate muscles. The grafted animals appear to survive longer.[41] This finding raises hopes that motoneuron replacement in the developing nervous system may be possible. In adult mice, co-transplantation of glial cells in the sciatic nerve to attract axonal growth from the motoneurons that are grafted to the spinal cord appears to occur,[39] indicative that motoneuron replacement in adults is not impossible.

Conclusion

Human stem cells, including hESCs and hiPSCs, can be efficiently differentiated into motoneurons and astrocytes, two of the main cell types that are targeted in motoneuron diseases. These cellular models offer an unprecedented tool for dissecting molecular mechanisms underlying motoneuron health and disease, thus complementing the existing transgenic animal models. While these cellular models have resulted in discoveries of developmental mechanisms, significant efforts are underway to create novel tools to simulate pathological processes in a dish and to translate findings obtained in the cellular models to treatment options for these devastating motoneuron diseases.

Acknowledgments

Studies from our laboratories described in the article have been supported by the NIH-NINDS (NS045926, NS046587, NS057778, NS061243), the ALS Association, partly from the NICHD (P30 HD03352), Ministry of Science and Technology, China (2006CB94700, 2006AA02A101), and Shanghai Municipality (06dj14001).

Conflicts of interest

The authors declare no conflicts of interest.

References

1. Li, X.J. *et al.* 2005. Specification of motoneurons from human embryonic stem cells. *Nat. Biotechnol.* **23:** 215–221.

2. Singh, R.N. *et al.* 2005. Enhancer-specified GFP-based FACS purification of human spinal motor neurons from embryonic stem cells. *Exp. Neurol.* **196:** 224–234.

3. Krencik, R., J.H. Weick, Z. Zhang & S.C. Zhang. 2009. Regional and functional specific astrocytes from human embryonic stem cells. *Society for Neuroscience Abstract* **808.9**.

4. Ebert, A.D. *et al.* 2009. Induced pluripotent stem cells from a spinal muscular atrophy patient. *Nature* **457:** 277–280.

5. Dimos, J.T. *et al.* 2008. Induced pluripotent stem cells generated from patients with ALS can be differentiated into motor neurons. *Science* **321:** 1218–1221.

6. Jessell, T.M. 2000. Neuronal specification in the spinal cord: inductive signals and transcriptional codes. *Nat. Rev. Genet.* **1:** 20–29.

7. Wichterle, H., I. Lieberam, J.A. Porter & T.M. Jessell. 2002. Directed differentiation of embryonic stem cells into motor neurons. *Cell* **110:** 385–397.

8. Zhang, S.C., M. Wernig, I.D. Duncan, *et al.* 2001. *In vitro* differentiation of transplantable neural precursors from human embryonic stem cells. *Nat. Biotechnol.* **19:** 1129–1133.

9. Pankratz, M.T. *et al.* 2007. Directed neural differentiation of human embryonic stem cells via an obligated primitive anterior stage. *Stem Cells* **25:** 1511–1520.

10. Lavaute, T.M. *et al.* 2009. Regulation of neural specification from human embryonic stem cells by BMP and FGF. *Stem Cells* **27:** 1741–1749.

11. Chambers, S.M. *et al.* 2009. Highly efficient neural conversion of human ES and iPS cells by dual inhibition of SMAD signaling. *Nat. Biotechnol.* **27:** 275–280.

12. Johnson, M.A., J.P. Weick, R.A. Pearce & S.C. Zhang. 2007. Functional neural development from human embryonic stem cells: accelerated synaptic activity via astrocyte coculture. *J. Neurosci.* **27:** 3069–3077.

13. Yan, Y. *et al.* 2005. Directed differentiation of dopaminergic neuronal subtypes from human embryonic stem cells. *Stem Cells* **23:** 781–790.

14. Zhang, S.C. 2006. Neural subtype specification from embryonic stem cells. *Brain Pathol.* **16:** 132–142.

15. Ullian, E.M., S.K. Sapperstein, K.S. Christopherson & B.A. Barres. 2001. Control of synapse number by glia. *Science* **291:** 657–661.

16. Barres, B.A. 2008. The mystery and magic of glia: a perspective on their roles in health and disease. *Neuron* **60:** 430–440.

17. Rowitch, D.H. 2004. Glial specification in the vertebrate neural tube. *Nat. Rev. Neurosci.* **5:** 409–419.

18. Zhang, S.C. 2001. Defining glial cells during CNS development. *Nat. Rev. Neurosci.* **2:** 840–843.

19. Bruijn, L.I. *et al.* 1997. ALS-linked SOD1 mutant G85R mediates damage to astrocytes and promotes rapidly progressive disease with SOD1-containing inclusions. *Neuron* **18:** 327–338.

20. Bruijn, L.I., T.M. Miller & D.W. Cleveland. 2004. Unraveling the mechanisms involved in motor neuron degeneration in ALS. *Annu. Rev. Neurosci.* **27:** 723–749.

21. Furukawa, Y., R. Fu, H.X. Deng, *et al.* 2006. Disulfide cross-linked protein represents a significant fraction of ALS-associated Cu, Zn-superoxide dismutase aggregates in spinal cords of model mice. *Proc. Natl. Acad. Sci. USA* **103:** 7148–7153.

22. Monani, U.R. *et al.* 2000. The human centromeric survival motor neuron gene (SMN2) rescues embryonic lethality in Smn(−/−) mice and results in a mouse with spinal muscular atrophy. *Hum. Mol. Genet.* **9:** 333–339.

23. Hsieh-Li, H.M. *et al.* 2000. A mouse model for spinal muscular atrophy. *Nat. Genet.* **24:** 66–70.

24. Oberheim, N.A. *et al.* 2009. Uniquely hominid features of adult human astrocytes. *J. Neurosci.* **29:** 3276–3287.

25. Zwaka, T.P. & J.A. Thomson. 2003. Homologous recombination in human embryonic stem cells. *Nat. Biotechnol.* **21:** 319–321.

26. Xia, X., Y. Zhang, C.R. Zieth & S.C. Zhang. 2007. Transgenes delivered by lentiviral vector are suppressed in human embryonic stem cells in a promoter-dependent manner. *Stem Cells Dev.* **16:** 167–176.

27. Du, Z.W., B.Y. Hu, M. Ayala, *et al.* 2009. Cre recombination-mediated cassette exchange for building versatile transgenic human embryonic stem cells lines. *Stem Cells* **27:** 1032–1041.

28. Hockemeyer, D. *et al.* 2009. Efficient targeting of expressed and silent genes in human ESCs and iPSCs using zinc-finger nucleases. *Nat. Biotechnol.* **27:** 851–857.

29. Takahashi, K. *et al.* 2007. Induction of pluripotent stem cells from adult human fibroblasts by defined factors. *Cell* **131:** 861–872.

30. Yu, J. *et al.* 2007. Induced pluripotent stem cell lines derived from human somatic cells. *Science* **318:** 1917–1920.

31. Hu, B., J.H. Weick, J. Yu, *et al.* 2010. Neural differentiation of human iPS cells is variable and less efficient than hESCs. *Proc. Natl. Acad. Sci. USA* **107:** 4335–4340.

32. Marchetto, M.C. *et al.* 2008. Non-cell-autonomous effect of human SOD1 G37R astrocytes on motor neurons derived from human embryonic stem cells. *Cell Stem Cell* **3:** 649–657.

33. Di Giorgio, F.P., G.L. Boulting, S. Bobrowicz & K.C. Eggan. 2008. Human embryonic stem cell-derived motor neurons are sensitive to the toxic effect of glial cells carrying an ALS-causing mutation. *Cell Stem Cell* **3:** 637–648.

34. Clement, A.M. *et al.* 2003. Wild-type nonneuronal cells extend survival of SOD1 mutant motor neurons in ALS mice. *Science* **302:** 113–117.

35. Bjorklund, A. & O. Lindvall. 2000. Cell replacement therapies for central nervous system disorders. *Nat. Neurosci.* **3:** 537–544.

36. Lepore, A.C. *et al.* 2008. Focal transplantation-based astrocyte replacement is neuroprotective in a model of motor neuron disease. *Nat. Neurosci.* **11:** 1294–1301.

37. Li, X.J. *et al.* 2008. Directed differentiation of ventral spinal progenitors and motor neurons from human embryonic stem cells by small molecules. *Stem Cells* **26:** 886–893.

38. Yohn, D.C., G.B. Miles, V.F. Rafuse & R.M. Brownstone. 2008. Transplanted mouse embryonic stem-cell-derived motoneurons form functional motor units and reduce muscle atrophy. *J. Neurosci.* **28:** 12409–12418.

39. Deshpande, D.M. *et al.* 2006. Recovery from paralysis in adult rats using embryonic stem cells. *Ann. Neurol.* **60:** 32–44.

40. Lee, H. *et al.* 2007. Directed differentiation and transplantation of human embryonic stem cell-derived motoneurons. *Stem Cells* **25:** 1931–1939.

41. Corti, S. *et al.* 2009. Motoneuron transplantation rescues the phenotype of SMARD1 (spinal muscular atrophy with respiratory distress type 1). *J. Neurosci.* **29:** 11761–11771.

42. Krencik, R. & S.C. Zhang. 2006. Stem cell neural differentiation: a model for chemical biology. *Curr. Opin. Chem. Biol.* **10:** 592–597.

Ann. N.Y. Acad. Sci. ISSN 0077-8923

Developmental regulation of subtype-specific motor neuron excitability

Rosa L. Moreno and Angeles B. Ribera

Department of Physiology and Biophysics, University of Colorado at the Anschutz Medical Center, Aurora, Colorado

Address for correspondence: Rosa L. Moreno, Department of Physiology and Biophysics, MS 8307, RC-1N, P18-7117, 12800 East 19th Avenue, P.O. Box 6511, Aurora, CO 80045. rosa.moreno@ucdenver.edu

At early embryonic stages, zebrafish spinal neuron subtypes can be distinguished and accessed for physiological studies. This provides the opportunity to determine electrophysiological properties of different spinal motor neuron subtypes. Such differences have the potential to then regulate, in a subtype-specific manner, activity-dependent developmental events such as axonal outgrowth and pathfinding. The zebrafish spinal cord contains a population of early born neurons. Our recent work has revealed that primary motor neuron (PMN) subtypes in the zebrafish spinal cord differ with respect to electrical properties during early important periods when PMNs extend axons to their specific targets. Here, we review recent findings regarding the development of electrical properties in PMN subtypes. Moreover, we consider the possibility that electrical activity in PMNs may play a cell nonautonomous role and thus influence the development of later developing motor neurons. Further, we discuss findings that support a role for a specific sodium channel isoform, Nav1.6, expressed by specific subtypes of spinal neurons in activity-dependent processes that impact axonal outgrowth and pathfinding.

Keywords: motor neuron subtype; potassium current; Rohon-Beard cell; sodium channel; zebrafish

Introduction

Whereas the molecular and morphological attributes of zebrafish primary motor neuron (PMN) subtypes have been the focus of many studies, less is known about PMN excitability properties. In view of the molecular and morphological features that distinguish PMNs, it is important to characterize electrical properties in terms of PMN subtypes. Moreover, little is known about molecular factors that direct differentiation of electrical excitability in neurons. Do the development of neuronal morphology and excitability share common molecular programs? Recently, studies using the *Drosophila* model have provided evidence that support (1) subtype-specific differentiation of electrical properties in motor neurons, and (2) a connection among molecular factors important for morphological development and those contributing to electrical differentiation.[1]

The zebrafish vertebrate model presents the opportunity to study the electrical properties of identifiable motor neurons. This is particularly important early in development when motor neuron excitability may influence activity-dependent processes. Zebrafish motor neurons are spontaneously active at early embryonic stages while their axons are navigating to specific muscle targets.[2] Periods of spontaneous activity occur during development of many nervous systems.[3] In some cases, the spontaneous activity occurs prior to synapse formation, whereas in the majority of instances, the activity patterns studied occur after initial synapse formation. Regardless of when the spontaneous activity occurs, activation of important developmental signaling mechanisms takes place, which affects properties such as axonal outgrowth, pathfinding, neurotransmitter expression, and synapse formation.[3–5] Whether subtype-specific patterns of electrical activity are present in zebrafish PMNs, and how they

doi: 10.1111/j.1749-6632.2009.05426.x

may differentially regulate axonal pathfinding in these neurons has yet to be explored.

Gene expression can be altered with relative ease in the zebrafish system, and this may aid in identifying molecular factors critical for neuronal electrical differentiation. Similar to mammalian spinal motor neurons, zebrafish PMNs express transcription factors, such as HB9, Islet1, Islet2, and Lim3.[6–9] Among these factors Islet1 and Islet2 show PMN subtype-specific patterns of expression.[8] Nonetheless, the molecular mechanisms directing subtype-specific differentiation remain obscure.

In this review, we discuss the maturation of electrical properties in two different PMN subtypes, during the first two days of embryonic development. We highlight differences in PMN electrical properties between the two subtypes and consider how this may suggest subtype-specific functions. Further, we discuss the role of the ion channel Nav1.6, expressed in many zebrafish primary spinal neurons, in activity-dependent pathways that impact axonal pathfinding.

Development of excitability in zebrafish primary spinal neurons

Many different types of spinal neurons show a developmental program for excitability consisting of delayed upregulation of potassium current with respect to inward currents.[3] However, for the most part, the molecular identity of ion channels that achieve these changes is not known. Moreover, it is not known if spinal neuron subtypes differ in the molecular mechanisms mediating their electrical differentiation. For example, the density, the kinetics, and/or the molecular identity of ion channels expressed may impart subtype-specific firing properties. As reviewed above, unique electrical properties could then, among other factors, contribute to the specification of axonal outgrowth, pathfinding, and neurotransmitter phenotype. Thus, understanding how specific spinal neuron subtypes differentiate electrically will allow us ultimately to understand better the role of electrical activity in neuronal development.

In *Xenopus, in vitro* and *in vivo* studies demonstrate that early spinal neuron excitability properties change dramatically within a day of development as evidenced by a substantial decrease in action potential duration.[10–12] Increases in the density of voltage-dependent inward and outward currents drive the maturation of the action potential waveform, with changes in voltage-dependent potassium current driving the decrease in duration of the impulse.[12,13]

Similarly, in *Ambystoma* spinal neurons the duration of action potentials is substantially decreased by changes in the amplitude and kinetics of voltage-dependent potassium currents.[14,15]

In rat lumbar motor neurons, inward and outward conductances increase substantially during the last week of embryonic development and the initial postnatal period, leading to increased amplitude and decreased duration of action potentials.[16,17] Additionally, in rat motor neurons the substantial changes in ionic currents bring about increased motor neuron excitability. Thus at postnatal stages these neurons are able to fire multiple action potentials.[16,17] Similarly, in the chick, firing properties of limb motor neurons change substantially as axons navigate to appropriate targets.[18]

Many studies have described the developmental sequence of electrical maturation of spinal neurons. However, only a few of these studies have focused on specific subtypes of spinal neurons, and the specific ion channels involved in their maturing electrical properties.[11,13,19–22] Several aspects of the zebrafish embryo model allow the opportunity to study the electrical development of specific neuronal types. Transgenic lines labeling specific neuronal populations and the ease with which neurons can be accessed *in situ* at very early embryonic stages both facilitate such studies (Fig. 1). Moreover, the ease for the manipulation of gene expression provides the opportunity to address the role that specific ion channels may serve in neuronal electrical differentiation and activity-dependent processes.

In the embryonic zebrafish spinal cord, PMNs exit the cell cycle at 11 hpf, and subsequently acquire subtype identity.[8,23] About 2 hs prior to axonal outgrowth (16–17 hpf), several properties reveal PMN subtype identities, including soma position within a hemisegment and homeodomain transcription factor expression.[8,23,24] The most caudal PMN (CaP) exits the cell cycle and initiates axonal outgrowth around 2 h prior to two other PMNs, MiP (middle), and RoP (rostral). All PMN axons exit the spinal cord via a common exit point just ventral to CaP's soma position. Upon spinal cord exit, all PMN axons initially follow a common path extending

Ann. N.Y. Acad. Sci. 1198 (2010) 201–207 © 2010 New York Academy of Sciences.

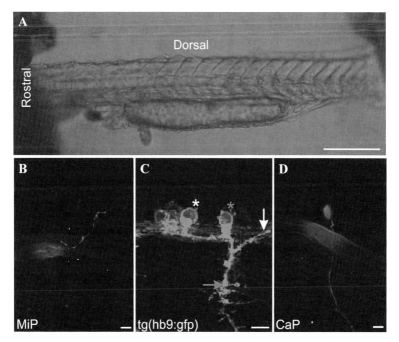

Figure 1. Primary motor neuron (PMN) subtypes can be identified by their expression of GFP in the Tg(hb9:gfp) zebrafish line allowing selection of specific motor neuron subtypes for *in situ* electrophysiological analysis. (**A**) Anesthetized and sacrificed embryos are glued to the bottom of a sylgard chamber where following skin removal blunt dissection of the muscle and tearing of the meninges exposes PMNs. (**B–D**) Tg(hb9:gfp) embryos (**C**) facilitate identification of CaPs (*gray*) and MiPs (*white*). However, some interneurons also express GFP in the Tg(hb9:gfp) transgenic line. Accordingly, MiPs (**B**) and CaPs (**D**) are further identified by dye filling during whole-cell patch recordings. Scale bars: (**A**) 200 μm; (**B–D**), 10 μm. (Used with permission from Moreno and Ribera, 2009.)

ventrally along the medial surface of the somites until they reach a choice point at the horizontal myoseptum after which axons follow subtype-specific trajectories.[23,24] Thus, PMN subtypes can be identified based on their specific ventral (CaP), dorsal (MiP), and medial (RoP) axon trajectories and targets (Fig. 2).

In addition to PMNs, the zebrafish spinal cord also has other early birth-date neurons, including sensory Rohon-Beard cells and various interneuron subtypes.[25] All primary spinal neurons initiate electrical development soon after cell cycle exits. Voltage-dependent outward currents are detected in PMNs prior to the initiation of axonal outgrowth (17 hpf), while voltage-dependent sodium currents develop simultaneously with or soon after the appearance of axons.[26]

Comparison of electrical development between CaP and MiP PMNs reveals subtype-specific differ-

ences (Fig. 3).[26] Prior to axon outgrowth (17 hpf) CaPs and MiPs differ substantially in the density of their outward currents. At later developmental stages, both inward and outward current densities in CaPs are greater than those in MiPs. Consequently, the firing properties of these PMN subtypes differ substantially at 24 and 48 hpf, particularly in the duration of evoked or spontaneous action potentials (Fig. 3).

Understanding the mechanisms that mediate motor neuron subtype-specific electrical development requires knowledge of the molecular identity of ion channels expressed and their developmental regulation. Electrical differences between CaP and MiP suggest that the number, function, or the molecular identity of channels expressed by the two PMN subtypes differ substantially. Developmental changes in PMN subtype-specific excitability likely arise from a combination of these factors.

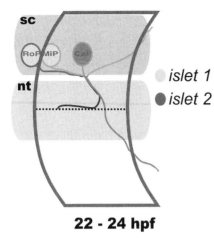

Figure 2. Three PMN subtypes are born by the end of gastrulation in the zebrafish spinal cord. Each PMN can be distinguished based on soma position within a hemisegment, axonal trajectories, muscle targets, and expression of *islet* transcription factor genes. RoP (*purple*) is the most rostral PMN and innervates medial muscle; MiP (*blue*) with medial soma position innervates dorsal muscle; CaP (*green*) is the most caudal and targets ventral muscle. By 18 hpf, PMN subtypes can also be distinguished by their characteristic *islet* expression patterns.

Developmental role of the sodium channel Nav1.6 in the zebrafish spinal cord

Little is known about the molecular identities of calcium and potassium ion channels expressed by zebrafish spinal neurons. However, for sodium channels, Novak *et al.* (2006) identified several genes that show an expression in the embryonic spinal cord.[27] Among the genes identified, the *scn8aa* gene, which encodes the Nav1.6a sodium channel α-subunit, has emerged as an important developmental player in the zebrafish spinal cord.[28–31]

The mammalian ortholgues of *scn8aa* and Nav1.6a are *SCN8A and* Nav1.6, respectively.[27] In mammals, the adult CNS and PNS show abundant expression of *SCN8A* transcripts and the encoded Nav1.6 protein.[32,33] In neurons, Nav1.6 protein distributes to several locations including the soma, dendrites, and axons, particularly in nodes of Ranvier.[33,34] The broad distribution of this channel across neurons and at several sub-cellular locations suggests that Nav1.6 plays an important role in excitability. In support of this notion, in mice ho-

mozygous for the "motor endplate disease" (*med*) allele, lack of Nav1.6 function results in abnormal neuromuscular junctions that show defective nerve sprouting and aberrant endplate distribution.[35] Additionally, this mutation is associated with reduced Purkinje cell excitability and degeneration.[36]

In zebrafish, the early embryo expresses the *scn8aa* gene.[27,29–31] As in mammals, *scn8aa* mRNA is broadly distributed in the CNS and PNS. The *scn8aa* transcript first appears at 16 hpf in Rohon-Beard neurons (RBs) and the trigeminal ganglia. By the second day of development, transcripts localize to the forebrain, midbrain, and hindbrain. Between 24 and 72 hpf, the *scn8aa* transcript is present in additional spinal neurons including PMNs, some secondary motor neurons (SMNs), and several interneurons.[27,29–31] The substantial changes in sodium current that occur in all RBs from 16 to 48 hpf are partly attributed to changes in Nav1.6a channel current density, which may result from increases in *scn8aa* transcript and consequent Nav1.6a expression, or to posttranslational regulatory mechanisms.[30]

Interestingly, in PMNs, *scn8aa* expression is subtype-specific and limited to CaPs.[30] It is not known whether the substantial upregulation in sodium current density occurring within the first 2 days of development in CaPs is mediated via increased Nav1.6a-dependent conductance as occurs in RBs. Nevertheless, other sodium channel transcripts such as *scn8ab*, *scn1Lab*, and *scn5Lab* are present at early embryonic stages in the ventral spinal cord and their contribution to sodium currents in CaPs remains uncharacterized.[27]

RBs function as a transient neuronal population involved in the response to tactile stimulation.[37,38] RBs participate in this response by virtue of their extensive peripheral projections innervating the skin, and their expression of mechanosensitive ion channels. Normal electrical development of RBs is critical for acquisition of tactile sensory function at early stages and Nav1.6a contributes significantly to these electrical properties.[30,39] This is best exemplified by the *macho* mutant, where decreased sodium currents in RBs leads to a defective touch response.[39] While the *macho* gene remains unidentified, it is clear that it is not the *scn8aa* gene, as *macho* and *scn8aa* belong to different linkage groups.[27,29] Nevertheless, this mutant line has revealed a critical role for Nav1.6a channels in the zebrafish behavior

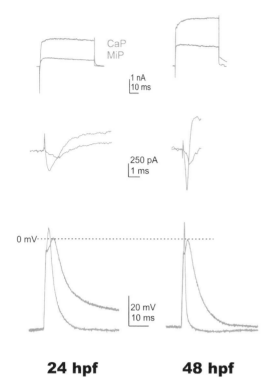

CaP
MiP

1 nA
10 ms

250 pA
1 ms

0 mV

20 mV
10 ms

24 hpf

48 hpf

Figure 3. PMN firing properties change substantially between the first 2 days of development. In both CaPs (*green traces*) and MiPs (*blue traces*), the amplitudes of outward (*top row*) and inward (*middle row*) currents increase significantly, resulting in briefer action potential durations (*bottom row*) at 48 (*right column*) compared 24 (*left column*) hpf. However, at any given stage, CaPs and MiP differ in their electrical properties. Notably, the amplitudes of outward and inward currents are greater in CaPs (*green traces*) compared to MiPs (*blue traces*).

and activity-dependent processes that have been further characterized by direct knockdown of this isoform.[28,30,39]

In the zebrafish spinal cord, *scn8aa* expression is important for the proper axonal outgrowth of specific populations of motor neurons.[30] Following direct knockdown of Nav1.6a via a morpholino approach, dorsally projecting SMNs fail to extend axons. Additionally, in ventrally projecting SMNs, axon branching and targeting to postsynaptic acetylcholine receptor clusters is altered.[30] The mechanisms by which Nav1.6s influences neuronal development are not fully understood. However, whereas the effects on dorsally projecting SMNs may involve cell-autonomous mechanisms, those on

ventrally projecting SMN axons clearly involve non-cell autonomous pathways.[30] These studies suggest that Nav1.6a-mediated excitability may be required for (a) responsiveness to cues needed for pathfinding, or (b) release of target derived factors important for proper axonal outgrowth.

Molecular factors important for neuronal electrical development

Only recently have transcription factors involved in motor neuron morphological differentiation been linked to their electrical development. *Drosophila* Even-skipped (Eve) is a homeodomain transcription factor important for proper axon guidance by specific populations of dorsally projecting motor neurons.[41,42] Manipulation of Eve expression affects the electrical properties of this subset of motor neurons via effects on the transcription of a potassium channel gene, *Slowpoke* (*slo*), belonging to the BK calcium-gated family. Eve plays a repressor function in the transcriptional regulation of *slo*, and thus Eve overexpression decreases potassium channel conductance via reduced transcription of *slo*, resulting in increased motor neuron excitability.[1]

Additionally, studies in the ascidian *Halocynthia roretzi* have demonstrated a link between the expression of the LIM homolog (Hrlim) and the expression of a motor neuron specific voltage-gated sodium channel. Misexpression of Hrlim induces the expression of the sodium channel *TuNa2* in epidermal cells.[43]

In zebrafish, all PMN subtypes express *islet1* (*isl1*) as they exit the cell cycle.[6–8] Prior to axogenesis, the expression of islet transcription factor genes is dynamic resulting in downregulation of *isl1* in all PMN subtypes. *Isl1* expression is later upregulated in MiPs and RoPs, but not in CaPs. During the downregulation of *isl1*, CaPs initiate expression of *islet2* (*isl2*) and by 16 hpf, CaPs only express the latter factor.[8] The transient expression of islet1 in some PMNs, such as CaP, is critical for motor neuron differentiation. Reduced *isl1* expression prevents ventral neuron axons from exiting the spinal cord, leading to a differentiation program more characteristic of interneurons. Interestingly, in the absence of *isl1*, *isl2* is able to induce proper motor neuron differentiation.[44]

It is clear that *isl1* expression is important for a commitment to motor neuron fate. However, the combinatorial expression of factors responsible for motor neuron subtype differentiation remains unidentified and represents an area of great interest in neurobiology. Moreover, how the combinatorial expression of *Islet* and other transcription factors results in the specific set of ion channels that bring about motor neuron subtype-specific excitability is an open question that has not yet been addressed.

Future directions

Understanding how combinatorial expression of specific transcription factors allows motor neurons to differentiate morphological and electrical properties represents an area of great interest. For example, to develop strategies aimed at inducing distinct motor neuron subtypes from neuronal stem cells, it is imperative that we first identify the specific molecular factors and pathways involved in both morphological and electrical differentiation.

In addition, it is not known whether the electrical differences between CaP and MiP persist to later larval, juvenile, and adult stages. It is also not clear whether PMN subtype-specific electrical properties may be functionally significant. Nevertheless, these differences occur during the period when axons navigate to their specific targets, a process that may be influenced by electrical activity. Moreover, it is possible that electrical activity may influence axonal pathfinding via a noncell autonomous pathway. In this regard, it is interesting that early ablation studies provide support for the idea that CaP and MiP serve different roles as pioneers of their respective trajectories.[40] CaP facilitates SMN pathfinding, but it is unnecessary for this process while MiP is required for proper guidance of later developing SMNs.[40] Thus studies of (1) how CaP and MiP electrical activity influences SMN axonal pathfinding, and (2) whether PMN subtype-specific electrical properties can be linked to specific pathways influencing axonal trajectories, are warranted.

Conflicts of interest

The authors declare no conflicts of interest.

References

1. Pym, E.C. *et al*. 2006. The homeobox transcription factor Even-skipped regulates acquisition of electrical properties in Drosophila neurons. *Neural Dev.* **1:** 3.

2. Saint-Amant, L. & P. Drapeau. 2000. Motoneuron activity patterns related to the earliest behavior of the zebrafish embryo. *J. Neurosci.* **20:** 3964–3972.

3. Moody, W.J. & M.M. Bosma. 2005. Ion channel development, spontaneous activity, and activity-dependent development in nerve and muscle cells. *Physiol. Rev.* **85:** 883–941.

4. Zhang, L.I. & M.M. Poo. 2001. Electrical activity and development of neural circuits. *Nat. Neurosci.* **4**(Suppl.): 1207–1214.

5. Hanson, M.G., L.D. Milner & L.T. Landmesser. 2008. Spontaneous rhythmic activity in early chick spinal cord influences distinct motor axon pathfinding decisions. *Brain Res. Rev.* **57:** 77–85.

6. Korzh, V., T. Edlund & S. Thor. 1993. Zebrafish primary neurons initiate expression of the LIM homeodomain protein Isl-1 at the end of gastrulation. *Development* **118:** 417–425.

7. Inoue, A. *et al*. 1994. Developmental regulation of islet-1 mRNA expression during neuronal differentiation in embryonic zebrafish. *Dev. Dyn.* **199:** 1–11.

8. Appel, B. *et al*. 1995. Motoneuron fate specification revealed by patterned LIM homeobox gene expression in embryonic zebrafish. *Development* **121:** 4117–4125.

9. Wendik, B., E. Maier & D. Meyer. 2004. Zebrafish mnx genes in endocrine and exocrine pancreas formation. *Dev. Biol.* **268:** 372–383.

10. Spitzer, N.C. & J.E. Lamborghini. 1976. The development of the action potential mechanism of amphibian neurons isolated in culture. *Proc. Natl. Acad. Sci. USA* **73:** 1641–1645.

11. Baccaglini, P.I. & N.C. Spitzer. 1977. Developmental changes in the inward current of the action potential of Rohon-Beard neurones. *J. Physiol.* **271:** 93–117.

12. O'Dowd, D.K., A.B. Ribera & N.C. Spitzer. 1988. Development of voltage-dependent calcium, sodium, and potassium currents in Xenopus spinal neurons. *J. Neurosci.* **8:** 792–805.

13. Desarmenien, M.G., B. Clendening & N.C. Spitzer. 1993. *In vivo* development of voltage-dependent ionic currents in embryonic Xenopus spinal neurons. *J. Neurosci.* **13:** 2575–2581.

14. Barish, M.E. 1985. A model of inward and outward membrane currents in cultured embryonic amphibian spinal neurons and reconstruction of the action potential. *J. Physiol. (Paris).* **80:** 298–306.

15. Barish, M.E. 1986. Differentiation of voltage-gated potassium current and modulation of excitability in cultured amphibian spinal neurones. *J. Physiol.* **375:** 229–250.

16. Fulton, B.P. & K. Walton. 1986. Electrophysiological properties of neonatal rat motoneurones studied *in vitro*. *J. Physiol.* **370:** 651–678.

17. Gao, B.X. & L. Ziskind-Conhaim. 1998. Development of ionic currents underlying changes in action potential waveforms in rat spinal motoneurons. *J. Neurophysiol.* **80:** 3047–3061.

18. McCobb, D.P., P.M. Best & K.G. Beam. 1990. The differentiation of excitability in embryonic chick limb motoneurons. *J. Neurosci.* **10:** 2974–2984.

19. Spitzer, N.C. & P.I. Baccaglini. 1976. Development of the action potential in embryo amphibian neurons *in vivo*. *Brain Res.* **107:** 610–616.

20. Spitzer, N.C. 1976. The ionic basis of the resting potential and a slow depolarizing response in Rohon-Beard neurones of Xenopus tadpoles. *J. Physiol.* **255:** 105–135.

21. Pineda, R.H., R.A. Heiser & A.B. Ribera. 2005. Developmental, molecular, and genetic dissection of INa *in vivo* in embryonic zebrafish sensory neurons. *J. Neurophysiol.* **93:** 3582–3593.

22. Pineda, R.H. & A.B. Ribera. 2008. Dorsal-ventral gradient for neuronal plasticity in the embryonic spinal cord. *J. Neurosci.* **28:** 3824–3834.

23. Myers, P.Z., J.S. Eisen & M. Westerfield. 1986. Development and axonal outgrowth of identified motoneurons in the zebrafish. *J. Neurosci.* **6:** 2278–2289.

24. Westerfield, M., J.V. McMurray & J.S. Eisen. 1986. Identified motoneurons and their innervation of axial muscles in the zebrafish. *J. Neurosci.* **6:** 2267–2277.

25. Kimmel, C.B. *et al.* 1995. Stages of embryonic development of the zebrafish. *Dev. Dyn.* **203:** 253–310.

26. Moreno, R.L. & A.B. Ribera. 2009. Zebrafish motor neuron subtypes differ electrically prior to axonal outgrowth. *J. Neurophysiol.* **102:** 2477–2484.

27. Novak, A.E. *et al.* 2006. Embryonic and larval expression of zebrafish voltage-gated sodium channel alpha-subunit genes. *Dev. Dyn.* **235:** 1962–1973.

28. Svoboda, K.R., A.E. Linares & A.B. Ribera. 2001. Activity regulates programmed cell death of zebrafish Rohon-Beard neurons. *Development* **128:** 3511–3520.

29. Tsai, C.W. *et al.* 2001. Primary structure and developmental expression of zebrafish sodium channel Na(v)1.6 during neurogenesis. *DNA Cell Biol.* **20:** 249–255.

30. Pineda, R.H. *et al.* 2006. Knockdown of Nav1.6a Na+ channels affects zebrafish motoneuron development. *Development* **133:** 3827–3836.

31. Wu, S.H. *et al.* 2008. Multiple regulatory elements mediating neuronal-specific expression of zebrafish sodium channel gene, scn8aa. *Dev. Dyn.* **237:** 2554–2565.

32. Schaller, K.L. *et al.* 1995. A novel, abundant sodium channel expressed in neurons and glia. *J. Neurosci.* **15:** 3231–3242.

33. Caldwell, J.H. *et al.* 2000. Sodium channel Na(v)1.6 is localized at nodes of ranvier, dendrites, and synapses. *Proc. Natl. Acad. Sci. USA* **97:** 5616–5620.

34. Krzemien, D.M., K.L. Schaller, S.R. Levinson & J.H. Caldwell. 2000. Immunolocalization of sodium channel isoform NaCh6 in the nervous system. *J. Comp. Neurol.* **420:** 70–83.

35. Burgess, D.L. *et al.* 1995. Mutation of a new sodium channel gene, Scn8a, in the mouse mutant 'motor endplate disease'. *Nat. Genet.* **10:** 461–465.

36. Dick, D.J., R.J. Boakes & J.B. Harris. 1985. A cerebellar abnormality in the mouse with motor end-plate disease. *Neuropathol. Appl. Neurobiol.* **11:** 141–147.

37. Roberts, A. & B.P. Hayes. 1977. The anatomy and function of 'free' nerve endings in an amphibian skin sensory system. *Proc. R Soc. Lond. B Biol. Sci.* **196:** 415–429.

38. Clarke, J.D., B.P. Hayes, S.P. Hunt & A. Roberts. 1984. Sensory physiology, anatomy, and immunohistochemistry of Rohon-Beard neurones in embryos of Xenopus laevis. *J. Physiol.* **348:** 511–525.

39. Ribera, A.B. & C. Nusslein-Volhard. 1998. Zebrafish touch-insensitive mutants reveal an essential role for the developmental regulation of sodium current. *J. Neurosci.* **18:** 9181–9191.

40. Pike, S.H., E.F. Melancon & J.S. Eisen. 1992. Pathfinding by zebrafish motoneurons in the absence of normal pioneer axons. *Development* **114:** 825–831.

41. Landgraf, M. *et al.* 1999. Even-skipped determines the dorsal growth of motor axons in Drosophila. *Neuron* **22:** 43–52.

42. Fujioka, M. *et al.* 2003. Even-skipped, acting as a repressor, regulates axonal projections in Drosophila. *Development* **130:** 5385–5400.

43. Okada, T., Y. Katsuyama, F. Ono & Y. Okamura. 2002. The development of three identified motor neurons in the larva of an ascidian, *Halocynthia roretzi*. *Dev. Biol.* **244:** 278–292.

44. Hutchinson, S.A. & J.S. Eisen. 2006. Islet1 and Islet2 have equivalent abilities to promote motoneuron formation and to specify motoneuron subtype identity. *Development* **133:** 2137–2147.

Ann. N.Y. Acad. Sci. ISSN 0077-8923

ANNALS OF THE NEW YORK ACADEMY OF SCIENCES
Issue: *Neurons and Networks in the Spinal Cord*

Serotonin controls the maturation of the GABA phenotype in the ventral spinal cord via 5-HT$_{1B}$ receptors

Anne-Emilie Allain, Louis Ségu, Pierre Meyrand, and Pascal Branchereau

Centre de Neurosciences Intégratives et Cognitives (CNIC), Université de Bordeaux, CNRS, Talence, France

Address for correspondence: Pascal Branchereau, Centre de Neurosciences Intégratives et Cognitives (CNIC), Université de Bordeaux & CNRS – UMR 5228, Av. des Facultés, 4ème étage Est, 33405 Talence, France. p.branchereau@cnic.u-bordeaux1.fr

Serotonin (5-hydroxytryptamine or 5-HT) is a pleiotropic neurotransmitter known to play a crucial modulating role during the construction of brain circuits. Descending bulbo-spinal 5-HT fibers, coming from the caudal medullary cell groups of the raphe nuclei, progressively invade the mouse spinal cord and arrive at lumbar segments at E15.5 when the number of ventral GABA immunoreactive (GABA-ir) interneurons reaches its maximum. We thus raised the question of a possible interaction between these two neurotransmitter systems and investigated the effect of 5-HT descending inputs on the maturation of the GABA phenotype in ventral spinal interneurons. Using a quantitative anatomical study performed on acute and cultured embryonic mouse spinal cord, we found that the GABAergic neuronal population matured according to a similar rostro-caudal gradient both *in utero* and in organotypic culture. We showed that 5-HT delayed the maturation of the GABA phenotype in lumbar but not brachial interneurons. Using pharmacological treatments and mice lacking 5-HT$_{1B}$ or 5-HT$_{1A}$, we demonstrated that the 5-HT repressing effect on the GABAergic phenotype was specifically attributed to 5-HT$_{1B}$ receptors.

Keywords: mouse embryonic development; serotonin receptors; spinal GABA interneurons; raphe descending inputs; transmitter specification

Introduction

The lumbar spinal cord contains neural networks generating rhythmic movements such as swimming and walking independently of central and peripheral inputs. In rodent, these networks that are called central pattern generators (CPGs) consist of neurons located in laminae VII, VIII, IX, and X endowed with rhythm-generating capabilities.[1–3] Serotonin (5-hydroxytryptamine, 5-HT) is extensively used to activate the CPGs in the *in vitro* spinal cord preparation, applied alone or in combination with *N*-methyl-D-aspartate (NMDA).[4–9] NMDA may also be employed as a neurochemical inducing rhythmic activity of the spinal lumbar networks but NMDA receptor-mediated oscillations appear to be 5-HT dependent.[10] These results highlight the importance of 5-HT in locomotion. However, if 5-HT appears as a key activator of mature spinal neural networks,

this neurotransmitter also plays crucial roles during the construction of these spinal networks as we will see in this paper.

Although locomotion can be elicited, in neonate rat spinal cord, in the presence of bicuculline or strychnine,[11,12] coordination between antagonistic muscles and left-right limbs likely depends on fast GABA and glycine synaptic inhibition.[13–15] This coordination develops during embryonic life as the neonate spinal cord exhibits clear left-right, flexor-extensor alternations.[16,17] Interestingly, it develops while bulbo-spinal 5-HT descending inputs reach the spinal cord.[18,19] In this paper, we will first recall the ontogeny of descending 5-HT fibers in the mouse spinal cord, second review our data on the development of the GABA and glycine phenotype in the mouse embryonic spinal cord, and third describe how 5-HT descending inputs control the GABA phenotype maturation.

doi: 10.1111/j.1749-6632.2010.05433.x

The ontogeny of the bulbo-spinal descending 5-HT inputs parallels the maturation of left-right alternation

We have traced 5-HT immunoreactivity in the mouse spinal cord from embryonic (E) day 11.5 (E11.5) to postnatal (PN) day 10 (PN10).[19] Our results indicated that by E11.5, descending 5-HT immunoreactive (5-HT-ir) fibers, originating from caudal raphe nuclei, were detected in the ventral and lateral funiculi, at anterior cervical spinal levels, but not at more caudal levels. Descending 5-HT-ir axons reached thoracic levels at E13.5 and lumbar levels at E15.5. Some 5-HT-ir fibers could be detected in the ventral and intermediate gray matter by E15.5, whereas the dorsal gray matter was not invaded before PN0.

In parallel with these anatomical experiments, we have determined when first lumbar left-right alternation can be induced following activation of CPGs by 5-HT.[17] We performed electrophysiological recordings from the ventral roots of isolated spinal cords of mouse embryos. From E11.5 to E14.5, motor bursts of mean duration 4.9 s and frequency 0.06 Hz could be induced after bath application of serotonin and most of the contralateral and ipsilateral bursts were closely coupled in a single-phase rhythm, suggesting that bilateral inhibitory interconnections between the immature left and right CPGs are absent or not synaptically active at these stages. Importantly, because descending 5-HT spinal pathways have not yet reached the lumbo-sacral part of the cord at E14.5, we concluded that left and right rhythm generators already possess functional 5-HT receptors. At E15.5–E16.5, 5-HT evoked a different activity that consisted of tonic firing followed by an episode of rhythmic motor bursting (3–7 s, 0.05–0.1 Hz). Although no convincing evidence for coupling between bilateral motor rhythms was revealed at this stage, the contralateral activity patterns seemed to interact in a complex manner. In the presence of strychnine this coupling became synchronous, suggesting that inhibitory glycinergic pathways between reciprocal CPGs are in the process of developing after E15.5, a stage that appears to be crucial in the development of lumbar locomotor-like pattern and that corresponds to the arrival of descending bulbo-spinal 5-HT descending inputs. A typical adult-like pattern was fully developed at E17.5, the frequency of this latter activity being higher (0.1–0.3 Hz) than that seen at E15.5–E16.5. Once established, this alternating pattern was the sole pattern seen until the end of gestation and after birth as also described in rat.[20]

Commissural interneurons that have axons crossing the midline are essential for left-right alternation and include, in the mouse and rat neonatal lumbar spinal cord, GABAergic and/or glycinergic interneurons.[14,21] Data have been published describing in rat[22,23] and chick[24,25] the embryonic maturation of the GABA and/or glycine system in the spinal cord. However, no systematic equivalent exists in mouse in relation to the maturation of the left-right alternation. A physiological study performed on rat spinal cord indicates that GABA is involved in left-right alternation at embryonic stages whereas around birth the left-right alternation becomes mainly dependent on glycine.[26]

Here we present the embryonic maturation of the GABAergic and glycinergic phenotype in the mouse spinal cord as previously described.[27,28]

Time course of the embryonic maturation of the GABA and glycine phenotype

As illustrated in Figure 1(A1,B1) (in green), the ontogeny of GABA immunoreactive (GABA-ir) cell bodies and fibers in the embryonic mouse spinal cord was analyzed at brachial and lumbar levels, from E11.5 to P0. GABA-ir somata were first detected at E11.5 exclusively at brachial level in the presumed ventral gray matter. By E13.5, the number of GABAergic neurons sharply increased throughout the extent of the ventral horn both at brachial and lumbar levels. Stained perikarya first appeared in the future dorsal horn at E15.5 and progressively invaded this area while they decreased in number in the ventral horn. GABA-ir fibers also appeared at the E11.5 stage in the presumptive lateral white matter at brachial level. At E12.5 and E13.5, GABA-ir fibers progressively invaded the ventral marginal zone and by E15.5 reached the dorsal marginal zone. At E17.5 and P0, the number of GABA-ir fibers declined in the white matter. Finally, by P0, GABA immunoreactivity that delineated somata was mainly restricted to the dorsal gray matter and declined in intensity and extent. The ventral gray matter exhibited very few GABA-ir cell bodies at this neonatal stage of development. A quantitative study of the GABA-ir

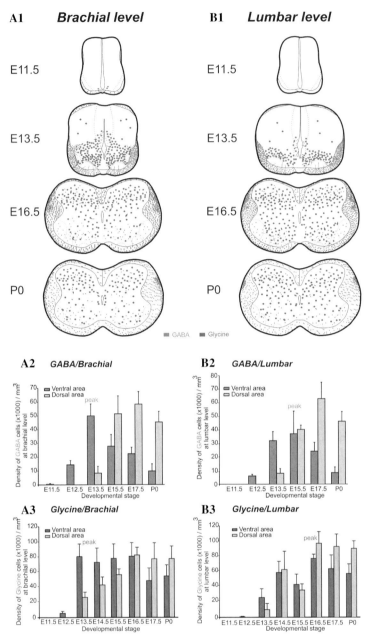

Figure 1. Evolution of the GABAergic and glycinergic system during embryonic development of the mouse spinal cord. Schematic representation of the GABA and glycine immunoreactivity from spinal cord sections performed at brachial (**A1**) and lumbar level (**B1**). Each drawing is consistent with representative confocal acquisition from corresponding stage of development. *Large dots* correspond to either GABA-ir (*green*) or glycine-ir (*red*) cell bodies, whereas *small dots* represent GABA or glycine fibers. *Black lines* in the spinal cord sections delineate the limit of the marginal zone and *dotted lines* the localization of the pools of somatic motor neurons. Quantitative analysis of GABA-ir and glycine-ir somata density in the ventral and dorsal horns during the course of development was performed at brachial level (**A2,A3**) and lumbar level (**B2,B3**). One can notice a rostro-caudal delay of the maximum density of GABA and glycine cells in the ventral area: peak of GABA occurring by E13.5 at brachial level and by E15.5 at lumbar level; peak of glycine at E13.5 at brachial level and E16.5 at lumbar level. Each histogram corresponds to four to six measurements. Error bars indicate SEM. (Modified from Refs. 27 and 28.)

perikarya density (Fig. 1(A2, B2)) evidenced a peak at E13.5 and E15.5 in the ventral area, at brachial and lumbar level, respectively.

As for the GABAergic system, the ontogeny of glycine immunoreactive (Gly-ir) somata and fibers system was studied, at brachial and lumbar levels, from E11.5 to P0 (Fig. 1(A1,B1), in red). Spinal Gly-ir somata appeared at E12.5 (1 day after first GABA-ir somata) in the ventral horn, with a higher density at brachial level. They were intermingled with numerous Gly-ir fibers reaching the border of the marginal zone. By E13.5, at brachial level, the number of Gly-ir perikarya sharply increased throughout the whole ventral horn and, in the dorsal horn first Gly-ir somata were then detected. From E13.5 to E16.5, at brachial level, the density of Gly-ir cells remained stable in the ventral horn and after E16.5 decreased to reach a plateau. In the dorsal horn, the density of Gly-ir cells increased and after E16.5 remained stable. At lumbar level, the maximum of expression was reached at E16.5 in both ventral and dorsal horn. The quantitative analysis (Fig. 1(A3,B3)) revealed that the density of the Gly-ir perikarya, in the ventral area, reached a peak at E13.5 at brachial and at E16.5 at lumbar level.

Our data show that the glycinergic system matures 1 day later than the GABAergic system and follows a parallel spatio-temporal evolution leading at P0 to a larger population of glycine cells in the ventral horn.

Putative interaction between 5-HT descending inputs and ontogeny of the GABA/glycine phenotype: analysis of the GABA phenotype

As described earlier, 5-HT descending fibers invade the spinal cord during the embryonic life. At lumbar level, they can be detected at E15.5, that is, when GABA-ir somata reach their maximum density. A 5-HT/GABA double-staining performed at lumbar part of the mouse spinal cord indicated that GABA perikarya were densely innervated by supra-spinal 5-HT fibers (illustrated at E17.5 in Fig. 2A). To study the interaction between the 5-HT descending system and intraspinal GABA phenotype, we used organotypic cultures of E11.5 spinal cord enriched or not with 5-HT.[29] In such organotypic cultures, we found that 5-HT descending inputs invaded the spinal cord and reached the lumbar enlargement

after 6–8 days in culture (DIC) (Fig. 2B). Using a quantitative confocal study performed on acute and cultured spinal cords, we found that the GABAergic population matured according to a similar rostro-caudal temporal gradient both *in utero* and in organotypic culture. Thereafter, as illustrated in Figure 3, we analyzed the maturation of GABA interneurons in spinal cords with endogenous 5-HT (presence of intraspinal 5-HT cell bodies when 5-HT inputs are removed[30]), exogenous 5-HT, or without 5-HT (p-chlorophenylalanine [pCPA] treatment with or without the medulla). Our data showed that in the absence of 5-HT, the GABAergic population matured 2 days earlier, whereas in the presence of exogenous 5-HT, this population matured 2 days later. Hence, 5-HT descending inputs postpone the appearance of the spinal GABAergic system at lumbar level compared to brachial level leading to a rostro-caudal delay.

The schematic drawing presented in Figure 4 summarizes, along the course of the mouse embryonic development, (1) the maturation of 5-HT-induced rhythmic activity, (2) the *in vivo* ontogeny of the GABA and glycine phenotype in parallel to the maturation of 5-HT raphe descending inputs, and (3) the corresponding maturation in organotypic cultures with or without 5-HT descending inputs. For information, neurotransmitters (Ach and GABA/glycine) involved in the genesis of the spontaneous activity at early stages are mentioned as is the switch from excitatory GABA/glycine to inhibitory that occurs after E15.5.[31]

Altogether, our data suggest that, during the course of the embryonic development, 5-HT descending inputs delay the maturation of lumbar spinal motor networks relative to brachial networks. It now remains to be determined whether descending 5-HT inputs also control the maturation of the glycine phenotype.

Which 5-HT receptors are involved in the downregulating effect of 5-HT on the GABA phenotype?

To identify which type of 5-HT receptor mediates the effects of 5-HT, we selectively blocked the different types of 5-HT receptors known to be present in ventral parts of the spinal cord[32] and analyzed the GABA expression at the brachial level in spinal cords maintained 4 DIC without the medulla.

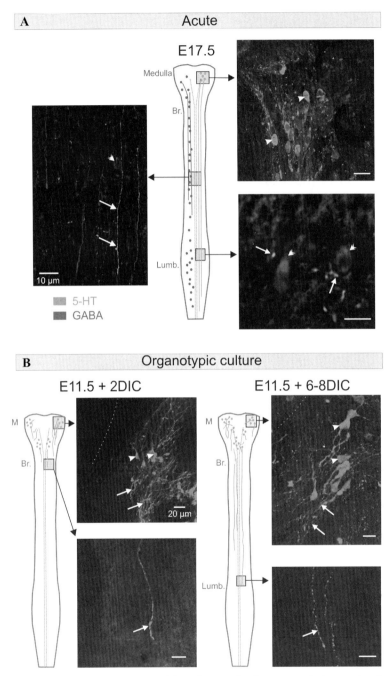

Figure 2. The organotypic preparation: a powerful tool to study the ontogenic interaction between the raphe descending 5-HT system and the intraspinal GABA phenotype. At E17.5 (**A**), caudal raphe nuclei express 5-HT-ir cells (*arrowheads*) and 5-HT descending inputs have reached the lumbar spinal level. Note that some descending 5-HT axons (*arrows*) are apposed to GABAergic cells (*double arrowheads*). (**B**) E11.5 spinal cords devoid of 5-HT innervation are cultured during 2–8 days (2–8 DIC). Serotonergic axons progressively invade the spinal cord in organotypic culture, as in acute preparation, and reach brachial level after 2 DIC, and lumber level after 6–8 DIC. M, medulla; Br, brachial; Lumb, lumbar. Scale bars correspond to 10 µm in (**A**) and 20 µm in (**B**).

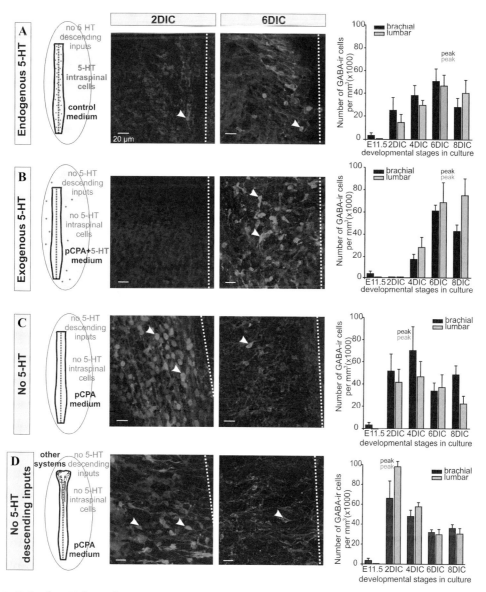

Figure 3. Role of 5-HT descending inputs on the maturation of the intraspinal GABAergic population: 5-HT delays the occurrence of the GABAergic system. All confocal images correspond to GABA immunoreactivity. In the presence of 5-HT, either endogenous 5-HT [(**A**) cultures maintained in a control medium without the medulla contain ectopic 5-HT cells [30]] or exogenous 5-HT [(**B**) addition of 5-HT to the medium in the presence of pCPA provides an exogenous source of 5-HT], a few or no GABA-ir interneurons (*arrowheads*) are detected after 2 DIC at brachial level whereas numerous stained cells are observed after 6 DIC. The quantitative analysis reveals that in the presence of 5-HT, the development of the GABAergic population is synchronous at brachial and lumbar level and exhibits a peak of GABA-ir interneurons at 6 DIC. In the absence of 5-HT and supra-spinal inputs [(**C**) spinal cord without the medulla maintained in culture with pCPA to eliminate 5-HT synthesis] or selective absence of 5-HT descending inputs [(**D**) spinal cord maintained in culture with the medulla in a pCPA medium to eliminate 5-HT synthesis], numerous GABA-ir cell bodies (*arrowheads*) and processes are stained at brachial level. After 6 DIC, the number of labeled cells has decreased. The quantification of the density of GABA cells indicates that GABA maturation is similar at brachial and lumbar levels, with an early peak of development (4 DIC in the absence of 5-HT in C and 2 DIC in the absence of 5-HT descending inputs in D). All scale bars are 20 μm. Error bars indicate SEM. (Modified from Ref. 29.)

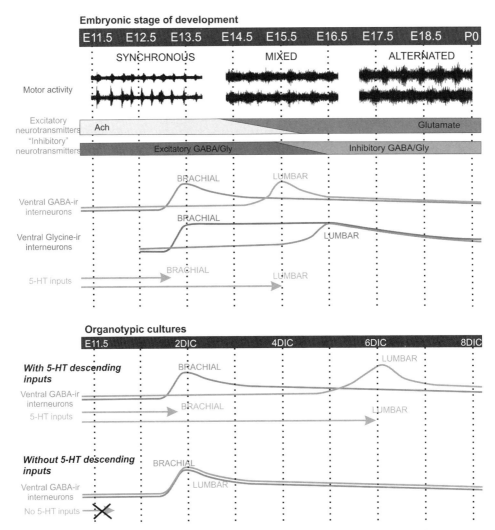

Figure 4. Schematic drawing that illustrates the maturation of the embryonic mouse spinal motor networks in parallel to the ontogeny of the GABA/glycine phenotype under the control of 5-HT descending inputs.

Addition of the 5-HT1A receptor antagonist (Fig. 5, WAY100635) to the pCPA/5-HT medium prevented the decrease of the density of GABA-ir cells observed in the pCPA/5-HT control medium. Similarly, chronic application of the 5-HT1B receptor antagonist (Fig. 5, SB224289) circumvented the reduction of the density of GABAergic cells. In contrast, neither the 5-HT2A/2C receptor antagonist (Fig. 5, ketanserin tartrate salt) nor the 5-HT3 receptor antagonist (Fig. 5, 3-TI-3-CM) prevented the inhibiting action of 5-HT on the maturation of the GABAergic population. This pharmacological demonstration indicates that 5-HT exerts its

downregulating effect on the GABAergic population through the 5-HT1 receptor family.

To further distinguish between a 5-HT1A or 5-HT1B receptor-related effect, we used genetically modified mice devoid of either 5-HT1A receptors ($1A^{-/-}$) or 5-HT1B receptors ($1B^{-/-}$). In wild-type animals (OF1, $1A^{+/+}$, and $1B^{+/+}$ mice), the analysis of the GABA expression at the brachial level, in spinal cords maintained 4 DIC without the medulla, confirmed the downregulating effect of 5-HT on the GABA phenotype (compare pCPA and pCPA/5-HT in Figs. 6A–C). KO animals revealed that 5-HT still exerts its repressive effect on the GABA

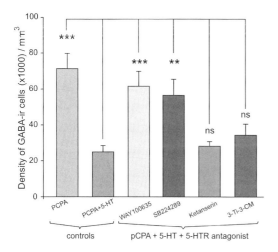

WAY 100635 : *5-HT1A receptor antagonist*
SB 224289 : *5-HT1B receptor antagonist*
Ketanserin tartrate salt (ketanserin) : 5-HT2 receptor antagonist
3-Tropanylindole-3-carboxylate methiodide (3-Ti-3-CM) : 5-HT3 receptor antagonist

Figure 5. Implication of the 5-HT1 receptor family in the downregulation of 5-HT on GABA phenotype: an *in vitro* pharmacological approach. Organotypic cultures were maintained 4 DIC without the medulla, in the presence of pCPA and the density of GABA-ir cells was quantified at brachial level. In control conditions, a high number of GABA-ir cells is observed in the absence of 5-HT (pCPA, *gray bar*), whereas the addition of 5-HT to the medium decreases the density of GABA-labeled cells (pCPA + 5-HT, *green histogram*). In the presence of 5-HT1A receptor antagonist (WAY 100635) or 5-HT1B receptor antagonist (SB 224289), the down-regulating effect of 5-HT is not prevented. In the presence of either 5-HT2 or 5-HT3 receptor antagonist, the inhibiting effect of 5-HT is still observed indicating that these 5-HT receptors are not involved. $*P < 0.05$, $**P < 0.01$, $***P < 0.001$; ns, not significant, drug treatment compared with control pCPA + 5-HT, unpaired *t*-test. Error bars indicate SEM. (Modified from Ref. 29.)

phenotype in $1A^{-/-}$ mice, this effect being prevented by 5-HT1B receptor antagonist (Fig. 6D) whereas in $1B^{-/-}$ mice, 5-HT was ineffective (Fig. 6E).

In summary, all these data demonstrate that 5-HT descending inputs exert a downregulating effect on the embryonic maturation of the GABA phenotype at lumbar level of the mouse spinal cord through a selective action on 5-HT1B receptors.

Is the downregulating effect of 5-HT activity dependent?

Serotonin is a neurochemical that activates the CPGs and exerts potent excitatory effect on embryonic spinal motoneurons,[33] leading to rhythmic $[Ca^{2+}]_i$ elevations.[34] Serotonergic neurons of the developing midline raphe system also play an excitatory role in initiating and propagating spontaneous activity throughout the hindbrain.[35,36] Thus, because of the well-known strong excitatory effect of 5-HT, we hypothesized that descending 5-HT inputs exert their repressive role on GABA phenotype through an activity-dependent mechanism. To test this hypothesis, again we analyzed the GABA expression at the brachial level in spinal cords maintained 4 DIC without the medulla, in control condition, in the presence of tetrodotoxin (TTX) that blocks voltage-dependent Na^+ channels, or in a medium containing an elevated concentration of K^+ (8 mM) to raise the excitability of the spinal networks maintained in culture. In each of the three conditions, the density of GABA-ir somata was compared with or without 5-HT (in a pCPA medium). These experiments revealed that neither TTX nor the high $[K^+]$ medium affected the downregulating effect of 5-HT on the maturation of the GABA phenotype (Fig. 7), indicating that the 5-HT action on the emergence of the GABA phenotype is likely nonactivity dependent.

Discussion

Most serotonergic neurons are found in the raphe nuclei that are divided into B1–B9 cell groups, B1–B5 corresponding to the caudal division (raphe pallidus, magnus, obscurus, and pontis), and B6–B9 to the rostral division (dorsal and medial raphe nuclei).[37] Although 5-HT nuclei include a small number of neurons (20,000 neurons in the rat [38]), serotonergic neurons modulate many aspects of embryonic development and adult behaviors.[39,40] Raphe serotonergic neurons are among the earliest neurons to be generated (E10–E12 in the mouse) and molecular mechanisms by which neural precursors become serotonergic are now elucidated.[41] Here we report that bulbo-spinal descending 5-HT fibers reach the lumbar mouse spinal cord at E15.5 and start to invade the gray matter. We also report that 5-HT downregulates the development of the GABA phenotype in intraspinal interneurons. At E15.5, the full 5-HT system is not complete and the

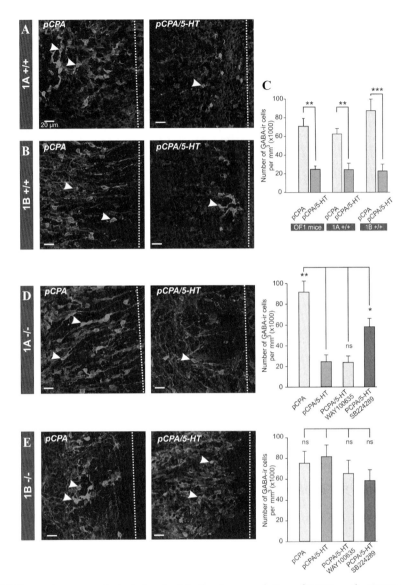

Figure 6. 5-HT1B receptors are exclusively involved in the downregulation of 5-HT on the GABAergic system: use of mice lacking either 5-HT1A or 5-HT1B receptors. In control experiments [(A) 5-HT$_{1A}$R$^{+/+}$ embryos and (B) 5-HT$_{1B}$R$^{+/+}$ embryos], spinal cords were maintained 4 DIC without the medulla in the presence of pCPA (high number of GABA-positive cells at this stage of *in vitro* development) or pCPA/5-HT (decreased number of GABA cells). Quantification of GABA-ir cell density at brachial level in 5-HT$_{1A}$R$^{+/+}$ and 5-HT$_{1B}$R$^{+/+}$ animals, shows that the down-regulating effect of 5-HT on the GABA phenotype occurs as in OF1 mice (our control strain, C). In 5-HT$_{1A}$R$^{-/-}$ spinal cords maintained in culture from E11.5 during 4 DIC without the medulla (D), numerous GABA-ir cells are detected in the absence of 5-HT (*pCPA*) whereas the number of GABA cells is decreased in the presence of 5-HT (*pCPA/5-HT*). 5-HT$_{1A}$R are thus not implicated in the repressive effect of 5-HT on the GABAergic system. Addition of 5-HT$_{1A}$R antagonist (WAY 100635) in pCPA/5-HT medium has no effect but when a 5-HT$_{1B}$R antagonist (SB 224289) is added to the pCPA/5-HT medium, 5-HT is no longer active. The use of 5-HT$_{1B}$R$^{-/-}$ mice (E) confirms the implication of the 5-HT$_{1B}$R in the down-regulating effect of 5-HT on the GABAergic population: neither 5-HT application nor the use of a 5-HT$_{1A}$R antagonist induce a decrease in the number of GABA-ir cells. Error bars indicate SEM. *$P < 0.05$, **$P < 0.01$, ***$P < 0.001$; ns, not significant, unpaired t-test.

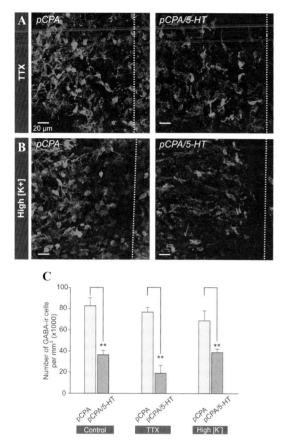

Figure 7. The ontogenic control of intraspinal GABA phenotype by 5-HT is not activity dependent. Organotypic preparations of embryonic spinal cords maintained 4 DIC without the medulla. Analysis was performed at the brachial level. In control conditions, a high number of GABA-ir cells is observed in the absence of 5-HT (*pCPA*), whereas exogenous 5-HT induces a clear drop of the GABA-ir cells density (*pCPA*/5-HT). In the presence of 1 µM TTX (A and C "TTX") or 8 mM K+ (B and C "High [K+]"), the inhibitory effect of 5-HT on the GABAergic cellular population is retained (*pCPA*/5-HT). Error bars indicate SEM. **$P < 0.01$, unpaired t-test.

dense plexus of 5-HT fibers that will be present in mature spinal cord is not formed. However, because 5-HT is released by growing axons as its neurotransmission is predominantly paracrine,[42] it is not surprising that the descending 5-HT exert such a potent role on GABA phenotype even though it is on process of maturation.

The use of genetically modified mice demonstrates that 5-HT1B receptors are involved while

our pharmacological data also highlight the involvement of 5-HT1A receptors. This discrepancy may be explained by the fact that the pharmacological blocker of 5-HT1A receptors that we used (WAY100635) looses its specificity when chronically applied (here during 4 DIC) and also antagonizes 5-HT1B receptors. The serotonin 1B receptors have been described as being presynaptically located on unmyelinated axons and terminals, but not on cell bodies[43,44] rendering difficult to interpret the implication of 5-HT1B receptors in the effect of descending 5-HT inputs on the GABA phenotype. However, a recent study based on electron microscopy indicates that a large percentage of 5-HT1B receptors in the hippocampus are postsynaptic, some of them being located on dendrites of GABAergic interneurons.[45] Therefore, it is likely that the 5-HT1B receptors that are involved in the ontogenic downregulating effect exerted by descending 5-HT fibers on the expression of the GABA phenotype involves 5-HT1B receptors located on proximal dendrites and/or somata of intraspinal GABAergic neurons. A confocal analysis, performed in our laboratory (data not shown), using antibodies directed against 5-HT1B receptors and GABA seems to reinforce this hypothesis but this remains to be unambiguously demonstrated using electron microscopy.

As a functional consequence, 5-HT descending inputs that regulate the expression of the GABA phenotype may also play a role on the switch between excitatory to inhibitory effects of GABA in motor networks. In fact, raphe descending 5-HT inputs reach the lumbar spinal cord at E15.5 when chloride-mediated GABA inhibitory (shunting) effects start to occur in spinal motoneurons.[31] A modulation of chloride homeostasis by endogenous 5-HT during maturation of locomotor networks has been demonstrated in zebrafish.[46]

Serotonergic descending inputs do not interfere with the establishment of the GABA population at brachial level but downregulate the GABA phenotype at lumbar level. This may be necessary for the delayed establishment of GABAergic inhibitory inputs in motor networks located at lumbar levels to match the arrival of proprioceptive afferents that develop during the embryonic life.[47] Interestingly, an interaction between sensory terminals and GABAergic interneurons mediating presynaptic inhibition has recently been demonstrated.[48] Hence, descending 5-HT inputs may play a differential role in such interaction during the construction of cervical and lumbar locomotor networks.

It has been shown in *Xenopus laevis* that modulating the electrical activity can modify the neuronal phenotype during ontogeny.[49] Because 5-HT strongly increases the excitability of the embryonic mouse spinal cord,[17] we may speculate that the downregulation of the GABA phenotype by 5-HT is activity dependent. Although our data show that this effect is preserved in the presence of TTX or high $[K^+]_e$, we cannot rule out the involvement of Ca^{2+}-dependent mechanisms. Further experiments remain to be performed to test this Ca^{2+} dependency.

Acknowledgments

This study was supported by grants from the Conseil Régional d'Aquitaine (#20040301202A) and the Institut pour la Recherche sur la Moelle épinière et l'Encéphale (IRME/2005/2006).

Conflicts of interest

The authors declare no conflicts of interest.

References

1. Kiehn, O. & O. Kjaerulff. 1998. Distribution of central pattern generators for rhythmic motor outputs in the spinal cord of limbed vertebrates. *Ann. N.Y. Acad. Sci.* **860:** 110–129.

2. Mentis, G.Z. *et al.* 2005. Noncholinergic excitatory actions of motoneurons in the neonatal mammalian spinal cord. *Proc. Natl. Acad. Sci. USA* **102:** 7344–7349.

3. Nishimaru, H. *et al.* 2005. Mammalian motor neurons corelease glutamate and acetylcholine at central synapses. *Proc. Natl. Acad. Sci. USA* **102:** 5245–5249.

4. Cazalets, J.-R., Y. Sqalli-Houssaini & F. Clarac. 1992. Activation of the central pattern generators for locomotion by serotonin and excitatory amino acids in neonatal rat. *J. Physiol. (Lond.)* **455:** 187–204.

5. Whelan, P., A. Bonnot & M.J. O'Donovan. 2000. Properties of rhythmic activity generated by the isolated spinal cord of the neonatal mouse. *J. Neurophysiol.* **84:** 2821–2833.

6. Cowley, K.C. & B.J. Schmidt. 1997. Regional distribution of the locomotor pattern-generating network in the neonatal rat spinal cord. *J. Neurophysiol.* **77:** 247–259.

7. Clarac, F. *et al.* 2004. The *in vitro* neonatal rat spinal cord preparation: a new insight into mammalian locomotor mechanisms. *J. Comp. Physiol. A Neuroethol Sens. Neural Behav. Physiol.* **190:** 343–357.

8. Jiang, Z., K.P. Carlin & R.M. Brownstone. 1999. An *in vitro* functionally mature mouse spinal cord preparation for the study of spinal motor networks. *Brain Res.* **816:** 493–499.

9. Whelan, P.J. 2003. Developmental aspects of spinal locomotor function: insights from using the *in vitro* mouse spinal cord preparation. *J. Physiol.* **553:** 695–706.

10. MacLean, J.N., K.C. Cowley & B.J. Schmidt. 1998. NMDA receptor-mediated oscillatory activity in the neonatal rat spinal cord is serotonin dependent. *J. Neurophysiol.* **79:** 2804–2808.

11. Cazalets, J.-R., Y. Sqalli-Houssaini & F. Clarac. 1994. GABAergic inactivation of the central pattern generators for locomotion in neonatal rat spinal cord. *J. Physiol. (Lond.)* **474:** 173–181.

12. Kremer, E. & A. Lev-Tov. 1997. Localization of the spinal network associated with generation of hindlimb locomotion in the neonatal rat and organization of its transverse coupling system. *J. Neurophysiol.* **77:** 1155–1170.

13. Cowley, K.C. & B.J. Schmidt. 1995. Effects of inhibitory amino acid antagonists on reciprocal inhibitory interactions during rhythmic motor activity in the *in vitro* neonatal rat spinal cord. *J. Neurophysiol.* **74:** 1109–1117.

14. Quinlan, K.A. & O. Kiehn. 2007. Segmental, synaptic actions of commissural interneurons in the mouse spinal cord. *J. Neurosci.* **27:** 6521–6530.

15. Hinckley, C., B. Seebach & L. Ziskind-Conhaim. 2005. Distinct roles of glycinergic and GABAergic inhibition in coordinating locomotor-like rhythms in the neonatal mouse spinal cord. *Neuroscience* **131:** 745–758.

16. Kudo, N., H. Nishimaru & K. Nakayama. 2004. Developmental changes in rhythmic spinal neuronal activity in the rat fetus. *Prog. Brain Res.* **143:** 49–55.

17. Branchereau, P. *et al.* 2000. Development of lumbar rhythmic networks: from embryonic to neonate locomotor-like patterns in the mouse. *Brain Res. Bull.* **53:** 711–718.

18. Rajaofetra, N. *et al.* 1989. Pre- and post-natal ontogeny of serotonergic projections to the rat spinal cord. *J. Neurosci. Res.* **22:** 305–321.

19. Ballion, B. *et al.* 2002. Ontogeny of descending serotonergic innervation and evidence for intraspinal 5-HT neurons in the mouse spinal cord. *Dev. Brain Res.* **137:** 81–88.

20. Nishimaru, H. & N. Kudo. 2000. Formation of the central pattern generator for locomotion in the rat and mouse. *Brain Res. Bull.* **53:** 661–669.

21. Weber, I. *et al.* 2007. Neurotransmitter systems of commissural interneurons in the lumbar spinal cord of neonatal rats. *Brain Res.* **1178:** 65–72.

22. Ma, W., T. Behar & J.L. Barker. 1992. Transient expression of GABA immunoreactivity in the developing rat spinal cord. *J. Comp. Neurol.* **325:** 271–290.

23. Tran, T.S., A. Alijani & P.E. Phelps. 2003. Unique developmental patterns of GABAergic neurons in rat spinal cord. *J. Comp. Neurol.* **456:** 112–126.

24. Antal, M. *et al.* 1994. Developmental changes in the distribution of gamma-aminobutyric acid-immunoreactive neurons in the embryonic chick lumbosacral spinal cord. *J. Comp. Neurol.* **343:** 228–236.

25. Berki, A.C., M.J. O'Donovan & M. Antal. 1995. Developmental expression of glycine immunoreactivity and its colocalization with GABA in the embryonic chick lumbosacral spinal cord. *J. Comp. Neurol.* **362:** 583–596.

26. Nakayama, K., H. Nishimaru & N. Kudo. 2002. Basis of changes in left-right coordination of rhythmic motor activity during development in the rat spinal cord. *J. Neurosci.* **22:** 10388–10398.

27. Allain, A.E. *et al.* 2004. Ontogenic changes of the GABAergic system in the embryonic mouse spinal cord. *Brain Res.* **1000:** 134–147.

28. Allain, A.E. *et al.* 2006. Expression of the glycinergic system during the course of embryonic development in the mouse spinal cord and its co-localization with GABA immunoreactivity. *J. Comp. Neurol.* **496:** 832–846.

29. Allain, A.E., P. Meyrand & P. Branchereau. 2005. Ontogenic changes of the spinal GABAergic cell population are controlled by the serotonin (5-HT) system: implication of 5-HT1 receptor family. *J. Neurosci.* **25:** 8714–8724.

30. Branchereau, P., J. Chapron & P. Meyrand. 2002. Descending 5-hydroxytryptamine raphe inputs repress the expression of serotonergic neurons and slow the maturation of inhibitory systems in mouse embryonic spinal cord. *J. Neurosci.* **22:** 2598–2606.

31. Delpy, A. *et al.* 2008. NKCC1 cotransporter inactivation underlies embryonic development of chloride-mediated inhibition in mouse spinal motoneuron. *J. Physiol.* **586:** 1059–1075.

32. Vergé, D. & A. Calas. 2000. Serotoninergic neurons and serotonin receptors: gains from cytochemical approaches. *J. Chem. Neuroanat.* **18:** 41–56.

33. Elliott, P. *et al.* 1999. Ionic mechanisms underlying excitatory effects of serotonin on embryonic rat motoneurons in long-term culture. *Neuroscience* **90:** 1311–1323.

34. Nakayama, K., H. Nishimaru & N. Kudo. 2004. Rhythmic motor activity in thin transverse slice preparations of the fetal rat spinal cord. *J. Neurophysiol.* **92:** 648–652.

35. Hunt, P.N., A.K. McCabe & M.M. Bosma. 2005. Midline serotonergic neurones contribute to widespread synchronized activity in embryonic mouse hindbrain. *J. Physiol.* **566:** 807–819.

36. Hunt, P.N. *et al.* 2006. Primary role of the serotonergic midline system in synchronized spontaneous activity during development of the embryonic mouse hindbrain. *J. Neurobiol.* **66:** 1239–1252.

37. Dahlstrom, A. & K. Fuxe. 1964. Localization of monoamines in the lower brain stem. *Experientia* **20:** 398–399.

38. Jacobs, B.L. & E.C. Azmitia. 1992. Structure and function of the brain serotonin system. *Physiol. Rev.* **72:** 165–229.

39. Whitaker-Azmitia, P.M. *et al.* 1996. Serotonin as a developmental signal. *Behav. Brain Res.* **73:** 19–29.

40. Lauder, J.M. 1993. Neurotransmitters as growth regulatory signals: role of receptors and second messengers. *Trends Neurosci.* **16:** 233–240.

41. Ding, Y.Q. *et al.* 2003. Lmx1b is essential for the development of serotonergic neurons. *Nat. Neurosci.* **6:** 933–938.

42. Bunin, M.A. & R.M. Wightman. 1999. Paracrine neurotransmission in the CNS: involvement of 5-HT. *Trends Neurosci.* **22:** 377–382.

43. Sari, Y. *et al.* 1999. Cellular and subcellular localization of 5-hydroxytryptamine1B receptors in the rat central nervous system: immunocytochemical, autoradiographic and lesion studies. *Neuroscience* **88:** 899–915.

44. Riad, M. *et al.* 2000. Somatodendritic localization of 5-HT1A and preterminal axonal localization of 5-HT1B serotonin receptors in adult rat brain. *J. Comp. Neurol.* **417:** 181–194.

45. Peddie, C.J. *et al.* 2008. Dendritic colocalisation of serotonin1B receptors and the glutamate NMDA receptor subunit NR1 within the hippocampal dentate gyrus: an ultrastructural study. *J. Chem. Neuroanat.* **36:** 17–26.

46. Brustein, E. & P. Drapeau. 2005. Serotoninergic modulation of chloride homeostasis during maturation of the locomotor network in zebrafish. *J. Neurosci.* **25:** 10607–10616.

47. Koo, S.J. & S.L. Pfaff. 2002. Fine-tuning motor neuron properties: signaling from the periphery. *Neuron* **35:** 823–826.

48. Betley, J.N. *et al.* 2009. Stringent specificity in the construction of a GABAergic presynaptic inhibitory circuit. *Cell* **139:** 161–174.

49. Borodinsky, L.N. *et al.* 2004. Activity-dependent homeostatic specification of transmitter expression in embryonic neurons. *Nature* **429:** 523–530.

Ann. N.Y. Acad. Sci. ISSN 0077-8923

ANNALS OF THE NEW YORK ACADEMY OF SCIENCES

Issue: *Neurons and Networks in the Spinal Cord*

Mechanisms regulating the specificity and strength of muscle afferent inputs in the spinal cord

George Z. Mentis,[1] Francisco J. Alvarez,[2] Neil A. Shneider,[1,3,4] Valerie C. Siembab,[2] and Michael J. O'Donovan[1]

[1]Developmental Neurobiology Section, National Institute of Neurological Disorders and Stroke, National Institutes of Health, Bethesda, Maryland. [2]Department of Neurosciences, Cell Biology and Physiology, Wright State University, Dayton, Ohio. [3]Department of Neurology, Columbia University, New York, New York. [4]Center for Motor Neuron Biology and Disease, Columbia University, New York, New York

Address for correspondence: George Z. Mentis, Center for Motor Neuron Biology and Disease, Columbia University, P & S Building, Room 4-450, 630 W 168th Street, New York, NY 10032. gzmentis@columbia.edu

We investigated factors controlling the development of connections between muscle spindle afferents, spinal motor neurons, and inhibitory Renshaw cells. Several mutants were examined to establish the role of muscle spindles, muscle spindle-derived NT3, and excess NT3 in determining the specificity and strength of these connections. The findings suggest that although spindle-derived factors are not necessary for the initial formation and specificity of the synapses, spindle-derived NT3 seems necessary for strengthening homonymous connections between Ia afferents and motor neurons during the second postnatal week. We also found evidence for functional monosynaptic connections between sensory afferents and neonatal Renshaw cells although the density of these synapses decreases at P15. We conclude that muscle spindle synapses are weakened on Renshaw cells while they are strengthened on motor neurons. Interestingly, the loss of sensory synapses on Renshaw cells was reversed in mice overexpresssing NT3 in the periphery, suggesting that different levels of NT3 are required for functional maintenance and strengthening of spindle afferent inputs on motor neurons and Renshaw cells.

Keywords: proprioceptor; muscle spindle; motor neuron; Renshaw; stretch reflex

Introduction

The monosynaptic spinal stretch reflex circuit is mediated by the synaptic connections between muscle spindle proprioceptive Ia afferents and spinal α-motor neurons. Ia afferents connect specifically with motor pools innervating homonymous muscles and establish weaker synapses with synergistic motor neurons, but avoid motor pools innervating strict antagonists. Because of its relative simplicity, this circuit has been the object of many developmental studies of synaptic specificity, patterns of connectivity and synaptic strength.[1,2] However, this simple circuit is embedded within a larger interneuronal network that patterns the motor output. Antagonistic motor neurons are not only excited by different sets of Ia afferents but also reciprocally inhibited via Ia inhibitory interneurons (IaINs) that receive input

from specific sets of Ia afferents and project to antagonists. Moreover, the output of each motor pool is controlled by Renshaw cells which provide recurrent inhibition to the same motor neurons and also to motor pools that are coupled through broad muscle synergies, frequently with similar Ia excitation.[2]

For this network to function as a balanced output module of the motor circuit, it is essential that Ia afferents establish specific connections with defined sets of motor neurons and interneurons. In addition, the relative strength of these synapses needs to be matched to the appropriate level of Ia afferent excitation or inhibition of homonymous, heteronymous and antagonistic motor neurons. Little is known about the mechanisms responsible for the establishment of specific connectivity and the regulation of appropriate synaptic strength in most elements of this circuit. To date, most studies have

doi: 10.1111/j.1749-6632.2010.05538.x

Ann. N.Y. Acad. Sci. 1198 (2010) 220–230 © 2010 New York Academy of Sciences.

focused on the development of specific, homonymous Ia-motor neuron connections,[1,2] Based on the extensive work of Frank and coworkers,[1,3–5] it is generally agreed that peripheral signals control the specificity of these connections in an activity-independent manner. The identity of these instructive signals is largely unknown, although a few recent studies have started to describe some aspects of the molecular mechanisms through which peripheral signals could specify Ia-motor neuron synaptic specifcity.[6,7] For example, neurotrophin-3 (NT3) has been shown to be important for the survival of Ia afferents[8,9] and in determining the strength of monosynaptic connections both chronically[10] and acutely.[11] Moreover, NT3 overexpression during development induces inappropriate synaptic strengthening and can result in loss of specificity of the Ia-motor neuron connection.[12]

Little is known about the formation, specificity or developmental strengthening of the connections between Ia afferents and interneurons. In this section, we review recent data from our laboratories analyzing the developmental maturation of central Ia connections on both motor neurons and interneurons. The results suggest that muscle spindles are not required for the specificity of the central connections of Ia afferents, but that spindle-derived NT3 is important in adjusting the final strength of central Ia synapses on motor neurons and interneurons. Moreover, NT3 actions are exerted at a relatively late postnatal period (second and third postnatal week in rodents) coincident with increased phasic and tonic firing in Ia afferents and the maturation of normal responses to muscle stretch.[13] Behaviorally this period is characterized by the beginning of coordinated, weight-bearing, adult-like locomotion.[14]

Functional specificity of connections between muscle spindle afferents and motor neurons does not depend on ErbB2 expression or muscle spindle integrity

In normal mice, proprioceptive afferents project monosynaptically to homonymous motor neurons, but do not make direct connections with functionally antagonist motor neurons.[15] To investigate the importance of muscle spindles in the establishment of these connections, we examined the strength and specificity of muscle afferent projections to identified motor neurons in mice whose muscle spindle

induction was inhibited by the conditional elimination of the neuregulin 1 (Nrg1) receptor ErbB2 from muscle spindle precursors.[16] Because neuronal induction of muscle spindle development depends on Nrg1 signaling[17] through the activation of ErbB2 receptors on primary myocytes,[18,19] conditional elimination of ErbB2 from intrafusal muscle precursors resulted in a 70% loss of muscle spindles and a 90% loss in the number of intrafusal fibers.[16] The remaining muscle spindles were rudimentary and never fully matured. Immunocytochemical analysis in the ErbB2 mutants using markers for proprioceptive central axons and synapses (VGluT1, parvalbumin)[20] revealed that the density of primary afferent boutons on motor neuron somata at P21 was reduced by ~30%. Thus, in the absence of normal spindle development, there is only a modest reduction in the normal density of VGluT1 contacts on motor neurons. This led us to examine whether the putative synaptic contacts between muscle afferents and motor neurons were functional and target specifically homonymous motor pools.

For this purpose, we compared the sensorimotor connections between the functionally antagonist motor neurons innervating the lateral gastrocnemius (LG) and the tibialis anterior (TA) muscles in wild type (age range: P3–P5) and ErbB2∆ mice (age range: P3–P5). In normal mice, intracellular recordings revealed that the latency of EPSPs evoked by antagonist nerve stimulation (presumed polysynaptic) was approximately 5 ms longer than that evoked by stimulation of the homonymous nerve (monosynaptic activation). In ErbB2 mutant animals, the difference in homonymous and antagonist latency was similar (Fig. 1D), indicating that: (i) monosynaptic inputs from muscle afferents are functional in the ErbB2 mutant animals and (ii) for the TA and LG motor neurons, the specificity of the connections is preserved.[16]

These results suggest that functional connections retained their specificity in the mutant animals, but we could not rule out the possibility that erroneous connections might be formed in the ErbB2 mice that were functionally silent or too weak to detect physiologically. To test this possibility, we used a morphological assay for specificity. Cholera Toxin B subunit (CTb) conjugated to either Alexa-488 or Alexa-647 was injected *in vivo* into the TA and LG muscles respectively to label both motor neurons and proprioceptive afferent boutons and the tissue

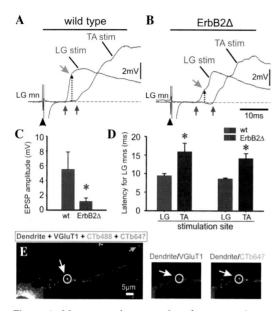

Figure 1. Monosynaptic connections between primary afferents and motor neurons are specific but reduced in strength in ErbB2Δ mice. (A) Comparison of the potentials recorded from a wild type (age: P4) LG motor neuron evoked by homonymous (*blue* trace, LG) and antagonist (*red* trace, TA) muscle nerve stimulation at 5× T intensity averaged from five stimuli applied once every 10 s. The blue and red arrows indicate the onset of the EPSPs. (B) Recordings of homonymous and antagonist evoked synaptic potentials in an ErbB2Δ LG motor neuron (age: P4). The conditions and stimulation parameters were the same as for the wild-type records in *A*. The *dotted lines with an arrow* point to the amplitude of the EPSP at 3 ms after the EPSP onset for both motoneurons. (C) Bar graph showing the average amplitude of the intracellularly recorded monosynaptic EPSP in wild-type (*blue bars*, n = 5 motor neurons) and ErbB2Δ animals (*red bars*, n = 6 motor neurons) in response to stimulation of a peripheral nerve (*P < 0.05, t-test). (D) Bar graph showing the average latency of the synaptic potential evoked in LG motor neurons by stimulation of the homonymous, LG nerve, and the antagonistic, TA nerve, for wild-type (*blue bars*) and ErbB2Δ (*red bars*) mice. Error bars are SEM. Age range: P3-P5. (E) Image is from a wild-type LG motor neuron labeled *in vivo* by LG muscle injection with CTb647 (in *white*) and retrogradely filled (3 days later) *in vitro* with Texas Red Dextran (in *red*) to reveal its somato-dendritic morphology. The CTb488 (in *green*) was injected *in vivo* into the TA muscle at the same time as CTb647 (see *green arrow* for a putative afferent fiber originating in the TA muscle). The

was later processed for VGlut1 immunoreactivity. Although the anterograde labeling methods we used do not label all afferent boutons, we failed to find any evidence in both normal and ErbB2Δ mice, of inappropriate projections either in the soma or proximal dendrites (∼50–100 μm in length) of LG afferents to TA motor neurons and vice versa (Fig. 1E). The results therefore, suggest that spindle-derived factors are not required for the initial formation or the specificity of the central connections of muscle afferents with motor neurons.

We found however that the amplitude of the monosynaptic EPSPs was reduced by ∼80% in the ErbB2Δ animals compared with wild-type animals (Figs. 1A and 1B) and this was paralleled by a similar reduction (80–85%) in the amplitude of ventral root potentials (from ErbB2Δ animals) generated in response to stimulation of the muscle nerves.[16] Thus in the ErbB2Δ mutant, a substantial number of specific Ia-motor neuron connections are formed (Figs. 1A, 1B, and 1D), but these synapses are weaker than normal. One possible mechanism to account for these findings is a lack of spindle-derived NT3.[10] Consistent with this idea, there was no detectable expression of NT3 mRNA in the muscles of Erb2Δ conditional mutants.

Effects of spindle-derived NT3 on the strength of monosynaptic Ia to motor neuron synapses

We studied the effects of selective elimination of NT3 expression from intrafusal fibers to investigate whether the reduction of the afferent evoked monosynaptic EPSPs in the ErbB2Δ mutant animals was due to the loss of spindle-derived NT3 rather than some other abnormality of spindle

motoneuron soma contains CTb647 (*white*) and Texas Red Dextran (*red*) confirming the identity of the motoneuron as LG. VGluT1-IR synaptic boutons were revealed immunohistochemically (shown in *blue*). The synaptic bouton circled in *yellow* (see *white arrow*) is shown in higher magnification on the right-hand side. The bouton is VGluT1+ (*blue*) and the CTb647+ (*white*) conferring its identity as a primary afferent bouton from the LG muscle. Each image is a single optical scan at 0.69 μm thickness. The *green arrow* points to a putative TA afferent bouton labeled with CTb488.

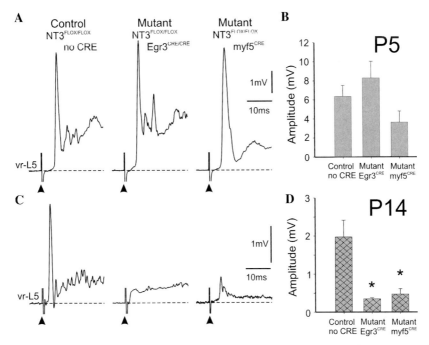

Figure 2. Muscle afferent-evoked monosynaptic ventral root potentials in animals deficient in muscle-spindle or muscle NT3 are not reduced at P5 but do show significant reductions at P14. (**A**) Averaged extracellular recordings from the L5 ventral root after stimulation of the L5 dorsal root at 5× T from three groups of animals (1 control and 2 mutants) at P5. The frequency of stimulation was 0.1 Hz. Note that the amplitude of the monosynaptic component the ventral root potential did not differ significantly between the controls (NT3$^{FLOX/FLOX}$; no Cre) and either of the two mutants (NT3$^{FLOX/FLOX}$/Egr3$^{CRE/CRE}$ or NT3$^{FLOX/FLOX}$/myf5^{CRE}). (**B**) Graph showing the average responses from three preparations from each group of animals. There was no significant difference between the groups ($P = 0.10$, ANOVA). (**C**) Recordings from the same groups as in A but at P14. Note that the monosynaptic reflex was greatly reduced in the mutants compared with the controls. (**D**) Graph showing the averaged amplitude of the monosynaptic response from three animals per group. There was a significant reduction in the monosynaptic reflex for both mutants compared with that of the control group (*$P < 0.01$, ANOVA Fisher's test). The latency of the onset of the responses was not significantly different between the mutant and control animals.

development. For this purpose, a novel transgenic mouse line carrying an *Egr3-IRES-CRE* allele was generated and crossed to animals with floxed alleles of NT3[21] to selectively eliminate NT3 expression from the intrafusal fibers of muscle spindles. In these animals, muscle spindle number and afferent innervation was normal.[16]

To monitor the strength of the afferent-motor neuron connections, we recorded the L5 ventral root responses following stimulation of the homonymous dorsal root. There was no difference between the amplitude of the ventral root potentials in the wild type and spindle-NT3 mutants in neonatal (P5) mice (Figs. 2A and 2B). However, in juveniles (P14), the amplitude of the monosynaptic reflex was significantly reduced (>80%) in animals

that lacked spindle-derived NT3 (Figs. 2C and 2D). To rule out the possibility that the reduction in monosynaptic activation was due to NT3 deletion in non-spindle structures that also express Egr3 (Schwann cells and peripheral vasculature), we also investigated the strength of sensory afferent-motor neuron connections in animals in which NT3 was selectively eliminated from all muscle fibers (intrafusal and extrafusal) using a *myf5^{CRE}* allele. The results were similar to those obtained with the selective elimination of NT3 expression from intrafusal fibers; there was no significant difference between *myf5^{CRE}* mutants and wild type at P5, but at P14 there was a dramatic reduction in ventral root reflex amplitude (Fig. 2) and no significant difference in the latency of the ventral root responses.

These results indicate that deficits of spindle derived NT3 cannot explain the reduction in the strength of the connections in the ErbB2Δ mutants during the first postnatal week. However, they reveal an important role for spindle-derived NT3 during later postnatal maturation. Interestingly, NT3 actions on the connections between Ia afferents and motor neurons coincides with the time that mice develop weight-bearing locomotion and maturation in the activity and responses of muscle spindle afferents.[13]

Previous work describing the presence of inappropriate connections in mice overexpressing NT3 in muscle proposed that a minor population of inappropriate but normally "silent" connections was strengthened by the excess NT3.[12] Although it has been previously reported that inappropriate afferent inputs on motoneurons are present during embryonic development in the rat spinal cord, these connections are greatly suppressed within a few days after birth.[22] One possibility is that non-specific connections are located in distal dendritic regions that are not accessible for analysis. Alternatively, inappropriate connectivity in these mutants may result from excessive NT3-induced branching and extension of Ia afferent central terminals arbors within the cord[23,24] and/or the retention of an excess of spindle afferents during development.[25] These NT3 effects are believed to result from overcoming inhibitory signals acting on sensory axon projections, particularly in the ventral part of the spinal cord[24,26,27] and preventing normal cell death of a proportion of Ia afferents during development.[25] A larger than normal sensory afferent projection into lamina IX could then overwhelm repulsive molecular mechanisms during synaptogenesis that normally prevent the formation of inappropriate monosynaptic connections.[7] Indeed, by P21, in mlc::NT3 animals we observed a very large increase (∼200%) in VGluT1+ contacts on motor neuron cell somata that was paralleled by a significant increase in the density of VGluT1-IR clusters in Laminae IX and VII.[28]

Primary afferents make functional monosynaptic contacts on Renshaw interneurons in the developing spinal cord

Ia afferents also make specific connections with Renshaw cells, Hb9 interneurons[29] and other interneu-rons but little is known about the development of these connections. Most of our knowledge on the organization of proprioceptive inputs to interneu-rons comes from experiments in the adult cat spinal cord.[30,31] For example, cat Ia inhibitory interneu-rons (IaINs), which mediate reciprocal inhibition between antagonistic pools, receive inputs from Ia muscle afferents that appear to be stronger and more specific than on other interneurons (i.e., Ia/Ib in-terneurons, group II interneurons). This conclu-sion is based on the strong coupling between IaINs and Ia afferent inputs, their ability to follow rela-tively high frequencies of Ia afferent discharge in response to muscle stretch, and the fact that they do not receive convergent inputs from other proprio-ceptors.[31–33] In contrast, cat Renshaw cells, which mediate recurrent inhibition of homonymous and synergistic motor neurons, do not appear to receive direct connections from Ia fibers or any other low-threshold afferent fibers in the adult spinal cord.[34,35] The mechanisms by which Ia afferents select spe-cific interneuronal targets within the ventral horn are unknown.

Although muscle afferent inputs to Renshaw cells cannot be detected functionally in the adult cat, work in the chick embryo demonstrated that muscle afferents make monosynaptic connections with R-interneurons, a class of avian embryonic inhibitory interneuron thought to be similar to the mammalian Renshaw cell.[36] However, because afferent inputs on mammalian Renshaw cells had not previously been studied in neonatal animals, it was not clear if these connections are also formed in mammalian devel-opment, or if they were unique to avians. To ad-dress this issue, we analyzed muscle afferent inputs to Renshaw cells in late embryonic, postnatal and adult rats and mice.[37]

Using a variety of morphological methods to de-fine proprioceptive primary afferents (VGluT1-IR, parvalbumin-IR, anterograde tracing from dorsal roots), we found that murine Renshaw cells receive few primary afferent inputs during late embryonic development when Ia afferent connections to mo-tor neurons became functional (∼E16–E17).[15,38] However, the fraction of Renshaw cells that receive spindle afferent inputs gradually increases to ∼50% at P0, 100% by P10, and these inputs are main-tained in all adult Renshaw cells (Fig. 3C). This re-sult was surprising because previous *in vivo* stud-ies from adult cat had reported that Renshaw cells

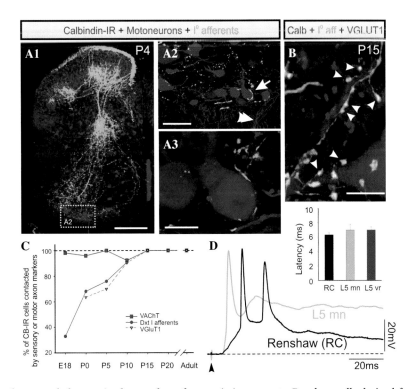

Figure 3. Developmental changes in the number of synaptic inputs onto Renshaw cells derived from dorsal root and motor axon afferents. (**A1**) Confocal image of a P4 hemicord containing primary afferent sensory fibers labeled with fluorescein dextran (*green*) and motor neurons and motor axons labeled with Texas Red Dextran (*red*). The section was also immunolabeled with calbindin antibody (*blue*). (**A2**) Higher magnification image of the area boxed in (**A1**). Renshaw cells are positioned at the exit of motoneuron axons from the cord (*double arrowhead*). Motor neurons (*red*) and calbindin-IR Renshaw cells (*blue*) are both surrounded and contacted by primary afferent axons (*green, arrow*). Renshaw cells are contacted in addition by motor axon varicosities (*red*). (**A3**) High magnification image of the Renshaw cell indicated with an *arrow* in (**A2**), receiving convergent contacts from motor axon (*red*) and primary afferent (*green*) varicosities. (**B**) High magnification images from a P15 spinal cord triple labeled to show primary afferents (dorsal root fill, in *green*), VGluT1-IR varicosities (*red*), and calbindin-IR Renshaw cells (*blue*). Superimposition of VGluT1-IR shows that all primary afferent varicosities, including those in contact with Renshaw cells, contain VGluT1-immunoreactivity. *Arrowheads* point to VGluT1-IR dorsal root afferent varicosities (*yellow*) in contact with a Renshaw cell calbindin-IR dendrite (*blue*). (**C**) Percentage of calbindin-IR cells (CB-IR; presumed Renshaw cells) receiving at least one contact from each of the markers used to identify dorsal and ventral root inputs. Almost all calbindin-IR Renshaw cells receive VAChT-IR contacts (motor axons) in embryo (age: E18). In contrast, dorsal root inputs are few in the embryo spreading to all Renshaw cells after birth. (**D**), Comparison of synaptic responses from a motor neuron (*green*) and a Renshaw cell (*black*) to a single dr-L5 stimulus at suprathreshold intensity. Both neurons responded robustly and fired action potentials superimposed on the EPSPs. Inset shows comparison of average latencies for Renshaw cells (*black*, $n = 10$), L5 motor neurons (*green*, $n = 5$), and the ventral root L5 extracellular recording (*blue*, $n = 4$) following stimulation of the dorsal root L5 (age range: P2–P3). There were no significant differences in the latencies among these groups ($P > 0.05$, One-way ANOVA). Error bars indicate SEM. Scale bars: A1: 200 μm; A2: 40 μm; A3: 10 μm; B: 10 μm.

cannot be monosynaptically activated by dorsal root stimulation.

To investigate whether the morphologically identified inputs were functional in newborn animals, we obtained whole cell recordings from identified Renshaw cells in the isolated spinal cord of the neonatal mouse. Most (11 of 12) Renshaw interneurons displayed a short-latency response following dorsal root stimulation (Fig. 3D). This response was determined to be monosynaptic because the onset of the evoked EPSP exhibited very little jitter during high frequency stimulation and the average latency of the response (~6 ms) was similar to the latency of monosynaptic afferent-evoked EPSPs recorded from motor neurons. In conclusion, our morphological evidence demonstrates the presence of functional sensory afferent synaptic inputs onto neonatal Renshaw cells.

Because Renshaw cells are located in the ventral most regions of laminae VII and IX, we assumed these projections must come from Ia afferents because no other sensory afferent class is known to project this ventrally in the spinal cord.[39] This raises the question of why Renshaw cells do not seem to have functional monosynaptic Ia afferent inputs in the adult cat. One possible explanation is that Ia afferent inputs do not make synaptic contacts on Renshaw cells in all species. To date most physiological studies of adult Renshaw cells have been conducted in the cat, while our findings were obtained in neonatal mice. However, one study conducted in fetal cats[40] provided evidence compatible with the presence of monosynaptic dorsal root inputs on embryonic Renshaw cells. Moreover, our morphological data revealed VGLUT1 sensory synapses on adult Renshaw cells in cats, similar to those found in rodents. Thus the available data seem to rule out the possibility of species differences. An alternative explanation is that Renshaw cells lose this functional input during postnatal development by weakening its synaptic effectiveness, despite maintaining a significant number of synaptic contacts.

Developmental changes in the primary afferent synaptic density on Renshaw cells

Electrophysiological recordings from interneurons during the second and third postnatal week are difficult to obtain in rodents, and for this reason we analyzed the postnatal maturation of sensory inputs onto the dendrites and somata of Renshaw cells in rat and mouse using VGluT1 as a marker of proprioceptive inputs.[37] We used synaptic density as an indirect estimate of input strength and investigated ultrastructural features[37] that are known to correlate with synaptic efficacy at Ia synapses.[41]

VGluT1+ contact densities changed with development on both dendrites and somata. However,

most VGluT1+ boutons were found on dendrites and therefore most of the analysis focused on three-dimensional reconstructions of the dendritic arbors.[37] On dendrites, VGluT1 densities increased five to sevenfold from P0 to P15 and then decreased to less than half the P15 density in the adult. This contrasted with the developmental maturation of VAChT bouton numbers, which we used as a marker of motor axon synapses. VAChT density increased during the first 2 weeks but then was maintained at the same density from P15 to adulthood. These results suggest that Renshaw cells shift from integrating sensory and motor inputs in neonates to predominantly motor inputs in the adult and raise the possibility that VGluT1 immunoreactive terminals on adult Renshaw cells may be functionally silent. Although we could not obtain electrophysiological evidence for the weakening of this input in mature mice spinal cords, we found (using electron microscopy) a partial regression of both the number and size of synaptic active zones in VGluT1+ synapses on Renshaw cells. A similar regression of the synaptic apparatus was not observed on other VGluT1 targets in the ventral spinal cord. These ultrastructural changes and the decreased synaptic density are consistent with a progressive weakening of VGluT1+ positive synapses on Renshaw cells during postnatal maturation.

Weakening or perhaps even silencing VGluT1+ inputs on Renshaw cells might be responsible for the deselection of these interneurons as a major target of Ia afferents in the adult spinal cord. The mechanisms by which this "late" developmental synaptic adjustment on Renshaw cells occurs are unknown. To investigate whether the loss of muscle spindle afferent inputs onto Renshaw cells could be reversed by NT3, we analyzed this connection in mlc::NT3 transgenic mice[25] in which exogenous NT3 is overexpressed in embryonic and postnatal muscle (Fig. 4). Using immunohistochemistry, we found that the density of VGluT1+ boutons on Neurolucida reconstructed Renshaw cell dendritic arbors increased by approximately 28% in mlc::NT3[+/−] animals with respect to controls at P15. More importantly, the densities of these contacts were maintained into adulthood, or even slightly increased (Fig. 4D). As a result, adult Renshaw cells displayed a large (99%) significant increase in VGluT1+ contact density compared to wild-types (in WT = 0.98 ± 0.03 contacts per

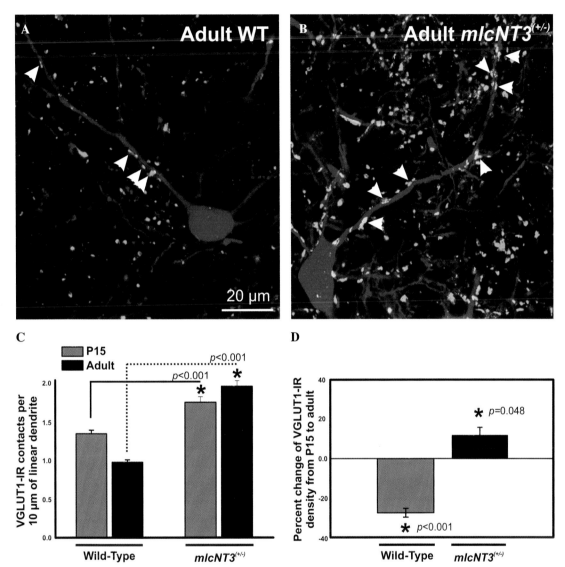

Figure 4. Density of VGluT1-immunoreactive contacts on postnatal Renshaw cells in the ventral horn of control and *mlcNT3*[(+/−)] mice. (A and B) High magnification images of VGluT1-immunoreactivity (FITC, *green*) on adult Calbindin-immunoreactive (CB-IR; Cy3, *red*) Renshaw cells (RCs) of control and *mlcNT3*[(+/−)] mice. *Arrowheads* indicate VGluT1-IR contacts on RC dendrites. There are fewer contacts on RCs from Ia afferents in control mice compared to *mlcNT3*[(+/−)] mice. (C) VGluT1-IR contacts per 10 μm of linear dendrite of P15 and adult CB-IR RCs in control and *mlcNT3*[(+/−)] mice. In control animals, VGluT1-IR density on RCs decreases significantly from P15 (1.35 ± 0.05 VGluT1+ contacts per 10 μm of linear dendrite, number of RCs = 57; number of animals = 5) to adult (0.98 ± 0.03, # RCs = 35, $N = 4$; $P < 0.001$, one-way ANOVA). In contrast, RCs in *mlcNT3*[(+/−)] mice showed a significant increase from P15 (1.76 ± 0.07, number of RCs = 40, $N = 3$) to adult (1.97 ± 0.10, number of RCs = 24, $N = 3$; $P = 0.041$, one-way ANOVA). At all ages analyzed, RCs from *mlcNT3*[(+/−)] mice showed significant increases in the density of VGluT1-IR contacts when compared to age-matched controls ($P < 0.001$, *t*-test). (D) Percentage change in the density of VGluT1-IR contacts on RCs from P15 to adult in control and *mlcNT3*[(+/−)] mice. VGluT1-IR contact density decreases by ∼30% from P15 to adult in control animals ($P < 0.001$, *t*-test). In contrast, in *mlcNT3*[(+/−)] animals, the density of VGluT1-IR contacts increases by ∼11% from P15 to adult. Therefore, it appears that increasing Ia afferent input density on RCs prevents their deselection. Scale bars: A and B (in A), 20 μm.

50 μm of dendrite; mlc::NT3$^{+/-}$ = 1.97 ± 0.1; $P <$ 0.001, t-test).

In summary, the late postnatal adjustment of input densities seen normally on Renshaw cells does not occur in mlc::NT3$^{+/-}$ animals, suggesting that the late postnatal weakening of central sensory afferent connections on Renshaw cells is controlled by processes that can be overcome by an excess supply of peripheral NT3.

Summary and conclusions

Our results suggest that spindle-derived factors are not responsible for specifying the connections between muscle spindle afferents and motor neurons, but that they do play a role in strengthening these connections during development. They also indicate that spindle-derived NT3 is important in this process when the animal begins to walk and afferent activity is significantly enhanced. Interestingly, during this time period, Ia synapses on Renshaw cells start to weaken, a process that can be overcome by excess NT3. It is therefore tempting to speculate that NT3-strengthening of Ia connections is differentially modulated depending on the target or its activity. For example, during postnatal maturation, Ia afferent activity might become tightly coupled with postsynaptic firing in motor neurons but not with Renshaw cells, leading to differential NT3-dependent strengthening on different targets. Normal levels of spindle-derived NT3 are adequate to strengthen and maintain spindle afferent synapses on motor neurons but not Renshaw cells. In this context, it would be of great interest to establish if homonymous or antagonistic Ia afferents project onto coupled motor neuron-Renshaw cell pairs.

Our studies also suggest that spindle-derived signals, including NT3, are not necessary for the development of specific connections between afferents and motor neurons. Other target-derived factors, for example glial cell-derived neurotrophic factor (GDNF) acting through the ETS transcription factor Pea3 have been shown to regulate connectivity between Ia afferents and motor neurons in particular motor pools.[6] Although the nature and source of the instructive signals that specify these connections remains unknown, recent work implicates semaphorin 3e and plexin D1 receptors in the read-out of these peripheral cues, which generate repulsive signals that restrict connectivity between certain forelimb spindle afferents and brachial motor pools.[7] As the molecular mechanism involved in Ia afferent-motor target specification become elucidated, it will be possible to test further the role of activity, target-derived factors and molecular recognition signals in the process. A model for activity-dependent modulation of genetic and molecular programs of axonal targeting was recently described for the case of motor neuron projections to specific peripheral targets.[42] Similar fine regulatory mechanisms might be necessary to precisely control the patterns of synaptic connectivity and strength within the spinal cord, even for the "simple" case of Ia afferent projections to ventral horn neurons.

Acknowledgments

This work was supported by the intramural program of NINDS (G.Z.M., N.A.S. and M.J.O'D) and by the National Institutes of Health Grant NS047357 (F.J.A.).

Conflicts of interest

The authors declare no conflicts of interest.

References

1. Ladle, D.R., E. Pecho-Vrieseling & S. Arber. 2007. Assembly of motor circuits in the spinal cord: driven to function by genetic and experience-dependent mechanisms. *Neuron.* **56:** 270–283.

2. Smith, C.L. & E. Frank. 1987. Peripheral specification of sensory neurons transplanted to novel locations along the neuraxis. *J. Neurosci.* **7:** 1537–1549.

3. Frank, E. & P. Wenner. 1993. Environmental specification of neuronal connectivity. *Neuron.* **10:** 779–785.

4. Wenner, P. & E. Frank. 1995. Peripheral target specification of synaptic connectivity of muscle spindle sensory neurons with spinal motoneurons. *J. Neurosci.* **15:** 8191–8198.

5. Chen, H.H. *et al.* 2003. Development of the monosynaptic stretch reflex circuit. *Curr. Opin. Neurobiol.* **13:** 96–102.

6. Vrieseling, E. & S. Arber. 2006. Target-induced transcriptional control of dendritic patterning and connectivity in motor neurons by the ETS gene Pea3. *Cell* **127:** 1439–1452.

7. Pecho-Vrieseling, E. *et al.* 2009. Specificity of sensory–motor connections encoded by Sema3e–Plxnd1 recognition. *Nature* **459:** 842–846.

8. Ernfors, P. *et al.* 1994. Lack of neurotrophin-3 leads to deficiencies in the peripheral nervous system and loss of limb proprioceptive afferents. *Cell* **77:** 503–512.

9. Fariñas, I. *et al.* 1994. Severe sensory and sympathetic deficits in mice lacking neurotrophin-3. *Nature* **369:** 658–661.

10. Chen, H.H., W.G. Tourtellotte & E. Frank. 2002. Muscle spindle-derived neurotrophin 3 regulates synaptic connectivity between muscle sensory and motor neurons. *J. Neurosci.* **22:** 3512–3519.

11. Arvanian, V.L. *et al.* 2003. Chronic neurotrophin-3 strengthens synaptic connections to motoneurons in the neonatal rat. *J. Neurosci.* **23:** 8706–8712.

12. Wang, Z. *et al.* 2007. Prenatal exposure to elevated NT3 disrupts synaptic selectivity in the spinal cord. *J. Neurosci.* **27:** 3686–3694.

13. Vejsada, R. *et al.* 1985. The postnatal functional development of muscle stretch receptors in the rat. *Somatosens Res.* **2:** 205–222.

14. Gramsbergen, A. 1998. Posture and locomotion in the rat: independent or interdependent development? *Neurosci. Biobehav. Rev.* **22:** 547–553.

15. Mears, S.C. & E. Frank. 1997. Formation of specific monosynaptic connections between muscle spindle afferents and motoneurons in the mouse. *J. Neurosci.* **17:** 3128–3135.

16. Shneider, N.A. *et al.* 2009. Functionally reduced sensorimotor connections form with normal specificity despite abnormal muscle spindle development: the role of spindle-derived neurotrophin 3. *J. Neurosci.* **29:** 4719–4735.

17. Hippenmeyer, S. *et al.* 2002. A role for neuregulin1 signaling in muscle spindle differentiation. *Neuron.* **36:** 1035–1049.

18. Andrechek, E.R. *et al.* 2002. ErbB2 is required for muscle spindle and myoblast cell survival. *Mol. Cell Biol.* **22:** 4714–4722.

19. Leu, M. *et al.* 2003. ErbB2 regulates neuromuscular synapse formation and is essential for muscle spindle development. *Development* **130:** 2291–2301.

20. Alvarez, F.J. *et al.* 2004. Vesicular glutamate transporters in the spinal cord, with special reference to sensory primary afferent synapses. *J. Comp. Neurol.* **472:** 257–280.

21. Bates, B. *et al.* 1999. Neurotrophin-3 is required for proper cerebellar development. *Nat. Neurosci.* **2:** 115–117.

22. Seebach, B.S. & L. Ziskind-Conhaim. 1994. Formation of transient inappropriate sensorimotor synapses in developing rat spinal cords. *J. Neurosci.* **14:** 4520–4528.

23. Bradbury, E.J. *et al.* 1999. NT-3 promotes growth of lesioned adult rat sensory axons ascending in the dorsal columns of the spinal cord. *Eur. J. Neurosci.* **11:** 3873–3883.

24. Ramer, M.S. *et al.* 2002. Neurotrophin-3-mediated regeneration and recovery of proprioception following dorsal rhizotomy. *Mol. Cell Neurosci.* **19:** 239–249.

25. Taylor, M.D. *et al.* 2001. Postnatal regulation of limb proprioception by muscle-derived neurotrophin-3. *J. Comp. Neurol.* **432:** 244–258.

26. Patel, T.D. *et al.* 2003. Peripheral NT3 signaling is required for ETS protein expression and central patterning of proprioceptive sensory afferents. *Neuron.* **38:** 403–416.

27. Li, L.Y. *et al.* 2006. Neurotrophin-3 ameliorates sensory-motor deficits in Er81-deficient mice. *Dev. Dyn.* **235:** 3039–3050.

28. Smith, C.A. *et al.* 2007. Influence of sensory afferents and motoneurons on the developmental regulation of calbindin and parvalbumin expression in spinal interneurons. *Soc. Neurosci. Abstracts* 132.22.

29. Ziskind-Conhaim, L. *et al.* 2010. Synaptic integration of rhythmogenic neurons in the locomotor circuitry: the case of Hb9 interneurons. *Ann. N.Y. Acad. Sci.* **1198:** 72–84.

30. Baldissera, F., H. Hultborn & M. Illert. 1981. Integration in spinal neuronal systems. In *Handbook of Physiology. The Nervous System* Vol. II. Brooks, V.B., Ed.: 509–595. Am. Physiol. Soc., Bethesda, Motor control. Part 1.

31. Jankowska, E. 1992. Interneuronal relay in spinal pathways from proprioceptors. *Prog Neurobiol.* **38:** 335–378.

32. Eccles, J.C., P. Fatt & S. Landgren. 1956. Central pathway for direct inhibitory action of impulses in largest afferent nerve fibres to muscle. *J. Neurophysiol.* **19:** 75–98.

33. Hultborn, H., E. Jankowska & S. Lindström. 1971. Recurrent inhibition of interneurones monosynaptically activated from group Ia afferents. *J. Physiol.* **215:** 613–636.

34. Renshaw, B. 1946. Central effects of centripetal impulses in axons of spinal central roots. *J. Neurophysiol.* **9:** 191–204.

35. Eccles, J.C., P. Fatt & K. Koketsu. 1954. Cholinergic and inhibitory synapses in a pathway from motor-axon collaterals to motoneurones. *J. Physiol.* **126:** 524–562.

36. Wenner, P. & M.J. O'Donovan. 1999. Identification of an interneuronal population that mediates recurrent inhibition of motoneurons in the developing chick spinal cord. *J. Neurosci.* **19:** 7557–7567.

37. Mentis, G.Z. *et al.* 2006. Primary afferent synapses on developing and adult Renshaw cells. *J. Neurosci.* **26:** 13297–13310.

38. Ziskind-Conhaim, L. 1990. NMDA receptors mediate poly- and monosynaptic potentials in motoneurons of rat embryos. *J. Neurosci.* **10:** 125–135.

39. Fyffe, R.E. 1984. Afferent fibers. In *Handbook of the Spinal Cord*. Vols 2 and 3, Anatomy and Physiology, Davidoff, R.A., Ed.: 79–135. New York: Dekker.

40. Naka, K.I. 1964. Electrophysiology of the fetal spinal cord. II. Interaction among peripheral inputs and recurrent inhibition. *J. Gen. Physiol.* **47:** 1023–1038.

41. Pierce, J.P., L.M. Mendell. 1993. Quantitative ultrastructure of Ia boutons in the ventral horn: scaling and positional relationships. *J. Neurosci.* **13:** 4748–4763.

42. Hanson, M.G., L.D. Milner & L.T. Landmesser. 2008. Spontaneous rhythmic activity in early chick spinal cord influences distinct motor axon pathfinding decisions. *Brain Res. Rev.* **57:** 77–85.

Ann. N.Y. Acad. Sci. ISSN 0077-8923

ANNALS OF THE NEW YORK ACADEMY OF SCIENCES
Issue: *Neurons and Networks in the Spinal Cord*

Permanent reorganization of Ia afferent synapses on motoneurons after peripheral nerve injuries

Francisco J. Alvarez, Katie L. Bullinger, Haley E. Titus, Paul Nardelli, and Timothy C. Cope

Department of Neurosciences, Cell Biology and Physiology, Wright State University, Dayton, Ohio

Address for correspondence: Francisco J. Alvarez, Department of Neurosciences, Cell Biology and Physiology, Wright State University, Boonshoft School of Medicine, Dayton, OH 45459. francisco.alvarez@wright.edu

After peripheral nerve injuries to a motor nerve, the axons of motoneurons and proprioceptors are disconnected from the periphery and monosynaptic connections from group I afferents and motoneurons become diminished in the spinal cord. Following successful reinnervation in the periphery, motor strength, proprioceptive sensory encoding, and Ia afferent synaptic transmission on motoneurons partially recover. Muscle stretch reflexes, however, never recover and motor behaviors remain uncoordinated. In this review, we summarize recent findings that suggest that lingering motor dysfunction might be in part related to decreased connectivity of Ia afferents centrally. First, sensory afferent synapses retract from lamina IX, causing a permanent relocation of the inputs to more distal locations and significant disconnection from motoneurons. Second, peripheral reconnection between proprioceptive afferents and muscle spindles is imperfect. As a result, a proportion of sensory afferents that retain central connections with motoneurons might not reconnect appropriately in the periphery. A hypothetical model is proposed in which the combined effect of peripheral and central reconnection deficits might explain the failure of muscle stretch to initiate or modulate firing of many homonymous motoneurons.

Keywords: stretch reflex; spinal cord; plasticity; motor control; adult

Introduction

Recovery of normal neural function after injury requires the regeneration of damaged axons and the reestablishment of synaptic connections between neurons. Although some compensation can be achieved as the result of redundancy and plasticity in the adult nervous system,[1,2] behavior cannot be normal if a significant number of connections are lost. This lends strong justification for the research effort to promote axonal regeneration, in particular after spinal cord injuries.[3–5] Axonal regrowth is only one step, however, in the recuperation of normal circuitry and unfortunately axonal regeneration is not synonymous with functional recovery. Failure to reestablish synapses of adequate strength together with nonadaptive secondary plasticity in surviving circuits could greatly interfere with normal function. This is best illustrated by the incomplete recovery of motor function that occurs after peripheral nerve injuries. Here we summarize recent findings on the plasticity of central synaptic connections between sensory afferents and spinal motoneurons that are triggered by injury to a peripheral nerve. These alterations are rather permanent and therefore likely contributors to the motor deficits that remain after normal regeneration in the periphery.

Peripheral regeneration does not fully restore motor function

In contrast to central axons, axons injured in the periphery readily regenerate and reconnect with denervated target tissues.[6] As a consequence, voluntary control over muscle contraction is restored and muscle strength is recovered.[7] Similarly, the flow of sensory information into the central nervous system from reinnervated skin or muscle is reestablished.[8] These gains assist functional recovery, which nonetheless remains incomplete. The most relevant data comes from experiments on muscles reinnervated by their own cut nerve (self-reinnervated) in which axon navigating errors are minimized

doi: 10.1111/j.1749-6632.2010.05459.x

and target reinnervation, at a macrolevel, is most successful. In this situation, muscle activity patterns and interjoint coordination after reinnervation are normal during certain kinds of locomotion.[9,10] Still, there is unmistakable disability outside the bounds of movements restricted to treadmill locomotion at low speed, over level ground, and in the absence of perturbations. Specifically, animals with reinnervated ankle extensor muscles exhibit abnormal ankle yield, lose coordination between ankle and the knee joints, and stumble during downhill walking.[10] In addition, changing the speed of locomotion brings out abnormalities in ankle–knee–hip coordination.[11] These global deficits in limb movement are made all the more impressive by the fact that experimental nerve damage in these cases involved only one or two muscles and that deficits persist long after peripheral reinnervation is completed.

Proprioceptive deficits after peripheral nerve regeneration

Ataxia expressed in limbs with reinnervated muscles prompted analysis of the proprioceptive system and, more specifically, the stretch reflex pathway after peripheral nerve injuries and surgical reunion. Surprisingly, after complete nerve transections, self-reinnervated muscles are absolutely unresponsive to stretch,[12,13] even though the reinnervated muscle is perfectly capable of contracting in response to other uninjured inputs, for example from cutaneous afferents. Muscle stretch superimposed on ongoing reflex activity yielded no additional force production highlighting two important conclusions. First, regenerated motoneurons are capable of responding to synaptic input. Second, stretch signals carried centrally by regenerated afferents are largely ineffective. Even a smaller than usual stretch synaptic input that is not strong enough to bring motoneurons from rest to firing threshold, should nevertheless exert some modulation of ongoing motoneuron firing.[14] Lack of modulation therefore suggests a complete failure of stretch signals to reach the motoneuron.

Possible explanations

One common explanation for lingering motor dysfunction after large peripheral nerve injuries is that the reconnection of regenerating sensory and motor axons with their targets is incomplete or nonspecific.[2,15,16] Incomplete regeneration in self-reinnervated muscles could result from injury induced cell death of the axotomized sensory or motor neurons. After injuries to major nerve branches, e.g., sciatic nerve, approximately 10% to 50% of dorsal root ganglia (DRG) neurons are lost, but large DRG neurons, including proprioceptive sensory neurons, are relatively spared and die only after long delays (several months) if regeneration is prevented.[17] Regarding motoneurons, their viability is not impaired after axotomy, even when regeneration is prevented,[18] as long as the injury does not happen in early life[19,20] (neonates) or occur very proximally to the motoneuron soma (for example, after ventral root avulsion[21]).

Physiological and anatomical evidence further suggests that after self-reinnervation of the medial gastrocnemius (MG) muscle there is a significant reinnervation of muscle spindle receptors (~75–84%[13,22]). Moreover, stretch-activated regenerated afferents display dynamic and static responses to stretch that are comparable to normal Ia afferents.[13,23] Similarly, motor unit properties recover after self-reinnervation quite successfully and only 10% of MG motoneurons fail to elicit a contraction.[24,25]

Despite this impressive recovery of peripheral connections, there are important questions about their specificity. Afferent and motor axons have the capacity to regenerate into wrong tissue and reinnervate wrong targets, for example muscle afferents can innervate cutaneous territories with some recovery of afferent firing properties and central connectivity with motoneurons.[26,27] Moreover, after lesions of major nerve trunks, many motoneurons indeed fail to reinnervate their parent muscle.[6,15] When muscles are self-reinnervated, i.e., reinnervated by their original nerve, failure of motor axons to reform neuromuscular junctions with their original muscle fibers is offset by respecification of muscle fiber properties, thereby restoring the normal proportion of motor unit types and sizes.[24,25] Thus, few differences are observed in force generation and motor unit recruitment is similar in self-reinnervated and normal muscle.[28]

More complex, however, is the situation involving sensory afferent peripheral reinnervation. Proprioceptive afferents in muscle can reinnervate the wrong receptor type (nonspecific reinnervation), but cannot respecify receptor structure.

Accordingly, Ib afferent fibers can successfully inner-vate muscle spindle receptors and replace the origi-nal Ia afferents with little difference in the resulting structure of the annulospiral endings or encoding properties to muscle stretch.[22,29] Therefore, group I afferents can change their peripheral apparatus and responses depending on the receptor type they in-nervate, but this afferent receptor switch seems not to be matched by respecification of their central pro-jections. In addition, a proportion of afferents fail to reinnervate any peripheral end organ and become unresponsive to natural stimuli. Thus, there are in-deed significant targeting failures during sensory re-connection in the periphery. Nevertheless, there is also substantial specific reinnervation, whereby re-generating spindle afferents reconnect with spindle receptors, making it difficult to envision how non-specific reinnervation alone could be responsible for the total collapse of the stretch reflex. One pos-sibility is that peripheral errors are accompanied by major reorganizations of central connectivity. It is well known that peripheral nerve injuries frequently result in profound structural and functional reorga-nizations of central synaptic circuits that can spread as far rostral as the cerebral cortex.[2,30] An obvious place to look for a functional deficit is then the cen-tral synapses established on spinal motoneurons by Ia afferent fibers.

Monosynaptic sensory inputs on motoneurons

Monosynaptic transmission between sensory affer-ents and motoneurons undergoes complex changes following peripheral nerve injuries. Within the first week and peaking at 3 days after nerve cut or crush, electrically evoked group I EPSPs increase substan-tially in size.[31–33] A few days later, however, there is a general decline in EPSP amplitude and an in-crease in time course.[13,34–39] There is also enhanced synaptic depression at high firing frequencies[27] that lasts for several weeks. These changes revert to-ward normal values following peripheral regener-ation and target reinnervation, such that electri-cally evoked group I EPSPs regain the ability to sustain nearly normal amplitudes during low or high-frequency stimulation.[13,34,38] Figure 1 shows no evidence of enhanced depression in regener-ated afferents using frequency-modulated electri-cal stimulation patterns that replicate the normal Ia firing in response to a ramp and hold stretch paradigm of the same muscle.[40] In other words,

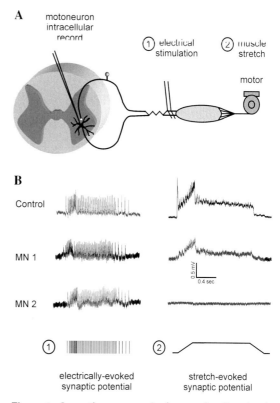

Figure 1. Synaptic responses in the stretch reflex circuit following peripheral nerve injuries. (**A**) Diagram depicts the monosynaptic stretch reflex circuit and elements of the experimental paradigm. Adult rats with muscles nor-mally innervated or reinnervated by a cut nerve were anesthetized for *in vivo* study wherein motoneuron mem-brane potential was recorded intracellularly during stim-ulation of afferents by either (1) electrical stimulation at group I strength or (2) ramp-hold-release stretch of the muscle by a motor. (**B**) Synaptic responses to affer-ent firing produced either mechanically (stretch-evoked synaptic potentials, SSP; *right column*) or electrically by trains designed to simulate the responses of single Ia af-ferents to the same ramp-hold-release stretch (train of group I EPSPs; *left column*), both recorded from each of three motoneurons: *top traces* from one control rat; *mid-dle traces* from two motoneurons in one rat with the MG muscle reinnervated 1 year after nerve section and surgi-cal reunion. Note the absence of a SSP in MN2 despite the presence of an electrically evoked EPSP and the presence of a smaller than normal SSP in MN1. Electrically evoked EPSPs were present in all control and in all reinnervating motoneurons, and showed no signs of amplitude depres-sion when firing at high frequencies. (Modified from data in Refs. 40 and 43.)

the regenerated group I afferent-motoneuron circuit operates normally when activated electrically. While consistent with reports of full recovery of the electrically evoked H-reflex,[41] these observations cannot explain the failure of muscle stretch to elicit any reflex activity or firing modulation of motoneurons.

Intriguingly, recuperation of electrically evoked EPSPs is not accompanied by the recovery of muscle stretch-evoked synaptic excitation of motoneurons. In normal animals, muscle stretch causes a motoneuron membrane depolarization that we call a stretch synaptic potential (SSP).[42] SSPs faithfully follow the time course and intensity of stretch-responsive spindle afferent firing. After peripheral regeneration in a rat model of MG self-reinnervation, SSPs are smaller than normal or completely absent in many motoneurons. This abnormality is observed even though normal electrically evoked group I EPSPs occur in every motoneuron[13,40] (Fig. 1). These observations raise the question of whether after peripheral injuries electrically evoked group I motoneuron EPSPs are evoked centrally by the same afferents that respond to stretch following reinnervation.

Spike triggered-averaging (STA) was used to test directly the central synaptic actions of individual regenerated afferents that responded with spindle-like firing to muscle stretch. From dorsal root filaments we discriminated action potentials of single regenerated afferents that fired identically to normal spindle afferents and tested their synaptic actions in homonymous regenerated motoneurons in control rats or in animals with regenerated medial gastrocnemius nerves.[43] In control rats we found that single group I spindle afferents activated by stretch produced STA EPSPs in nearly all homonymous motoneurons, just as is observed for control cats.[44] In contrast, after nerve injury and successful regeneration in the periphery, sensory afferents displaying normal responses to muscle stretch failed to generate STA EPSPs in nearly all homonymous motoneurons tested. More surprisingly, these same motoneurons displayed relatively normal sensory afferent EPSPs after electrical stimulation of the peripheral nerve.[43] Two potential explanations can be put forward. First, that after regeneration the population of afferent fibers activated by stretch is different from the afferent inputs responsible for generating monosynaptic electrically evoked EPSPs on motoneurons. Second, that stretch-evoked impulses entering the spinal cord lead to central suppression of the afferent synaptic input in a manner that does not occur after electrical stimulation. The following studies on the central structural remodeling of Ia afferent connections provide some support for the first explanation; however these data do not exclude the alternative possibility.

Central reorganization of synaptic connections after peripheral injury

One possible explanation for the reduction of SSPs is profound and permanent reorganization of central synapses as a consequence of peripheral nerve injury. This reorganization could weaken or suppress Ia synapses and/or change the balance between inhibition and excitation during the arrival of stretch-evoked signals into the spinal cord. There is indeed evidence for such possibilities. Synapses become detached ("stripped") from somata and proximal dendrites of motoneurons that are axotomized after nerve injuries.[45–49] This appears to be a relatively general phenomenon that is reproduced on other central and peripheral neurons after they become disconnected from their targets by either axotomy or excitotoxic lesions.[50–52] The purpose of synaptic stripping has been frequently explained as a switch in the axotomized postsynaptic cell from "signaling" to "regenerative" function. Unfortunately, this hypothesis has never been experimentally tested nor does it explain why motoneurons need to lose proximal synapses to switch on a "regeneration" mode. Therefore, it is an open question whether synaptic stripping is a well-adapted response necessary for neurons to regenerate their axons or an unfortunate outcome of target disconnection that is a possible source of functional abnormalities after peripheral regeneration is completed.

In early studies, it was argued that synaptic stripping explained the changes in amplitude and time course of sensory afferent-evoked EPSPs in motoneurons after nerve injury.[39,53,54] Indeed, the functional recovery of electrically evoked group I EPSPs coincides temporally with the recovery of central synapses after motoneurons reinnervate peripheral targets.[55–58] Later studies, however, discredited the early view of synaptic detachment as a relatively homogenous phenomenon that similarly affects all synapses. In fact, the degree of synaptic depletion after injury and recovery after regeneration depends on the type of synaptic input. For example, inhibitory terminals are more resistant to stripping[55,59–61] and recover even in the absence of peripheral regeneration.[60,62] One possible reason for their differential behaviors is that each synaptic input seems preferentially dependent on different trophic factor signals that can originate in the target or other sources. Brain-Derived Neurotrophic Factor (BDNF) is more effective in maintaining inhibitory and tonic inputs, while neurotrophin-3 (NT3) is best related to excitatory and phasic inputs including Ia afferent synapses.[61,63,64] Major sources of NT3 and BDNF are (in addition to the motoneuron), respectively, the muscle spindle and spinal glia, which exhibit distinct regulation and relationships to regenerating afferents and central synapses after injury. As a result, imbalances in the excitatory/inhibitory ratio or synaptic composition are usually created during recovery of central synapses on motoneurons that have reconnected with muscle.[55,56,60,61] In summary, despite significant recovery of central synapses after peripheral reconnection there seems to be also important changes in synaptic composition that have not yet been studied in enough detail. What is then the exact behavior of Ia afferent synapses during synaptic stripping and recovery?

Ia afferents

Despite earlier assumptions, it is difficult to extrapolate data gathered on stripping of excitatory synapses in general to the Ia synapses in particular. Ia synapses represent a small proportion (~2%) of all synapses on the motoneuron surface[65,66] and their contributions during central synaptic remodeling are likely diluted in overall quantitative analyses of all synapses. Moreover, Ia synapses mostly target the dendritic arbor (5–10% of Ia synapses target motoneuron somata[65,66]), while most studies on synaptic stripping have concentrated the analysis on the proximal somatodendritic region. Finally, a different behavior for Ia synapses should not be too surprising. This is because of all motoneuron inputs, they alone belong to presynaptic axons that are directly injured in the periphery.

Until recently, the main obstacle to uncover the fate of Ia afferent synapses after peripheral nerve injuries has been the lack of appropriate markers.

Fortunately, the vesicular glutamate transporter isoform 1 (VGLUT1) was recently found enriched in the central terminals of proprioceptive primary afferents including the central synapses of Ia afferents.[67–69] After peripheral nerve injuries, VGLUT1 content in these central synapses is rapidly reduced.[70] We therefore investigated the extent of recovery following reinnervation. To our surprise, depletions of VGLUT1 varicosities in lamina IX and around motoneuron cell bodies (Fig. 2A) were rather permanent and similar in intensity and time course after nerve injuries in which peripheral nerve regeneration was allowed or prevented. In both situations, VGLUT1 synapses that were lost in lamina IX were not recovered.[69] VGLUT1 contacts on motoneuron cell bodies remained depleted by more than 90% six months after the injury and following successful regeneration (Figs. 2B and C).[69] Depletions on dendrites were also permanent and concentrated to the proximal regions (viewed in a transverse plane). VGLUT1 contacts were significantly depleted by 40–50% in the first 100 μm of dendrite, but no significant differences were detected beyond this point (Fig. 2D, unpublished results). It is possible that these data underestimated the real amount of VGLUT1 detachment from motoneuron dendrites because rostrocaudally oriented dendrites receive the maximum percentage of Ia afferent inputs (60% of all Ia synapses received by single motoneurons[65]) and these dendritic branches distribute within lamina IX, the region showing the maximal depletion in VGLUT1 varicosities. Unfortunately, rostrocaudally oriented dendrites could not be analyzed in the transverse plane of sectioning used. Independent of the exact amount of depletion, it is evident that a significant number of Ia afferent central synapses are lost as a consequence of peripheral injuries and these are not recovered even long after regeneration has been completed in the periphery.

Overall, the data strongly suggest a significant removal of Ia afferent synapses from lamina IX. This possibility was further confirmed by intraaxonal recording and labeling of individual regenerated afferents that were activated by stretch and showed responses typical of normal Ia afferents. In good agreement with the VGLUT1 data, of five identified stretch-activated regenerated afferents recorded intraaxonally and filled with neurobiotin to trace their central terminations, only one displayed a terminal

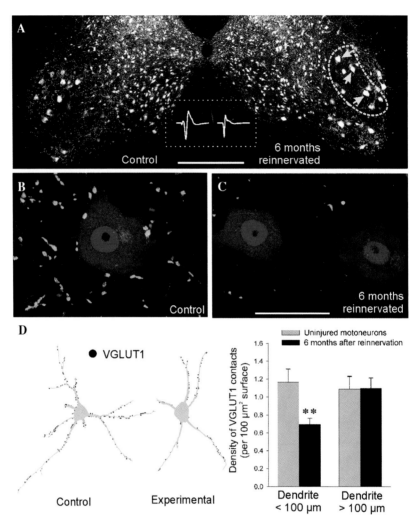

Figure 2. Permanent depletion of VGLUT1 contacts after peripheral nerve injuries. (**A**) Low magnification confocal image of control and experimental ventral horns in an animal in which the left tibial nerve was completely resectioned and immediately surgically rejoined and then allowed to regenerate for 6 months. *Middle inset* (inside the *dashed rectangle*) shows electrically evoked EMGs from the control and recovered MG muscles demonstrating peripheral reconnection. The section was dual immunostained for VGLUT1 (FITC, *green*) and NeuN (a general neuronal marker, Cy3, *white*). In this section from the lumbar five segment most motoneurons are distributed in lateral pools (large NeuN-labeled cell bodies). In the ventral horn and particularly in lamina IX, VGLUT1 punctae preferentially label presynaptic vesicle clusters of proprioceptive afferent synapses. The *yellow dashed outline* indicates the location of motor pools sending axons through the tibial nerve in the injured side. Compared to the contralateral side there is diminished density of VGLUT1 punctae in the experimental side. As a result many cell bodies (*yellow arrows*) are VGLUT1 denervated. (**B, C**) High-magnification confocal images of one control (**B**) and two experimental motoneurons (**C**) (four or five confocal planes at 1 μm z-steps and through the mid-region of each motoneuron are shown). Even 6 months after the injury and following successful reinnervation in the periphery, motoneurons in the injured side do not recover their somatic VGLUT1 contacts. Similarly the surrounding lamina IX neuropil shows diminished density of VGLUT1 punctae and these are usually of smaller size than in the control side. (**D**) VGLUT1 losses preferentially occur in the proximal somatodendritic regions. Neurolucida reconstructions of two MG motoneurons, one in the control and one in the injured side, that were retrogradely labeled from the MG muscle with cholera-toxin b subunit coupled to Alexa-555 (Ctb-555) one week before the analysis and 5.5 months after the

collateral in lamina IX with a few varicosities.[69] In contrast, all control afferents (n — 14) profusely send branches into lamina IX that were studded with many varicosities. Synaptic varicosities on regenerated afferents were mainly found in branches terminating in lamina V and to a lesser extent in lamina VII.

The data lead us to propose the working model depicted in Figure 3 to explain the lack of stretch-evoked afferent information reaching some motoneurons. After peripheral nerve injury and disconnection of Ia afferents from muscle spindles, there is a significant retraction of central Ia afferent collaterals projecting into lamina IX. These central branches are not regrown following peripheral reconnection. As a result, a large number of Ia synapses are removed from the proximal region of motoneurons. The retention of synapses on distal dendritic branches might explain why all regenerated motoneurons display electrically evoked compound monosynaptic EPSPs. But normally intact uninjured individual Ia afferents establish relatively few synapses on single motoneurons. For homonymous connections, each single Ia afferent establishes, on average, only 10 contacts per motoneuron. Moreover, the exact number is highly variable depending on the exact location of motoneurons within the pool and with respect to the entry rootlet of the Ia afferent.[65,66] Therefore, a significant reduction of proximal synapses, as observed using VGLUT1 as a marker, might result in a large number of disconnections of Ia afferent-motoneuron pairs. On the other hand, a proportion of Ia afferents that remain connected to motoneurons might incorrectly regenerate in the periphery. In the self-reinnervated medial gastrocnemius muscle of the cat, approximately 50% of Ia afferents are unsuccessful reconnecting with muscle spindle receptors,

some of which were reinnervated by other afferents including Ib afferents.[22]

The combined effect of fewer Ia afferents connected peripherally to muscle spindle receptors after regeneration (some of which could be Ib afferents not monosynaptically connected to motoneurons, Fig. 3) compounded with a significant reduction in the number of central synapses and central Ia-motoneuron connectivity might explain the lack of stretch-evoked responses in a significant proportion of motoneurons despite the presence of enough connectivity from dorsal root afferents to elicit monosynaptic EPSPs on most of the regenerated motoneurons that reconnect with muscle.

If the above-proposed hypothesis is correct, restorative actions could be taken to favor Ia afferent regrowth centrally in order to ensure that motoneurons retain innervation from at least a few afferents correctly innervating peripherally muscle spindles. We predict that manipulations intended to facilitate the proliferation of central afferent arborizations could contribute to the recovery of the lost stretch reflex and diminish the coordination deficits that impair motor function after peripheral nerve injuries and regeneration. Presently it is unknown if the failure of central axons from sensory afferents to repopulate lamina IX with VGLUT1 varicosities is due to lack of, or diminished peripheral signals that promote or maintain these central connections (for example spindle-derived NT3[64,71,72]) or if alternatively, the presence of negative factors in the adult spinal cord impair the regrowth of central sensory afferent synaptic arborizations.[5,73]

Acknowledgments

This work was supported by NIH grant P01NS057228. We also wish to thank Mrs. Eileen

---

injury (thus demonstrating peripheral connectivity in both cases). The distribution of VGLUT1 contacts was then plotted on their dendritic trees (*black filled circles*). A large depletion in VGLUT1 contacts is apparent in the cell body and proximal dendrite of MG motoneurons in the regenerated side compared to the uninjured side. Histograms show quantification of VGLUT1 contact density in dendritic segments within 100 μm distance from the cell body or beyond that point. Ten Ctb-555 labeled and reconstructed MG motoneurons were analyzed in the control and injured side. A significant 41% average depletion in VGLUT1 density was found in proximal dendrites (*asterisks*, $P = 0.01$, *t*-test; error bars indicate SEM) while no significant differences were detected in more distal dendrites. Scale bars, 500 μm in A; 50 μm in C (B at the same magnification as C). (*Panels A, B*, and *C* are modified from Ref. 69; *panel D* includes data from unpublished materials from HET, FJA, and TC.)

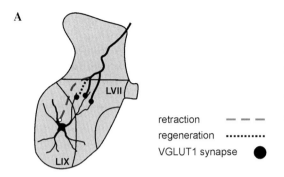

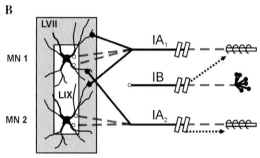

Figure 3. Working model consistent with available data including those described here for spinal motoneurons and their synaptic associations with muscle proprioceptors after muscle nerve cut and regeneration. (**A**) Depicts retraction of afferent axon (***dashed line***) and the loss of afferent synapses from proximal somatodendritic regions located in lamina IX while contacts on more distal dendrites located in LVII are retained. It is possible that local sprouting (regeneration) in this region might add some synapses (***dotted black line***), however these never reach the more proximal somatodendritic regions. (**B**) Model: severing peripheral nerve cuts both motor and sensory axons, which undergo Wallerian degeneration peripherally and synaptic stripping (decreased VGLUT1) and presynaptic axon retraction centrally (***dashed gray lines***). With peripheral regeneration there is: (**a**) nonspecific reinnervation of some spindle receptors (Ib afferents, ***top dotted black arrow***), (**b**) specific reinnervation of some spindle receptors by Ia afferents (Ia₂, ***bottom dotted black arrow***), and (**c**) no reinnervation of spindle receptors by some Ia afferents (Ia₁). Centrally Ia afferents fail to regain axonal projections into LIX on motoneuron soma and proximal dendrites; Ib afferent projections remain remote to LIX and not monosynaptically connected with motoneurons. The functional results are that stretch evoked synaptic potentials (SSPs) are lost in some motoneurons (MN 2) and reduced in others (MN 1), yet group I electrical stimulation of the whole nerve evokes EPSPs in every motoneuron. (Modified from Ref. 43.)

Kantanmeni (formerly Fitzsimons) for her efforts during the early stages of this project and Mrs. Lori L. Goss, RVT, for her invaluable help during animal surgeries, handling, and preparation.

Conflicts of interest

The authors declare no conflicts of interest.

References

1. Stein, D.G. & S.W. Hoffman. 2003. Concepts of CNS plasticity in the context of brain damage and repair. *J. Head Trauma Rehabil.* **18:** 317–341.

2. Navarro, X., M. Vivo & A. Valero-Cabre. 2007. Neural plasticity after peripheral nerve injury and regeneration. *Prog. Neurobiol.* **82:** 163–201.

3. Buchli, A. D. & M.E. Schwab. 2005. Inhibition of Nogo: a key strategy to increase regeneration, plasticity and functional recovery of the lesioned central nervous system. *Ann. Med.* **37:** 556–567.

4. Deumens, R., G.C. Koopmans & E.A. Joosten. 2005. Regeneration of descending axon tracts after spinal cord injury. *Prog. Neurobiol.* **77:** 57–89.

5. Fawcett, J.W. 2006. Overcoming inhibition in the damaged spinal cord. *J. Neurotrauma.* **23:** 371–383.

6. Bisby, M. 1995. Regeneration of peripheral nervous system axons. In *The Axon: Structure, Function and Pathophysiology*. S.G. Waxman, J.D. Kocsis & P.K. Stys, Eds.: 579–589. Oxford University Press. Oxford.

7. Thomas, C.K. *et al.* 1987. Patterns of reinnervation and motor unit recruitment in human hand muscles after complete ulnar and median nerve section and resuture. *J. Neurol. Neurosurg. Psychiatry.* **50:** 259–268.

8. Mackel, R. *et al.* 1983. Reinnervation of mechanoreceptors in the human glabrous skin following peripheral nerve repair. *Brain Res.* **268:** 49–65.

9. O'Donovan, M.J. *et al.* 1985. Kinesiological studies of self- and cross-reinnervated FDL and soleus muscles in freely moving cats. *J. Neurophysiol.* **54:** 852–866.

10. Abelew, T.A. *et al.* 2000. Local loss of proprioception results in disruption of interjoint coordination during locomotion in the cat. *J. Neurophysiol.* **84:** 2709–2714.

11. Chang, Y.H., J.P. Scholtz & T.R. Nichols. 2003. Hindlimb control during cat locomotion after loss of stretch reflexes. *Integr. Comp. Biol.* **43:** 987.

12. Cope, T.C., S.J. Bonasera & T.R. Nichols. 1994. Reinnervated muscles fail to produce stretch reflexes. *J. Neurophysiol.* **71:** 817–820.

13. Haftel, V.K. *et al.* 2005. Central suppression of regenerated proprioceptive afferents. *J. Neurosci.* **25:** 4733–4742.

14. Cope, T.C., E.E. Fetz & M. Matsumura. 1987. Cross-correlation assessment of synaptic strength of single Ia fibre connections with triceps surae motoneurones in cats. *J. Physiol.* **390:** 161–188.

15. Sumner, A.J. 1990. Aberrant reinnervation. *Muscle Nerve.* **13:** 801–803.

16. Johnson, R.D. & J.B. Munson. 1992. Specificity of regenerating sensory neurons in adult mammals. In *Sensory Neurons: Diversity, Development and Plasticity.* S.S. Scott, Ed.: 384–403. Oxford University Press. Oxford.

17. Tandrup, T., C.J. Woolf & R.E. Coggeshall. 2000. Delayed loss of small dorsal root ganglion cells after transection of the rat sciatic nerve. *J. Comp. Neurol.* **422:** 172–180.

18. Vanden Noven, S. *et al.* 1993. Adult spinal motoneurons remain viable despite prolonged absence of functional synaptic contact with muscle. *Exp. Neurol.* **123:** 147–156.

19. Kashihara, Y., M. Kuno & Y. Miyata. 1987. Cell death of axotomized motoneurones in neonatal rats, and its prevention by peripheral reinnervation. *J. Physiol.* **386:** 135–148.

20. Schmalbruch, H. 1984. Motoneuron death after sciatic nerve section in newborn rats. *J. Comp. Neurol.* **224:** 252–258.

21. Koliatsos, V. E. *et al.* 1994. Ventral root avulsion: an experimental model of death of adult motor neurons. *J. Comp. Neurol.* **342:** 35–44.

22. Collins, W.F., 3rd, L.M. Mendell & J.B. Munson. 1986. On the specificity of sensory reinnervation of cat skeletal muscle. *J. Physiol.* **375:** 587–609.

23. Brown, M.C. & R.G. Butler. 1976. Regeneration of afferent and efferent fibres to muscle spindles after nerve injury in adults cats. *J. Physiol.* **260:** 253–266.

24. Foehring, R.C., G.W. Sypert & J.B. Munson. 1986. Properties of self-reinnervated motor units of medial gastrocnemius of cat. II. Axotomized motoneurons and time course of recovery. *J. Neurophysiol.* **55:** 947–965.

25. Foehring, R.C., G.W. Sypert & J.B. Munson. 1986. Properties of self-reinnervated motor units of medial gastrocnemius of cat. I. Long-term reinnervation. *J. Neurophysiol.* **55:** 931–946.

26. Johnson, R.D. *et al.* 1995. Rescue of motoneuron and muscle afferent function in cats by regeneration into skin. I. Properties of afferents. *J. Neurophysiol.* **73:** 651–661.

27. Mendell, L.M. *et al.* 1995. Rescue of motoneuron and muscle afferent function in cats by regeneration into skin. II. Ia-motoneuron synapse. *J. Neurophysiol.* **73:** 662–673.

28. Cope, T.C. & B.D. Clark. 1993. Motor-unit recruitment in self-reinnervated muscle. *J. Neurophysiol.* **70:** 1787–1796.

29. Banks, R.W. & D. Barker. 1989. Specificities of afferents reinnervating cat muscle spindles after nerve section. *J. Physiol.* **408:** 345–372.

30. Lundborg, G. 2003. Richard P. Bunge memorial lecture. Nerve injury and repair–a challenge to the plastic brain. *J. Peripher. Nerv. Syst.* **8:** 209–226.

31. Bichler, E.K. *et al.* 2007. Enhanced transmission at a spinal synapse triggered in vivo by an injury signal independent of altered synaptic activity. *J. Neurosci.* **27:** 12851–12859.

32. Manabe, T., S. Kaneko & M. Kuno. 1989. Disuse-induced enhancement of Ia synaptic transmission in spinal motoneurons of the rat. *J. Neurosci.* **9:** 2455–2461.

33. Miyata, Y. & H. Yasuda. 1988. Enhancement of Ia synaptic transmission following muscle nerve section: Dependence upon protein synthesis. *Neurosci. Res.* **5:** 338–346.

34. Eccles, J.C. *et al.* 1962. Experiments utilizing monosynaptic excitatory action on motoneurons for testing hypotheses relating to specificity of neuronal connections. *J. Neurophysiol.* **25:** 559–580.

35. Eccles, J.C., K. Krnjevic & R. Miledi. 1959. Delayed effects of peripheral severance of afferent nerve fibres on the efficacy of their central synapses. *J. Physiol.* **145:** 204–220.

36. Gallego, R. *et al.* 1979. Disuse enhances synaptic efficacy in spinal mononeurones. *J. Physiol.* **291:** 191–205.

37. Gallego, R. *et al.* 1980. Enhancement of synaptic function in cat motoneurones during peripheral sensory regeneration. *J. Physiol.* **306:** 205–218.

38. Goldring, J.M. *et al.* 1980. Reaction of synapses on motoneurones to section and restoration of peripheral sensory connexions in the cat. *J. Physiol.* **309:** 185–198.

39. Mendell, L.M. 1988. Physiological aspects of synaptic plasticity: the Ia/motoneuron connection as a model. *Adv. Neurol.* **47:** 337–360.

40. Cope, T.C. & K.L. Bullinger. 2008. Synaptic responses to high frequency activation of regenerated Ia afferents. *Soc. Neurosci.* **74:** 12.

41. Valero-Cabre, A. & X. Navarro. 2001. H reflex restitution and facilitation after different types of peripheral nerve injury and repair. *Brain Res.* **919:** 302–312.

42. Westbury, D.R. 1972. A study of stretch and vibration reflexes of the cat by intracellular recording from motoneurones. *J. Physiol.* **226:** 37–56.

43. Bullinger, K.L. & T.C. Cope. 2009. Connectivity of individual Ia-motoneuron synapses after peripheral nerve regeneration. *Soc. Neurosci.* **442:** 7.

44. Mendell, L.M. & E. Henneman. 1971. Terminals of single Ia fibers: location, density, and distribution within a pool of 300 homonymous motoneurons. *J. Neurophysiol.* **34:** 171–187.

45. Blinzinger, K. & G. Kreutzberg. 1968. Displacement of synaptic terminals from regenerating motoneurons by microglial cells. *Z. Zellforsch. Mikrosk Anat.* **85:** 145–157.

46. Chen, D.H. 1978. Qualitative and quantitative study of synaptic displacement in chromatolyzed spinal motoneurons of the cat. *J. Comp. Neurol.* **177:** 635–664.

47. Kerns, J.M. & E.J. Hinsman. 1973. Neuroglial response to sciatic neurectomy. II. Electron microscopy. *J. Comp. Neurol.* **151:** 255–280.

48. Sumner, B.E. 1975. A quantitative analysis of the response of presynaptic boutons to postsynaptic motor neuron axotomy. *Exp. Neurol.* **46:** 605–615.

49. Sumner, B.E. & F.I. Sutherland. 1973. Quantitative electron microscopy on the injured hypoglossal nucleus in the rat. *J. Neurocytol.* **2:** 315–328.

50. Chen, D.H., W.W. Chambers & C.N. Liu. 1977. Synaptic displacement in intracentral neurons of Clarke's nucleus following axotomy in the cat. *Exp. Neurol.* **57:** 1026–1041.

51. de la Cruz, R.R., A.M. Pastor & J.M. Delgado-Garcia. 1994. Effects of target depletion on adult mammalian central neurons: morphological correlates. *Neuroscience* **58:** 59–79.

52. Purves, D. 1975. Functional and structural changes in mammalian sympathetic neurones following interruption of their axons. *J. Physiol.* **252:** 429–463.

53. Kuno, M. & R. Llinas. 1970. Alterations of synaptic action in chromatolysed motoneurones of the cat. *J. Physiol.* **210:** 823–838.

54. Titmus, M.J. & D.S. Faber. 1990. Axotomy-induced alterations in the electrophysiological characteristics of neurons. *Prog. Neurobiol.* **35:** 1–51.

55. Brannstrom, T. & J.O. Kellerth. 1998. Changes in synaptology of adult cat spinal alpha-motoneurons after axotomy. *Exp. Brain Res.* **118:** 1–13.

56. Brannstrom, T. & J.O. Kellerth. 1999. Recovery of synapses in axotomized adult cat spinal motoneurons after reinnervation into muscle. *Exp. Brain Res.* **125:** 19–27.

57. Cull, R.E. 1974. Role of nerve-muscle contact in maintaining synaptic connections. *Exp. Brain Res.* **20:** 307–310.

58. Sumner, B.E. 1976. Quantitative ultrastructural observations on the inhibited recovery of the hypoglossal nucleus from the axotomy response when regeneration of the hypoglossal nerve is prevented. *Exp. Brain Res.* **26:** 141–150.

59. Linda, H., S. Cullheim & M. Risling. 1992. A light and electron microscopic study of intracellularly HRP-labeled lumbar motoneurons after intramedullary axotomy in the adult cat. *J. Comp. Neurol.* **318:** 188–208.

60. Linda, H. *et al.* 2000. Ultrastructural evidence for a preferential elimination of glutamate-immunoreactive synaptic terminals from spinal motoneurons after intramedullary axotomy. *J. Comp. Neurol.* **425:** 10–23.

61. Novikov, L.N. *et al.* 2000. Exogenous brain-derived neurotrophic factor regulates the synaptic composition of axonally lesioned and normal adult rat motoneurons. *Neuroscience* **100:** 171–181.

62. Guntinas-Lichius, O. *et al.* 1994. Differences in glial, synaptic and motoneuron responses in the facial nucleus of the rat brainstem following facial nerve resection and nerve suture reanastomosis. *Eur. Arch. Otorhinolaryngol.* **251:** 410–417.

63. Davis-Lopez de Carrizosa, M.A. *et al.* 2009. Complementary actions of BDNF and neurotrophin-3 on the firing patterns and synaptic composition of motoneurons. *J. Neurosci.* **29:** 575–587.

64. Mendell, L.M., R.D. Johnson & J.B. Munson. 1999. Neurotrophin modulation of the monosynaptic reflex after peripheral nerve transection. *J. Neurosci.* **19:** 3162–3170.

65. Burke, R.E. & L.L. Glenn. 1996. Horseradish peroxidase study of the spatial and electrotonic distribution of group Ia synapses on type-identified ankle extensor motoneurons in the cat. *J. Comp. Neurol.* **372:** 465–485.

66. Fyffe, R.E.W. 2001. Spinal motoneurons: synaptic inputs and receptor organization. In *Motor Neurobiology of the Spinal Cord.* T.C. Cope, Ed.: 21–46. Boca Raton, FL.

67. Alvarez, F.J. *et al.* 2004. Vesicular glutamate transporters in the spinal cord, with special reference to sensory primary afferent synapses. *J. Comp. Neurol.* **472:** 257–280.

68. Todd, A.J. *et al.* 2003. The expression of vesicular glutamate transporters VGLUT1 and VGLUT2 in neurochemically defined axonal populations in the rat spinal cord with emphasis on the dorsal horn. *Eur. J. Neurosci.* **17:** 13–27.

69. Alvarez, F.J. *et al.* 2008. VGLUT1 content in central synapses of normal and regenerated Ia afferents *Soc. Neurosci.* **74:** 1.

70. Hughes, D.I. *et al.* 2004. Peripheral axotomy induces depletion of the vesicular glutamate transporter VGLUT1

in central terminals of myelinated afferent fibres in the rat spinal cord. *Brain Res.* **1017:** 69–76.

71. Li, L.Y. *et al.* 2006. Neurotrophin-3 ameliorates sensory-motor deficits in Er81-deficient mice. *Dev. Dyn.* **235:** 3039–3050.

72. Wang, Z. *et al.* 2007. Prenatal exposure to elevated NT3 disrupts synaptic selectivity in the spinal cord. *J. Neurosci.* **27:** 3686–3694.

73. Harvey, P.A. *et al.* 2009. Blockade of Nogo receptor ligands promotes functional regeneration of sensory axons after dorsal root crush. *J. Neurosci.* **29:** 6285–6295.

Ann. N.Y. Acad. Sci. ISSN 0077-8923

ANNALS OF THE NEW YORK ACADEMY OF SCIENCES

Issue: *Neurons and Networks in the Spinal Cord*

Deconstructing locomotor networks with experimental injury to define their membership

Andrea Nistri,[1,2] Giuliano Taccola,[1,2] Miranda Mladinic,[1,2] Gayane Margaryan,[1] and Anujaianthi Kuzhandaivel[1]

[1]International School for Advanced Studies, Trieste, Italy. [2]SPINAL Laboratory, Institute of Physical Medicine and Rehabilitation, Udine, Italy

Address for correspondence: Andrea Nistri, SISSA, Via Beirut 2-4, 34151 Trieste, Italy. Voice: 39-040-375 6518; fax: 39-40-375 6502. nistri@sissa.it

Although spinal injury is a major cause of chronic disability, the mechanisms responsible for the lesion pathophysiology and their dynamic evolution remain poorly understood. Hence, current treatments aimed at blocking damage extension are unsatisfactory. To unravel the acute spinal injury processes, we have developed a model of the neonatal rat spinal cord *in vitro* subjected to kainate-evoked excitotoxicity or metabolic perturbation (hypoxia, aglycemia, and free oxygen radicals) or their combination. The study outcome is fictive locomotion one day after the lesion and its relation to histological damage. Excitotoxicity always suppresses locomotor network activity and produces large gray matter damage, while network bursting persists supported by average survival of nearly half premotoneurons and motoneurons. Conversely, metabolic perturbation simply depresses locomotor network activity as damage mainly concerns white rather than gray matter. Coapplication of kainate and metabolic perturbation completely eliminates locomotor network activity. These results indicate distinct cellular targets for excitotoxic versus dysmetabolic damage with differential consequences on locomotor pattern formation. Furthermore, these data enable to estimate the minimal network membership compatible with expression of locomotor activity.

Keywords: excitotoxicity; oxygen glucose deprivation; reactive oxygen species; spinal injury; central pattern generator; rhythmogenesis

Introduction

The lumbar region of the spinal cord contains extensive neuronal networks which can generate coordinated locomotion independently from supraspinal or peripheral inputs.[1–3] Operationally this network arrangement is termed central pattern generator (CPG).[4]

The locomotor program consists of a series of motor commands (expressed by motoneurons) to flexor and extensor limb muscles to provide the swing and stance alternating pattern essential for over-ground gait. This is, indeed, a complex program that involves correct timing and phasing of the neuronal signals with rhythmic excitation and inhibition of reciprocal motor units. In fact, when synaptic excitation is blocked, locomotion is arrested,[5] whereas block of synaptic inhibition converts locomotor patterns into synchronous, slow disinhibited bursting.[6] The latter activity is believed to express basic network excitability and is useful to monitor the persistence of elementary functional connectivity within the circuitry.

Locomotion requires the activation of the CPG by descending inputs, for example from the mesencephalic locomotor centre, or from appropriate sensory inputs, often supplemented by drugs.[7,8] Because the locomotor CPG is believed to be fully contained in the lumbar spinal cord, *in vitro* preparations of the baby mouse or rat spinal cord produce rhythmically alternating motor patterns (readily recorded from ventral roots) when activated by neurochemicals (typically NMDA and serotonin, 5HT)[1] or dorsal root stimuli.[9] The observed pattern is termed "fictive locomotion" and is a very useful model to investigate the properties of the locomotor CPG.

doi: 10.1111/j.1749-6632.2009.05427.x

Ann. N.Y. Acad. Sci. 1198 (2010) 242–251 © 2010 New York Academy of Sciences.

In quadruped mammals considerable advance in our understanding of the CPG operation has been obtained by combining experimental data with a model in which the CPG is thought to comprise two main components, namely a "clock" that starts the program, sets its locomotor frequency and is hierarchically above the "pattern" formation responsible for producing the correct phase and sequence activation of motoneurons.[2]

Molecular genetics have recently identified important classes of interneuron that provide a powerful contribution to the locomotor program.[1,3] Their role has been investigated with direct imaging and/or genetically manipulated disruption or activation.[10–12] It is, however, difficult to identify the full membership (and their wiring) of the locomotor CPG since, to date, none of such cells has been proven to be absolutely essential to produce the full locomotor program. A clear understanding of the CPG structure remains an ambitious goal that is especially important to elucidate the pathophysiology of spinal injury. Once the blueprint of the locomotor CPG is obtained, strategies for repairing it or replacing lost elements can be better targeted to combat paralysis.

Pathophysiology of spinal injury

The damage occurring to the spinal cord can be temporally divided into various phases that start with the primary damage at the site of the lesion, followed by secondary damage spreading to uninjured areas and slowly evolving into a chronic condition.[13–15] Once the lesion is chronic, it is often accompanied by histopathological alterations like gliosis and formation of cysts that, in addition to aberrant network plasticity, make it difficult to repair the damage. It is, therefore, a more attainable target to try to block the negative evolution of the secondary damage.

Current theories propose that, regardless of its initial cause (traumatic, vascular, infective, etc.), the secondary damage develops because of a chain of deleterious cell processes that comprise, among the main players, excitotoxicity,[16–18] namely cell destruction because of excessive glutamate release and overactivation of glutamate receptors, and severe metabolic perturbation with generation of toxic reactive oxygen species and free radicals.[15,19–21] The basic pathophysiology of such events is difficult to investigate in patients as well as in animal mod-

els because of the need to continuously monitor the locomotor deficit and to correlate it with cell damage during a time frame of minutes, hours, and days without additional complicating factors arising from anesthesia, cardiovascular changes, and intensive care support.

In vitro model of spinal cord injury

In the attempt to clarify these important issues, we thought that using an *in vitro* model of acute spinal injury might help to understand the early dynamics of this process. In particular, this model should enable us to correlate the ability to produce fictive locomotion with the extent of network histological damage and should, ideally, represent a simple test system to screen neuroprotective agents. Furthermore, it should be possible to compare the relative contribution of excitotoxicity versus metabolic perturbation. Finally, a focal lesion *in vitro* should allow studying the consequences for spinal segments remote from the primary injury site. Of course, an *in vitro* model has limitations intrinsic to the experimental protocol, namely the lack of any vascular supply and the use of a neonatal preparation. Unfortunately, adult spinal cord preparations *in vitro* do not usually show survival beyond a few hours and are taken from nonlocomotor (sacral) regions.[22]

Clinical reports indicate that the shortest hospital admission time after acute spinal injury is under 3 h.[16,23,24] In the hospital the first goal of intensive care medicine is to stabilize the patient and to correct his metabolic state prior to any surgical or pharmacological intervention. To try to mimic this series of events *in vitro*, we applied a toxic solution (either locally or to the whole isolated spinal cord preparation) for 1 h and then washed it out with standard oxygenated-buffered saline for 24 h.[25,26] The outcome of each experiment was whether fictive locomotion was still present 24 h after the lesion. To this end, we performed electrophysiological recording from various ventral roots to collect information from rear limb flexor and extension motor pools (namely, at L2 and L5 segmental level) during and after the lesion protocol, and correlated it with histological and histochemical analysis.

Preliminary tests done by inserting (for a few min) a blunt (50 μm diameter) glass micropipette into one lumbar segment (L1 or L2) to simulate focal mechanical injury failed to induce long-lasting suppression of fictive locomotion as preparations spontaneously recovered their activity 24 h later. This observation led us to devise chemically evoked spinal lesions as this approach also provided a method to examine the cellular and molecular mechanisms underlying the acute injury.

Three main lesion protocols were, therefore, investigated: (1) intense neurotoxicity evoked by the powerful glutamate agonist kainate; (2) metabolic perturbation induced by a pathological medium (thereafter termed PM) with hypoxia, aglycemia, H_2O_2, sodium nitroprussiate, hypo-osmotic, Mg^{2+} free medium, and acid medium; (3) coapplication of kainate and PM. The solution recipes can be found in refs. 25 and 26.

We further refined our model by creating (with transverse plastic barriers) leak-proof compartments separately superfused with saline or toxic solution. This approach enabled us to restrict the application of the toxic medium (comprising kainate and PM) to 2–3 segments at the lower thoracic and upper lumbar segments (T12-L1), thus sparing the main L2-L5 segments containing the locomotor CPG. This experimental arrangement allowed us to study the downstream consequences of a lesion on apparently unaffected locomotor networks.

Excitotoxic damage to locomotor networks

Excitotoxicity stems from excessive activation of glutamate receptors with deleterious early and delayed effects on neuronal and glial survival. This process is thought to be important for a large number of pathological brain conditions like stroke, trauma, and neurodegenerative diseases.[27–29] Likewise, in the case of spinal injury, excitotoxicity is considered to be an important component.

We investigated the effect of a saturating concentration of kainate (1 h application) on locomotor networks of the neonatal rat spinal cord *in vitro*.[25] Several considerations led to the choice of kainate: its stability in solution, lack of transport by glutamate carriers and ability to produce excitotoxicity.[30] Because of previous reports on the need to apply high doses of kainate to lesion the rat spinal cord *in vivo*,[31,32] we used a high concentration (1 mM) of this drug that exceeds the one required for maximal depolarization of spinal neurons,[33] and approaches the glutamate levels detected after spinal trauma.[34]

Figure 1 summarizes the protocol employed for the kainate-evoked lesion of the lumbar spinal cord *in vitro* and its consequences for the rat spinal cord. First, typical fictive locomotion with alternating ventral roots discharges was induced by continuously applied (see horizontal green bar) NMDA (5 μM) and 5HT (10 μM). After washout and return to control saline solution (blue bar), kainate was applied (red bar) to generate a large depolarization of motor pools (with transient oscillations) that persisted to a stable plateau throughout the application time. After washout, synaptic responses recorded from ventral roots following dorsal root stimulation were severely depressed. Fictive locomotion was not observed either on the same day after extensive kainate washout or the day after (see Fig. 1). It was, however, possible to evoke disinhibited bursting (magenta bar) after pharmacological block of synaptic inhibition with a combination of strychnine and bicuculline, suggesting that basic network rhythmicity and excitability were retained.

Histological analysis indicated a substantial number of pyknotic nuclei (Fig. 1), showing cell death in the four selected regions (dorsal and ventral horns, area around the central canal, and lateral white matter). Examination of immunoreactive neurons and motoneurons with NeuN and SMI-32, respectively, demonstrated that, in the ventral horn area, essential for the rat locomotor CPG,[35] there was 43% neuronal loss and 37% motoneuronal loss.

To clarify the molecular mechanisms underlying the acute spinal cord dysfunction, we analyzed mRNA and protein content of the neonatal rat spinal cord at 4 and 24 h following 1 h application of kainate. Gene expression levels of different cell type markers (GFAP for astroglia, NeuN for neurons), the neuronal injury marker ATF-3,[36] and various genes involved in neuroinflammation (interleukin 1b, IL-1b;[37] serpine-1),[38] and cell proliferation (Egr-1)[39] were studied using Real-Time PCR or large-scale Superarrays. Preliminary data indicate that, already at 4 h from treatment, there was upregulation of ATF-3, Egr-1, IL-1b, and serpine-1 expression.

Metabolic perturbation induced by pathological medium

In addition to early excitotoxic damage due to massive release of glutamate, the acute stage of spinal

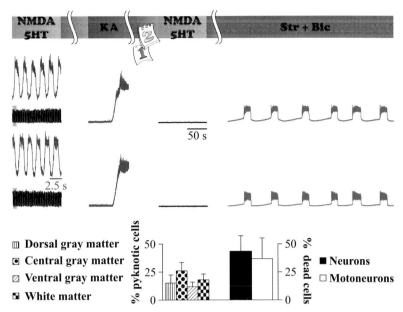

Figure 1. Kainate induced damage to lumbar locomotor networks. The *top panel* shows the scheme for the experimental protocol that includes control tests for fictive locomotion evoked by NMDA and 5HT, 1 h application of kainate, and subsequent wash with retesting of fictive locomotion the day after. In control condition, NMDA (5 μM) and 5HT (10 μM) elicit alternating oscillations recorded from L2 and L5 lumbar roots of the same side. The traces are also shown at faster time base to reveal the oscillation pattern. Kainate (1 mM) produces strong depolarization of motor pools which is followed by inability to evoke fictive locomotion the day after, although disinhibited bursting (caused by 1 μM strychnine and 10 μM bicuculline administration) is observed. Histograms indicate extent of cell death (*left*; estimated as percent of pyknotic nuclei) in four regions of the lumbar spinal cord 24 h after kainate application, or number of dead premotoneurons and motoneurons (*right*). Further details in ref. 25.

cord injury is believed to comprise a pathological cascade that includes generation of nitric oxide (NO),[16] free oxygen radicals, and metabolic dysfunction due to ischemia/hypoxia, energy store collapse, acidosis, and edema triggered by loss of vascular tone autoregulation.[16,19,20] Thus, we tested a medium containing a free oxygen radical donor (H_2O_2), a NO precursor (sodium nitroprussiate) and metabolic perturbations (low Mg^{2+}, low osmolarity, acid pH, hypoxia, aglycemia) typically associated with spinal (and brain) lesions. This solution was termed PM and its effects are exemplified in Figure 2. After obtaining standard fictive locomotion with NMDA and 5HT (green bar), application of PM (red bar) induced a slowly developing depolarization with irregular ventral root discharges. After approximately 1 h washout, fictive locomotion could be observed again although with smaller cycle amplitude and slower period.[25] This pattern was present also 24 h later, together with the ability to produce disinhibited bursting (magenta bar). PM

elicited extensive damage to the lateral white matter with relatively modest damage to interneurons and motoneurons (Fig. 2). In keeping with white matter damage we were unable to evoke fictive locomotion by electrical stimulation of dorsal root afferents.

While the results after either kainate or PM application showed some preservation of spinal networks, when kainate plus PM were applied together for 1 h, all electrophysiological responses were always lost and did not recover even one day later despite sustained washout. In this case, histological examination (24 h later) indicated widespread damage with large neuronal loss throughout the gray matter, substantial damage to the white matter, and strong loss of motoneurons. These data show that extensive damage to white matter, premotoneurons, and motoneurons was likely responsible for the suppression of electrophysiological responses.[25]

Furthermore, we unexpectedly found that the relatively restricted neuronal lesion produced by PM was largely intensified when the PM solution

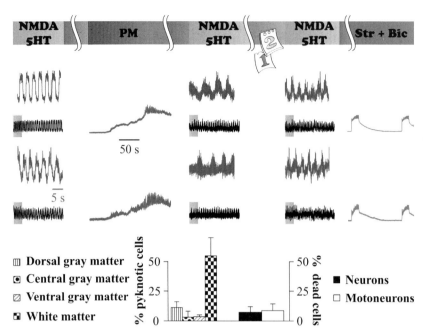

Figure 2. Pathological medium induced damage to lumbar locomotor networks. The *top panel* shows the scheme for the experimental protocol that includes control tests for fictive locomotion evoked by NMDA and 5HT, 1 h application of PM, and subsequent wash with retesting of fictive locomotion the day after. In control condition, NMDA (5 μM) and 5HT (10 μM) elicit alternating oscillations recorded from L2 and L5 lumbar roots of the same side. The traces are also shown at faster time base to reveal the oscillation pattern. PM depolarizes motor pools. After 1 h washout, fictive locomotion can be evoked by NMDA and 5HT even if cycle amplitude and periodicity have deteriorated: this pattern is detected also the day after together with disinhibited bursting (caused by 1 μM strychnine and 10 μM bicuculline administration). Histograms indicate extent of cell death (*left*; estimated as percent of pyknotic nuclei) in four regions of the lumbar spinal cord 24 h after PM application, or number of dead premotoneurons and motoneurons (*right*). Further details in ref. 25.

contained 1 or 2 mM Mg^{2+} (see ref. 26). In fact, fictive locomotion was fully and irreversibly suppressed together with enhanced neuronal loss chiefly affecting premotoneurons of the ventral horn (decreased by approximately 50%) against a relatively unchanged population of motoneurons. The damage to the white matter remained extensive. The mechanisms responsible for the deleterious action of Mg^{2+} are currently unknown, but they closely resemble the negative outcome of Mg^{2+} i.v. infusion in patients with acute brain trauma or stroke.[40–42]

Focal lesion induces remote effects on locomotor networks

The *in vitro* model of the neonatal rat isolated spinal cord is also suitable to investigate the process of sec-

ondary damage following acute experimental spinal injury. In fact, as indicated in Figure 3, transverse barriers placed at the low thoracic-upper lumbar region allowed focal superfusion (1 h) of kainate plus PM to these segments only. In this way, the spinal lesion was restricted as shown by average histological data in Figure 3: the number of cells with pyknotic nucleus was large in all areas of the segments located within the barriers, yet minimal in the segments below.

Figure 3 shows the results of functional tests to explore locomotor network activity with this arrangement. Fictive locomotion evoked by NMDA and 5HT from L2 and L5 segments was present in control conditions prior to the application of kainate and PM that generated a large and sustained ventral root depolarization of the L1 segment (between the barriers) and less intense and transient

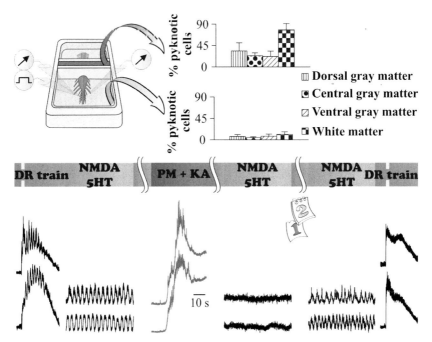

Figure 3. Focal application of toxic solution produces secondary damage to locomotor networks. *Top:* scheme indicating experimental arrangement whereby transverse barriers restricted the application of kainate plus PM to the T9-L1 area. Twenty-four h later, in the lesioned area (*top histograms*), there was substantial damage to all cell types, especially in the lateral white matter. Conversely, the *bottom histograms* indicate minimal damage to region topographically below the barrier placement. *Bottom panels* show the experimental protocol (see also Fig. 1 legend) and corresponding records from lumbar ventral roots outside the area affected by the toxic solution. After induction of fictive locomotion by NMDA and 5HT, application of kainate plus PM elicits strong depolarization. After 1 h washout, it is not possible to replicate fictive locomotion, although this pattern recovers one day later. Note that 1 Hz pulse trains applied to a dorsal root below the lesion evoke cumulative depolarization recorded from ventral roots but lacking fictive locomotion-like oscillations.

depolarization in segments above or below the barriers (not shown). Despite baseline recovery, L2 and L5 segments did not produce fictive locomotion 1 h later after washing out the kainate plus PM solution (Fig. 3). Nevertheless, after one day *in vitro*, recovery of fictive locomotion by NMDA and 5HT was observed as demonstrated in Figure 3, although trains of stimuli applied via dorsal root afferents failed to elicit this pattern in spite of a large cumulative depolarization recorded from the L5 ventral root. The causes for the loss of electrically induced fictive locomotion remain unclear especially in the absence of significant cell loss and suggest long-lasting plasticity changes perhaps triggered by neuromodulators like endocannabinoids and NO[43] released during the strong depolarization evoked

by the toxic solution that possibly led to persistent downregulation of certain synapses.[44,45]

Basic processes of acute spinal injury

While our *in vitro* model suggests distinct roles (and cell targets) of excitotoxicity and metabolic dysfunction in the acute injury to locomotor networks, it is clear that synergy of action between the powerful excitotoxic agent kainate and deranged metabolism leads to irreversible damage.[25]

It is interesting to compare the consequences of kainate or PM: kainate always abolished fictive locomotion, while PM induced only a deterioration of locomotor patterns (slow periodicity, small cycle size) observable when locomotor networks were directly activated by NMDA and 5HT. Electrical pulses, however, failed to produce fictive locomotion. Perhaps the strong loss of white matter elements elicited by PM led to impaired polysynaptic transmission that functionally isolated spinal networks from external inputs or reduced their ability to process them.

These results raise issues of potential relevance to the management of spinal injuries. In fact, if the early excitotoxicity could be pharmacologically blocked during the most acute phase, the metabolic perturbation developing as a consequence of trauma or vascular collapse might leave a network with enough structure for locomotion and whose potential further deterioration might be prevented once the cellular mechanisms are fully elucidated.

The toxic solutions used for the present investigation comprised a variety of substances and factors whose relative contribution will have to be studied in the future. It is, however, clear that, if kainate-evoked excitotoxicity caused generation of toxic metabolites, the latter process must have been of limited extent (or generated substances not included in the cocktail employed for our tests) because of the obvious differences in the effects due to kainate or PM.

The focal lesion protocol allowed us to reproduce the transient loss of locomotor activity which is typically seen immediately after an acute lesion in man ("spinal shock").[46] Our data indicate that, below the lesion, the locomotor network output was regained when the CPG was activated by neurochemicals, and that 24 h after the primary lesion, neuronal cell loss in those segments was minimal. However, like in the case of lesions affecting the whole spinal preparation, there was a persistent inability to produce fictive locomotion with dorsal root stimuli: the loss of integration of sensory afferent signals into the locomotor CPG may pose a major challenge to gait recovery and to neurorehabilitation. We propose that this is a novel observation so far unavailable from *in vivo* animal experiments in which the general anesthesia used together with the lesion protocol inevitably compounds the network synaptic transmission properties.

Elementary architecture of locomotor networks

Integrating our electrophysiological data with histological and immunohistochemical observations enables us to work out some estimates of the network size sufficient for locomotor pattern generation. Previous studies have shown that fictive locomotion requires at least three intact segments of the most rhythmogenic spinal region (i.e., the upper lumbar one).[47] The present study expands this information by estimating, in a standard cross section of the lumbar spinal cord, the minimum number of surviving neurons and glia compatible with fictive locomotion.

Following application of PM, intersegmental coupling responsible for fictive locomotion induced by NMDA and 5HT was still operational even with the loss of approximately 50% of the lateral white matter (though electrically evoked patterns were absent), suggesting that most intrinsic connectivity amongst cells of the locomotor CPG normally relied on proprioceptive wiring. The challenge will, therefore, be how to direct activation signals to the CPG when the sensory input integration is made inoperative by a lesion.

Focussing on gray matter elements and starting from the simplest form of synchronized rhythmicity, the network structure required the presence of at least 55% premotoneurons and 40% motoneurons to generate disinhibited bursting as indicated by the results with kainate.[25] This estimate is likely to be near the lowest sustainable membership because residual bursts were small and slow. Experiments with extracellular Mg^{2+} changes[26] show that fictive locomotion required a more complex circuitry including at least 65% ventral horn premotoneurons and a nearly intact motoneuron population. It is noteworthy that the margin between neuronal numbers necessary for locomotor pattern expression and neuronal numbers for synchronized bursting is rather narrow.

Because the locomotor CPG appears to be contained within the ventral/central area of the lumbar spinal cord,[35] the role played by dorsal horn neurons is probably less fundamental to the generation of this motor pattern. However, the large kainate-induced damage to the cells around the central canal (lamina X) which are part of the neuronal network generating locomotor activity[48] is likely to be an important contributing factor to the loss of fictive locomotion after excitotoxicity. Of course, our interpretation should be tempered by the fact that it derives from histological analysis and it does not include functional damage without obvious cell losses. In keeping with this notion, we also observed enhanced expression of genes involved in neuroinflammation (IL-1b; Serpine-1), cell proliferation (Egr-1), and motoneuron stress (ATF-3). Hence, the operational damage might even be more extensive than the one measured histologically, suggesting urgency of any postlesional intervention to inhibit further network deterioration. Furthermore, these data indicate the minimal objective in terms of network numbers that any attempt for repair or regeneration should attain in order to recover locomotion.

In conclusion, the *in vitro* acute injury model offers novel data potentially interesting to the pathophysiology of spinal injury and its treatment/repair. In the future, more emphasis should perhaps be placed on how to reinstate the function of the locomotor CPG especially when its basic structure remains viable after a lesion such as the one due to dysmetabolic insult. Motoneuron losses, even if slight, have strong, negative impact on the locomotor program and leave little room for redundancy and compensation. Preserving their integrity or replacing them may be a daunting challenge. The large premotoneuronal network (which undoubtedly includes a significant number of cells unrelated to the locomotor CPG) may better tolerate damage, leaving thus open the possibility to recover function through targeted repair and neurorehabilitation as long as motoneuron numbers are adequate. Future studies should investigate the possibility that the operation of this network depends on few crucial cells, whose identification might become strategically important to diagnose spinal damage and to monitor recovery progress and prospects.

Acknowledgments

This work was supported by the government of the Friuli Venezia Giulia region, the Italian Ministry of Universities and Research (PRIN grant), and the Vertical Foundation.

Conflicts of interest

The authors declare no conflicts of interest.

References

1. Kiehn, O. 2006. Locomotor circuits in the mammalian spinal cord. *Annu. Rev. Neurosci.* **29:** 279–306.

2. McCrea, D.A. & I.A. Rybak. 2008. Organization of mammalian locomotor rhythm and pattern generation. *Brain Res. Rev.* **57:** 134–146.

3. Goulding, M. 2009. Circuits controlling vertebrate locomotion: moving in a new direction. *Nature Revs. Neurosci.* **10:** 507–518.

4. Grillner, S. 2006. Biological pattern generation: the cellular and computational logic of networks in motion. *Neuron* **52:** 751–766.

5. Beato, M., E. Bracci & A. Nistri. 1997. Contribution of NMDA and non-NMDA glutamate receptors to locomotor pattern generation in the neonatal rat spinal cord. *Proc. Roy. Soc. London B.* **264:** 877–884.

6. Bracci, E., L. Ballerini & A. Nistri. 1996. Localization of rhythmogenic networks responsible for spontaneous bursts induced by strychnine and bicuculline in the rat isolated spinal cord. *J. Neurosci.* **16:** 7063–7076.

7. Gerasimenko, Y., R.R. Roy & V.R. Edgerton. 2008. Epidural stimulation: comparison of the spinal circuits that generate and control locomotion in rats, cats and humans. *Exp. Neurol.* **209:** 417–425.

8. Rossignol, S. *et al.* 2008. Plasticity of locomotor sensorimotor interactions after peripheral and/or spinal lesions. *Brain Res. Rev.* **57:** 228–240.

9. Marchetti, C., M. Beato & A. Nistri. 2001. Alternating rhythmic activity induced by dorsal root stimulation in the neonatal rat spinal cord in vitro. *J. Physiol.* **530:** 105–112.

10. Hinckley, C.A. *et al.* 2005. Locomotor-like rhythms in a genetically distinct cluster of interneurons in the mammalian spinal cord. *J. Neurophysiol.* **93:** 1439–1449.

11. Gosgnach, S. *et al.* 2006. V1 spinal neurons regulate the speed of vertebrate locomotor outputs. *Nature* **440:** 215–219.

12. Brownstone, R.M. & J.M. Wilson. 2008. Strategies for delineating spinal locomotor rhythm-generating networks and the possible role of Hb9 interneurones in rhythmogenesis. *Brain Res. Rev.* **57:** 64–76.

13. McDonald, J.W. & C. Sadowsky. 2002. Spinal-cord injury. *Lancet* **359:** 417–425.

14. Klussmann, S. & A. Martin-Villalba. 2005. Molecular targets in spinal cord injury. *J. Mol. Med.* **83:** 657–671.

15. Schwab, J.M. *et al.* 2006. Experimental strategies to promote spinal cord regeneration—an integrative perspective. *Prog. Neurobiol.* **78:** 91–116.

16. Hall, E.D. & J.E. Springer. 2004. Neuroprotection and acute spinal cord injury: a reappraisal. *NeuroRx.* **1:** 80–100.

17. Park, E., A.A. Velumian & M.G. Fehlings. 2004. The role of excitotoxicity in secondary mechanisms of spinal cord injury: a review with an emphasis on the implications for white matter degeneration. *J. Neurotrauma* **21:** 754–774.

18. Rossignol, S., M. Schwab, M. Schwartz & M.G. Fehlings. 2007. Spinal cord injury: time to move? *J. Neurosci.* **27:** 11782–11792.

19. Dumont, R.J. *et al.* 2001. Acute spinal cord injury, Part I. Pathophysiologic mechanisms. *Clin. Neuropharmacol.* **24:** 254–264.

20. Norenberg, M.D., J. Smith & A. Marcillo. 2004. The pathology of human spinal cord injury: defining the problems. *J. Neurotrauma* **21:** 429–440.

21. Xiong, Y., Rabchevsky & E.D. Hall. 2007. Role of peroxynitrite in secondary oxidative damage after spinal cord injury. *J. Neurochem.* **100:** 639–649.

22. Long, S.K., R.H. Evans & F. Krijzer. 1989. Effects of depressant amino acids and antagonists on an in vitro spinal cord preparation from the adult rat. *Neuropharmacology* **28:** 683–688.

23. Bracken, M.B. *et al.* 1990. A randomized, controlled trial of methylprednisolone or naloxone in the treatment of acute spinal-cord injury. Results of the Second National Acute Spinal Cord Injury Study. *N. Engl. J. Med.* **322:** 1405–1411.

24. Pointillart, V. *et al.* 2000. Pharmacological therapy of spinal cord injury during the acute phase. *Spinal Cord* **38:** 71–76.

25. Taccola, G., G. Margaryan, M. Mladinic & A. Nistri. 2008. Kainate and metabolic perturbation mimicking spinal injury differentially contribute to early damage of locomotor networks in the in vitro neonatal rat spinal cord. *Neuroscience* **155:** 538–555.

26. Margaryan, G., M. Mladinic, C. Mattioli & A. Nistri. 2009. Extracellular magnesium enhances the damage to locomotor networks produced by metabolic perturbation mimicking spinal injury in the neonatal rat spinal cord in vitro. *Neuroscience* **163:** 669–682.

27. Besancon, E. *et al.* 2008. Beyond NMDA and AMPA glutamate receptors: emerging mechanisms for ionic imbalance and cell death in stroke. *Trends Pharmacol. Sci.* **29:** 268–275.

28. Rowland, J.W., G.W. Hawryluk, B. Kwon & M.G. Fehlings. 2008. Current status of acute spinal cord injury pathophysiology and emerging therapies: promise on the horizon. *Neurosurg. Focus* **25:** 1–17.

29. Greve, M.W. & B.J. Zink. 2009. Pathophysiology of traumatic brain injury. *Mt. Sinai J. Med.* **76:** 97–104.

30. Vincent, P. & C. Mulle. 2009. Kainate receptors in epilepsy and excitotoxicity. *Neuroscience* **158:** 309–323.

31. Magnuson, D.S. *et al.* 1999. Comparing deficits following excitotoxic and contusion injuries in the thoracic and lumbar spinal cord of the adult rat. *Exp. Neurol.* **156:** 191–204.

32. Sun, H.Y. *et al.* 2006. Slow and selective death of spinal motor neurons in vivo by intrathecal infusion of kainic acid: implications for AMPA receptor-mediated excitotoxicity in ALS. *J. Neurochem.* **98:** 782–791.

33. Nistri, A. & A. Constanti. 1979. Pharmacological characterization of different types of GABA and glutamate receptors in vertebrates and invertebrates. *Prog. Neurobiol.* **13:** 117–235.

34. Liu, D., G.Y. Xu, E. Pan & D.J. McAdoo. 1999. Neurotoxicity of glutamate at the concentration released upon spinal cord injury. *Neuroscience* **93:** 1383–1389.

35. Taccola, G. & A. Nistri. 2006. Oscillatory circuits underlying locomotor networks in the rat spinal cord. *Crit. Rev. Neurobiol.* **18:** 25–36.

36. Tsujino, H. *et al.* 2000. Activating transcription factor 3 (ATF3) induction by axotomy in sensory and motoneurons: a novel neuronal marker of nerve injury. *Mol. Cell. Neurosci.* **15:** 170–182.

37. Fogal, B. & S.J. Hewett. 2008. Interleukin-1beta: a bridge between inflammation and excitotoxicity? *J. Neurochem.* **106:** 1–23.

38. Docagne, F. *et al.* 1999. Transforming growth factor-beta1 as a regulator of the serpins/t-PA axis in cerebral ischemia. *FASEB J.* **13:** 1315–1324.

39. Beck, H. *et al.* 2008. Egr-1 regulates expression of the glial scar component phosphacan in astrocytes after experimental stroke. *Am. J. Pathol.* **173:** 77–92.

40. Ikonomidou, C. & L. Turski. 2002. Why did NMDA receptor antagonists fail clinical trials for stroke and traumatic brain injury? *Lancet Neurol.* **1:** 383–386.

41. IMAGES. 2004. Magnesium for acute stroke (Intravenous Magnesium Efficacy in Stroke Trial): randomised controlled trial. *Lancet* **363:** 439–445.

42. Temkin, N.R. *et al.* 2007. Magnesium sulfate for neuroprotection after traumatic brain injury: a randomised controlled trial. *Lancet Neurol.* **6:** 29–38.

43. Kyriakatos, A. & A. El Manira. 2007. Long-term plasticity of the spinal locomotor circuitry mediated by endocannabinoid and nitric oxide signaling. *J. Neurosci.* **27:** 12664–12674.

44. Chevaleyre, V., K.A. Takahashi & P.E. Castillo. 2006. Endocannabinoid-mediated synaptic plasticity in the CNS. *Annu. Rev. Neurosci.* **29:** 37–76.

45. Massey, P.V. & Z.I. Bashir. 2007. Long-term depression: multiple forms and implications for brain function. *Trends Neurosci.* **30:** 176–184.

46. Ditunno, J.F., J.W. Little, A. Tessler & A.S. Burns. 2004. Spinal shock revisited: a four-phase model. *Spinal Cord* **42:** 383–395.

47. Kjaerulff, O. & O. Kiehn. 1996. Distribution of networks generating and coordinating locomotor activity in the neonatal rat spinal cord in vitro. a lesion study. *J. Neurosci.* **16:** 5777–5794.

48. Kjaerulff, O., I. Barajon & O. Kiehn. 1994. Sulphorhodamine-labelled cells in the neonatal rat spinal cord following chemically induced locomotor activity in vitro. *J. Physiol.* **478:** 265–273.

Ann. N.Y. Acad. Sci. ISSN 0077-8923

ANNALS OF THE NEW YORK ACADEMY OF SCIENCES
Issue: *Neurons and Networks in the Spinal Cord*

Spinal plasticity following intermittent hypoxia: implications for spinal injury

Erica A. Dale-Nagle, Michael S. Hoffman, Peter M. MacFarlane, Irawan Satriotomo, Mary Rachael Lovett-Barr, Stéphane Vinit, and Gordon S. Mitchell

Department of Comparative Biosciences, University of Wisconsin, Madison, Wisconsin

Address for correspondence: Gordon S. Mitchell, Department of Comparative Biosciences, University of Wisconsin, School of Veterinary Medicine, 2215 Linden Avenue, Madison, WI 53706. mitchell@svm.vetmed.wisc.edu

Plasticity is a fundamental property of the neural system controlling breathing. One frequently studied model of respiratory plasticity is long-term facilitation of phrenic motor output (pLTF) following acute intermittent hypoxia (AIH). pLTF arises from spinal plasticity, increasing respiratory motor output through a mechanism that requires new synthesis of brain-derived neurotrophic factor, activation of its high-affinity receptor, tropomyosin-related kinase B, and extracellular-related kinase mitogen-activated protein kinase signaling in or near phrenic motor neurons. Because intermittent hypoxia induces spinal plasticity, we are exploring the potential to harness repetitive AIH as a means of inducing functional recovery in conditions causing respiratory insufficiency, such as cervical spinal injury. Because repetitive AIH induces phenotypic plasticity in respiratory motor neurons, it may restore respiratory motor function in patients with incomplete spinal injury.

Keywords: spinal cord injury; intermittent hypoxia; plasticity

Introduction

Because breathing is a critical homeostatic control system essential for life, the neural system controlling breathing is often inappropriately thought of as autonomic. To the contrary, breathing shares features with somatic motor behaviors, such as lifting, locomotion, or visual saccades (i.e., it exhibits volitional control, and is mediated by spinal alpha motor neurons acting on striated skeletal muscle). As with other motor control systems, respiratory motor control exhibits considerable plasticity, meaning a change in future system performance based on experience,[1] and *meta*plasticity, or plastic plasticity.[2–4] In recent years, considerable progress has been made toward an understanding of cellular mechanisms giving rise to *spinal* respiratory plasticity.[1] One frequently studied model of spinal respiratory plasticity is phrenic long-term facilitation (pLTF), a prolonged increase in phrenic nerve activity following exposure to acute intermittent hypoxia (AIH).[5–8]

Spinal cord injury (SCI) disrupts motor output and causes paralysis below the site of injury.

Thus, ventilatory failure is the most frequent cause of death following cervical spinal injury.[9] An important goal of SCI research is to harness plasticity, restoring respiratory (and somatic) motor function via enhancement of spared synaptic pathways to motor neurons below the site of injury.[10] Using a similar approach, it may be possible to restore breathing capacity in cases of ventilatory compromise arising from diverse etiologies including spinal injury, motor neuron disease, and obstructive sleep apnea.[11] Despite differences in the pathogenesis of these disorders, each shares a common therapeutic goal: increased synaptic strength onto respiratory motor neurons via spontaneous and/or induced neuroplasticity.[11]

Considerable effort in our laboratory is focused on strengthening synaptic pathways to respiratory motor neurons via physiological or pharmacological approaches. We have recently come to realize that multiple, distinct signaling pathways give rise to long-lasting phrenic motor facilitation (PMF) via spinal mechanisms.[12–15] The most frequently studied model of PMF has been AIH-induced pLTF.[7,8,16]

doi: 10.1111/j.1749-6632.2010.05499.x

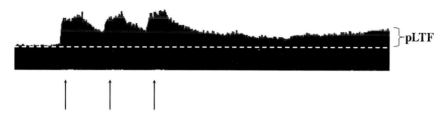

Figure 1. Compressed phrenic neurogram showing phrenic long-term facilitation (pLTF; *bracket*) following acute intermittent hypoxia. Compressed 1.5 h time scale shows the short-term hypoxic responses (dramatic increase in phrenic amplitude) during three hypoxic episodes (*arrows*). pLTF results from these intermittent hypoxic episodes and is an example of the Q pathway to PMF.

In brief, pLTF requires spinal serotonin type 2 receptor activation, new synthesis of BDNF, activation of the high-affinity BDNF receptor, TrkB, and then ERK MAP kinase signaling.[12,17] We refer to this signaling cascade as the "Q pathway" to PMF because serotonin type 2 receptors are metabotropic receptors coupled to Gq proteins, and other Gq protein coupled metabotropic receptors elicit similar PMF.[15]

In contrast, activation of Gs protein coupled metabotropic receptors, such as adenosine 2A or serotonin type 7 receptors, elicits long-lasting PMF via a unique mechanism independent of BDNF synthesis. This mechanism requires new synthesis of an immature TrkB isoform, and phosphoinositide 3 (PI3) kinase/protein kinase B signaling.[13,17] We refer to this signaling cascade as the "S pathway" because multiple metabotropic receptors coupled to Gs proteins elicit the same effect.[15] The S pathway does not contribute to AIH-induced pLTF under normal circumstances.[14] In fact, the S pathway appears to inhibit the Q pathway following AIH, attenuating AIH-induced pLTF via cross-talk inhibition.[14]

Both the S and Q pathways to PMF have potential to induce functional recovery following SCI via pharmacological interventions.[11] However, in this review, we focus on the potential for intermittent hypoxia (and therefore the Q pathway) to enhance ventilatory capacity following chronic cervical spinal injury since it has been investigated more thoroughly.

Phrenic long-term facilitation

pLTF was originally described as a persistent increase in phrenic motor output following repeated stimulation of the carotid sinus nerve.[18,19] Similar pLTF is also observed following repeated hypoxic episodes (see Fig. 1).[7,16] pLTF requires spinal serotonin type 2 receptor activation for its induction, but not maintenance.[12,20] Conversely, intra-spinal injections of serotonin or 5-HT2 receptor agonists are sufficient to elicit PMF without hypoxia.[21] Downstream from (type 2) serotonin receptor activation, pLTF requires new BDNF synthesis,[22] activation of its high-affinity receptor (TrkB),[22] and the activation of ERK MAP kinases.[17,23] Events downstream from TrkB/ERK activation are unclear, but may involve phosphorylation and insertion of glutamate receptors at the synapse between premotor and respiratory motor neurons,[7,24–26] changes in motor neuron excitability,[1] or effects on spinal interneurons.[27] Aspects of our working cellular model of pLTF are shown in Figure 2.

pLTF is pattern-sensitive since intermittent, but not sustained, hypoxia elicits its underlying mechanism.[28] Details of the intermittent hypoxia protocol seem relatively unimportant because the magnitude of pLTF is similar with hypoxic episodes ranging from 15 sec to 5 min in duration,[29,30] and from 28 to nearly 70 mmHg arterial PO_2.[8,24,30] Thus, the intermittent pattern is more important than the duration or severity of hypoxia. Serotonin receptor activation is both necessary and sufficient to elicit PMF,[12,21] and serotonin-induced PMF exhibits pattern sensitivity similar to hypoxia.[21] Thus, pLTF pattern-sensitivity may arise "downstream" from serotonin receptor activation versus hypoxia per se. Similar pattern sensitivity is characteristic of other models of serotonin-dependent neuroplasticity, including serotonin-induced facilitation of *Aplysia* sensory-motor synapses[31,32] and *in vitro* LTF in neonatal XII motor neurons.[26]

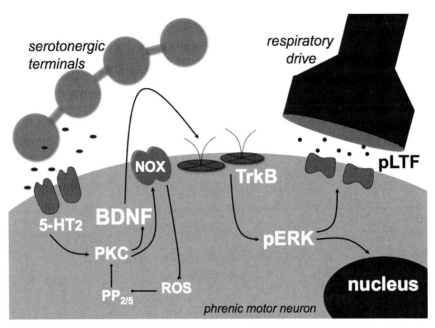

Figure 2. Working model of cellular mechanisms giving rise to pLTF. Intermittent activation of serotonergic 5-HT2 receptors during hypoxic episodes activates protein kinase C (PKC). This, in turn, initiates new BDNF protein synthesis and increases NADPH oxidase (NOX) activity. After BDNF binds its high-affinity receptor, TrkB, downstream signaling molecules include ERK MAP kinases. Although less clear, we suggest that ERK activity increases synaptic strength between descending respiratory pre-motor neurons and phrenic motor neurons, thereby expressing pLTF. Protein phosphatases (PP2A/5) normally constrain pLTF. However, ROS formation via NADPH oxidase activity inhibits these phosphatases and relieves their inhibitory constraint to pLTF. When this pathway is activated chronically, we propose that increased gene transcription occurs (i.e., in the cell nucleus), enhancing the expression of elements critical in this form of plasticity. For further detail, see text.

Although we do not yet have a complete understanding of mechanisms giving rise to pattern sensitivity in AIH-induced pLTF or serotonin-induced PMF, considerable progress has been made in recent years.[33–37] Our working model is that repetitive serotonin release in the phrenic motor nucleus activates nicotinamide adenine dinucleotide phosphate (NADPH) oxidase, thereby increasing reactive oxygen species (ROS) formation. ROS, in turn, inhibit the activity of okadaic acid-sensitive serine/threonine protein phosphatases that normally constrain pLTF expression.[21,34,35] NADPH oxidase and protein phosphatase 2A appear to constitute a "regulatory cassette" that regulates pLTF expression and confers its pattern sensitivity because: (1) okadaic acid-sensitive phosphatases constrain pLTF during sustained, but not intermittent hypoxia[36]; (2) ROS[34,35] and NADPH oxidase activity[37] are necessary for pLTF; and (3) pLTF can be rescued in

rats with suppressed ROS levels by spinal okadaic acid administration.[36] The relevant ROS production arises from repeated serotonin receptor activation, because serotonin-induced PMF requires NADPH oxidase activity.[21]

Collectively, these data demonstrate that intermittent (versus sustained) hypoxia and/or spinal serotonin receptor activation have the requisite properties to initiate spinal plasticity of potential relevance in the treatment of SCI. However, unique properties become apparent following repeated exposure to intermittent hypoxia.

Repetitive intermittent hypoxia

Considerable research has focused on extreme protocols of intermittent hypoxia (frequent episodes for ~8–12 h per day over many days to weeks) due to interest in the pathophysiological consequences of

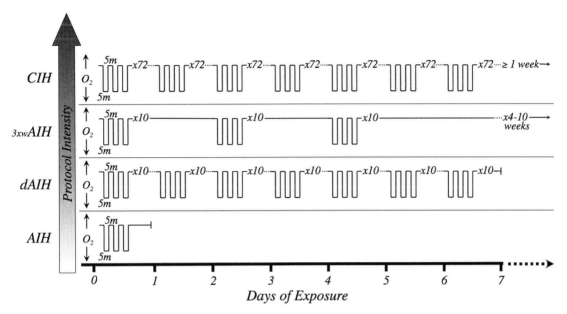

Figure 3. Experimental protocols of intermittent hypoxia vary in their duration and intensity. The most limited protocol, acute intermittent hypoxia (AIH), elicits pLTF in short-time domains. Daily AIH (dAIH) involves 10 hypoxic episodes per day for 7 days. Thrice weekly AIH (3×wAIH) involves 10 episodes per day, 3 days per week for 4–10 weeks. These intermediate protocols of repetitive AIH upregulate key "plasticity proteins" involved in pLTF and confer metaplasticity to phrenic motor output. Whereas chronic intermittent hypoxia (CIH) also elicits spinal plasticity and metaplasticity, its intensity (72 episodes of hypoxia per day for 7–14 days) causes deleterious side effects such as hypertension and learning disabilities.

sleep disordered breathing.[38] Although such chronic intermittent hypoxia (CIH) protocols elicit robust spinal plasticity,[39] pathophysiological effects make CIH unsuitable as a therapeutic tool in cases of spinal injury. More modest protocols of intermittent hypoxia (Fig. 3) may trigger spinal plasticity without adverse side effects.

Acute intermittent hypoxia (AIH; 3–10 hypoxic episodes in <2 h) elicits spinal plasticity of relatively short duration (see discussion of pLTF earlier). To prolong and enhance AIH effects, we use repetitive AIH, including daily exposure for 1 week (dAIH)[23] or three times per week for 4–10 weeks (3×wAIH).[40,41] Although the optimal protocols are not yet known, dAIH and 3×wAIH both elicit spinal plasticity without obvious adverse consequences and, thus, may be useful in the treatment of chronic SCI.[42]

Chronic intermittent hypoxia

CIH elicits plasticity at multiple sites of the respiratory control system, including increased: (1) carotid body chemosensitivity,[29,43] (2) synaptic strength in the nucleus tractus solitarius,[44] and (3) synaptic strength in spinal pathways to phrenic motor neurons.[39] Pretreatment with CIH also elicits metaplasticity, or plastic plasticity.[2–4] Examples of respiratory metaplasticity include: (1) enhanced AIH-induced pLTF[45,46] and (2) revelation of a unique form of sensory long-term facilitation in carotid chemo-afferent neurons, an effect not expressed in naïve rats.[29,47] Although each of these forms of plasticity/metaplasticity may enhance respiratory function, only spinal plasticity has the potential to elicit functional recovery below the site of injury because "upstream" regions (e.g., medulla) are effectively blocked from communication due to the injury itself.

Offsetting the potential benefits of CIH-induced spinal plasticity, deleterious side effects may result from such severe protocols including hypertension,[48] impaired baroreflex control of heart rate,[49] neurocognitive deficits,[50] and metabolic syndrome.[51]

Repetitive acute intermittent hypoxia

dAIH consists of 10, 5-min hypoxic episodes with 5-min intervals per day for 7 days.[23,52,53] dAIH increases ventral cervical BDNF protein levels, particularly within phrenic motor neurons, and increases ERK phosphorylation following AIH,[23] an effect associated with spinal plasticity. These effects were observed without evidence of hypertension.[23] 3×wAIH consists of 10 episodes per day, 3 days per week for 10 weeks. 3×wAIH also upregulates proteins critical for plasticity in phrenic motor neurons, including BDNF, TrkB, phospho-ERK1/2, and phospho-Akt.[54] 3×wAIH increases serotonin terminal density within the phrenic motor nucleus and serotonin 2A receptor expression on presumptive phrenic motor neurons.[54] In association, 3×wAIH enhances AIH-induced pLTF, similar to CIH (threefold increase),[41] demonstrating that repetitive AIH elicits spinal plasticity *and* metaplasticity.

Collectively, these observations in normal rats are consistent with the possibility that repetitive AIH may be an effective treatment to improve respiratory function following cervical spinal injury. However, of considerable interest, we observed similar changes in nonrespiratory motor neurons from regions of the spinal cord not associated with respiratory motor control.[40] Thus, intermittent hypoxia may also enable plasticity in nonrespiratory motor neurons and, potentially, improve nonrespiratory motor function following chronic SCI.

Intermittent hypoxia and SCI

Upper cervical SCI affects both respiratory and somatic motor systems. Because SCI is generally not complete, there is considerable potential to strengthen spared spinal synaptic pathways as a therapeutic approach.[10] One frequently studied experimental model of SCI is C2 cervical hemisection (C2HS), which enables study of normally "silent" crossed-spinal synaptic pathways to phrenic motor neurons.[55] Following C2HS, some spontaneous recovery of phrenic (and diaphragm) activity below the injury is observed over weeks or months, an effect known as the "crossed phrenic phenomenon."[55] However, spontaneous recovery is limited, and therapeutic strategies that further strengthen these pathways would be of considerable benefit.[11,42] Thus, intermittent hypoxia has considerable potential as a

therapeutic approach in persons with high cervical SCI.

Acute intermittent hypoxia

Two weeks following C2HS, rats exposed to AIH do not express pLTF on the side of injury.[56] However, by 8 weeks postinjury, robust AIH-induced pLTF is observed.[56] Because serotonergic innervation of the phrenic motor nucleus decreases dramatically 2 weeks post-C2HS, but substantially recovers by 8 weeks, the capacity to express pLTF may be limited by this phenomenon. On the side opposite C2HS, limited capacity for pLTF is observed, even 8 weeks post-C2HS,[57] suggesting that compensatory responses to unilateral cervical SCI prevent pLTF expression in contralateral phrenic motoneurons. However, the capacity to express contralateral pLTF is restored by pretreatment with dAIH.[58] One important point from these studies is that the ability to induce spinal plasticity via intermittent hypoxia is limited shortly after SCI, but recovers progressively with serotonergic innervation below the site of injury. Thus, intermittent hypoxia may be most effective therapeutically in cases of chronic (versus acute) SCI. On the other hand, spontaneous compensation may limit the capacity for induced plasticity in fully intact motor pools (e.g., side opposite C2HS).

Chronic intermittent hypoxia

Even 2 weeks post-C2HS, CIH strengthens crossed-spinal synaptic pathways to phrenic motor neurons.[39] Thus, more robust protocols of intermittent hypoxia may overcome limitations caused by reduced serotonergic innervation within the phrenic motor nucleus. CIH may induce spinal plasticity through "brute force" due to the greater number of hypoxic episodes, but this ability may also relate to an upregulation of relevant serotonin receptors (5-HT2A) within the phrenic motor pool.[59]

Repetitive AIH

We have treated rats with dAIH beginning 1 week post-C2HS and demonstrated considerable potential for induced functional recovery of breathing capacity.[52,53] Specifically, dAIH nearly restored the capacity to increase tidal volume during hypercapnia,[52] increased spontaneous phrenic motor output at graded levels of hypercapnia, and increased spinally evoked potentials ipsilateral and contralateral to injury.[53] Similarly, in rats treated with dAIH 1 week post-C2HS, AIH-induced pLTF was observed contralateral to injury, suggesting that repetitive AIH can restore ventilatory capacity (i.e., plasticity) and enhance the potential for additional plasticity (i.e., metaplasticity). We have not yet performed $3\times$wAIH on rats with cervical spinal injury; such experiments are currently under way.

In addition to respiratory plasticity, preliminary observations suggest that intermittent hypoxia also induces plasticity in nonrespiratory motor behaviors in persons with incomplete, chronic, cervical spinal injuries.[60] Collectively, the demonstrated ability of intermittent hypoxia to induce functional recovery of breathing capacity (and possibly limb movements) following cervical spinal injury is exciting, and suggests that further exploration of this area is warranted.

The S pathway and SCI

Although our best evidence to date indicates that the S pathway inhibits the Q pathway to PMF following AIH,[14] these interactions may change during chronic disturbances, such as repetitive AIH or SCI. It remains to be explored if the S pathway contributes to plasticity induced by repetitive AIH in normal rats, or if it plays a greater role following SCI. From another perspective, knowledge that both the Q and S pathways are capable of inducing PMF suggests additional therapeutic strategies for patients with SCI. For example, drugs known to activate the S pathway may be of benefit, restoring respiratory, and/or nonrespiratory motor function following acute or chronic SCI.[13]

Conclusion

Because plasticity is an important feature of the respiratory control system, we are interested in understanding and harnessing these intrinsic mechanisms to strengthen synaptic connections and induce functional recovery following spinal injury. We have only recently come to realize that intermittent hypoxia increases phrenic motor output via spinal plasticity, and that this plasticity may restore breathing capacity in rodents with impaired breathing function.[11] This exciting line of research has considerable potential to develop novel therapeutic approaches to devastating ventilatory control disorders with few effective treatments and no known cures (e.g., spinal injury, ALS, or obstructive sleep apnea).

Acknowledgments

This work was supported by grants from NIH HL69064, HL80209, and NS05777. Trainee support was provided by NIH training grants (T32 HL07654 to MRLB and F31 HL092785 to MSH), the Francis Family Foundation (PM), and the Craig H. Neilsen Foundation (SV).

Conflicts of interest

The authors declare no conflicts of interest; NIH funded.

References

1. Mitchell, G.S. & S.M. Johnson. 2003. Neuroplasticity in respiratory motor control. *J. Appl. Physiol.* **94:** 358–374.

2. Abraham, W.C. & M.F. Bear. 1996. Metaplasticity: the plasticity of synaptic plasticity. *Trends Neurosci.* **19:** 126–130.

3. Byrne, J.H. 1997. Plastic plasticity. *Nature* **389:** 791–792.

4. Kim, J.J. & K.S. Yoon. 1998. Stress: metaplastic effects in the hippocampus. *Trends Neurosci.* **21:** 505–509.

5. Mitchell, G.S. *et al.* 2001. Invited review: intermittent hypoxia and respiratory plasticity. *J. Appl. Physiol.* **90:** 2466–2475.

6. Feldman, J.L., G.S. Mitchell & E.E. Nattie. 2003. Breathing: rhythmicity, plasticity and chemosensitivity. *Ann. Rev. Neurosci.* **26:** 239–266.

7. Mahamed, S. & G.S. Mitchell. 2007. Is there a link between intermittent hypoxia-induced respiratory plasticity and obstructive sleep apnoea? *Exp. Physiol.* **92:** 27–37.

8. Baker-Herman, T.L. & G.S. Mitchell. 2008. Determinants of frequency long-term facilitation following acute intermittent hypoxia in vagotomized rats. *Respir. Physiol. Neurobiol.* **162:** 8–17.

9. Frankel, H.L. *et al.* 1998. Long-term survival in spinal cord injury: a fifty year investigation. *Spinal Cord* **36:** 266–274.

10. Ramer, M.S., G.P. Harper & E.J. Bradbury. 2000. Progress in spinal cord research—a refined strategy for the International Spinal Research Trust. *Spinal Cord* **38:** 449–472.

11. Mitchell, G.S. 2007. Respiratory plasticity following intermittent hypoxia: a guide for novel therapeutic approaches to ventilatory control disorders. In *Genetic Basis for Respiratory Control Disorders.* C. Gaultier, Ed.: Springer Publishing Company. New York.

12. Baker-Herman, T.L. & G.S. Mitchell. 2002. Phrenic long-term facilitation requires spinal serotonin receptor activation and protein synthesis. *J. Neurosci.* **22:** 6239–6246.

13. Golder, F.J. *et al.* 2008. Spinal adenosine A2a receptor activation elicits long-lasting phrenic motor facilitation. *J. Neurosci.* **28:** 2033–2042.

14. Hoffman, M.S. *et al.* 2009. Spinal adenosine 2A receptor inhibition enhances phrenic long term facilitation following acute intermittent hypoxia. *J. Physiol.* [Epub ahead of print, November 9, 2009, doi: 10.1113/jphysiol.2009.180075].

15. Dale-Nagle, E.A. *et al.* 2010. Multiple pathways to long-lasting phrenic motor facilitation. *Adv. Exp. Med. Biol.* In press.

16. Bach, K.B. & G.S. Mitchell.1996. Hypoxia-induced long-term facilitation of respiratory activity is serotonin dependent. *Respir. Physiol.* **104:** 251–260.

17. Hoffman, M.S. & G.S. Mitchell. 2009. Spinal 5-HT7 receptor agonist induced phrenic motor facilitation requires TrkB signaling. *FASEB J.* **23:** 607.4.

18. Millhorn, D.E., F.L. Eldridge & T.G. Waldrop. 1980. Prolonged stimulation of respiration by a new central neural mechanism. *Respir. Physiol.* **41:** 87–103.

19. Millhorn, D.E., F.L. Eldridge & T.G. Waldrop. 1980. Prolonged stimulation of respiration by endogenous central serotonin. *Respir. Physiol.* **42:** 171–188.

20. Fuller, D.D. *et al.* 2001. Physiological and genomic consequences of intermittent hypoxia: selected contribution: phrenic long-term facilitation requires 5-HT receptor activation during but not following episodic hypoxia. *J. Appl. Physiol.* **90:** 2001–2006.

21. MacFarlane, P.M. & G.S. Mitchell. 2009. Episodic serotonin receptor activation elicits long-lasting phrenic motor facilitation by an NADPH oxidase-dependent mechanism. *J. Physiol.* **587**(Pt 22): 5469–5481.

22. Baker-Herman, T.L. *et al.* 2004. BDNF is necessary and sufficient for spinal respiratory plasticity following intermittent hypoxia. *Nat. Neurosci* **7:** 48–55.

23. Wilkerson, J.E. & G.S. Mitchell. 2009. Daily intermittent hypoxia augments spinal BDNF levels, ERK phosphorylation and respiratory long-term facilitation. *Exp. Neurol.* **217:** 116–123.

24. Fuller, D.D. *et al.* 2000. Long term facilitation of phrenic motor output. *Respir. Physiol.* **121:** 135–146.

25. McGuire, M. *et al.* 2008. Formation and maintenance of ventilatory long term facilitation requires NMDA but not non-NMDA receptors in awake rats. *J. Appl. Physiol.* **105:** 942–950.

26. Bocchiaro, C.M. & J.L. Feldman. 2004. Synaptic activity-independent persistent plasticity in endogenously active

27. Lane, M.A. *et al.* 2009. Spinal circuitry and respiratory recovery following spinal cord injury. *Resp. Phys. Neurobiol.* **169:** 123–132.

28. Baker, T.L. & G.S. Mitchell. 2000. Episodic but not continuous hypoxia elicits long-term facilitation of phrenic motor output in rats. *J. Physiol.* **529:** 215–219.

29. Peng, Y.J. & N.R. Prabhakar. 2004. Effect of two paradigms of chronic intermittent hypoxia on carotid body sensory activity. *J. Appl. Physiol.* **96:** 1236–1242.

30. Mahamed, S. & G.S. Mitchell. 2008. Respiratory long-term facilitation: too much or too little of a good thing? *Adv. Exp. Med. Biol.* **605:** 224–227.

31. Mauelshagen, J., C.M. Sherff & T.J. Carew. 1998. Differential induction of long-term facilitation by spaced and massed applications of serotonin at sensory neuron synapses of *Aplysia californica. Learn. Mem.* **5:** 246–256.

32. Michael, D. *et al.* 1998. Repeated pulses of serotonin required for long-term facilitation activate mitogen activated protein kinase in sensory neurons of *Aplysia. Proc. Natl. Acad. Sci. USA* **95:** 1864–1869.

33. Wilkerson, J.E. *et al.* 2007. Respiratory plasticity following intermittent hypoxia: roles of protein phosphatases and reactive oxygen species. *Biochem. Soc. Trans.* **35:** 1269–1272.

34. MacFarlane, P.M. *et al.* 2008. Reactive oxygen species and respiratory plasticity following intermittent hypoxia. *Respir. Physiol. Neurobiol.* **164:** 263–271.

35. MacFarlane, P.M. & G.S. Mitchell. 2008b. Respiratory long-term facilitation following intermittent hypoxia requires reactive oxygen species formation. *Neuroscience* **152:** 189–197.

36. Wilkerson, J.E. *et al.* 2008. Okadaic acid-sensitive protein phosphatases constrain phrenic long-term facilitation after sustained hypoxia. *J. Neurosci.* **28:** 2949–2958.

37. MacFarlane, P.M. *et al.* 2009. NADPH oxidase activity is necessary for acute intermittent hypoxia-induced phrenic long-term facilitation. *J. Physiol.* **587**(Pt 9): 1931–1942.

38. Gauda, E.B. 2009. Introduction: Sleep-disordered breathing across the life span: exploring human disorder using animal models. *ILAR J.* **50:** 243–247.

39. Fuller, D.D. *et al.* 2003. Synaptic pathways to phrenic motoneurons are enhanced by chronic intermittent hypoxia after cervical spinal cord injury. *J. Neurosci.* **23:** 2993–3000.

40. Satriotomo, I. *et al.* 2009. Repetitive acute intermittent hypoxia increases neurotrophic and growth factor

mammalian motoneurons. *Proc. Nat. Acad. Sci. USA* **101:** 4292–4295.

expression in non-respiratory motor neurons. *FASEB J.* **23:** 791.7.

41. Vinit, S., I. Satriotomo, P.M. MacFarlane & G.S. Mitchell. 2010. Enhanced phrenic long-term facilitation (pLTF) following repetitive acute intermittent hypoxia. *FASEB J.* In press.

42. Vinit, S., M.R. Lovett-Barr & G.S. Mitchell. 2009. Intermittent hypoxia induces functional recovery following cervical spinal injury. *Resp. Phys. & Neurobiol.* **169:** 210–217.

43. Peng, Y. *et al.* 2001. Chronic intermittent hypoxia enhances carotid body chemoreceptor response to low oxygen. *Adv. Exp. Med. Biol.* **499:** 33–38.

44. Kline, D.D., A. Ramirez-Navarro & D.L. Kunze. 2007. Adaptive depression in synaptic transmission in the nucleus of the solitary tract after in vivo chronic intermittent hypoxia: evidence for homeostatic plasticity. *J. Neurosci.* **27:** 4663–4673.

45. Ling, L. *et al.* 2001. Chronic intermittent hypoxia elicits serotonin-dependent plasticity in the central neural control of breathing. *J. Neurosci.* **21:** 5381–5388.

46. McGuire, M. *et al.* 2003. Chronic intermittent hypoxia enhances ventilatory long-term facilitation in awake rats. *J. Physiol.* **95:** 1499–1508.

47. Peng, Y.J. *et al.* 2003. Induction of sensory long-term facilitation in the carotid body by intermittent hypoxia: implications for recurrent apneas. *Proc. Natl. Acad. Sci. USA* **100:** 10073–10078.

48. Fletcher, E.C. *et al.* 1992. Repetitive, episodic hypoxia causes diurnal elevation of blood pressure in rats. *Hypertension* **19:** 555–561.

49. Gu, H. *et al.* 2007. Selective impairment of central mediation of baroreflex in anesthetized young adult Fischer 344 rats after chronic intermittent hypoxia. *Am. J. Physiol. Heart. Circ. Physiol.* **293:** H2809–H2818.

50. Row, B.W. 2007. Intermittent hypoxia and cognitive function: implications from chronic animal models. *Adv. Exp. Med. Biol.* **618:** 51–67.

51. Tasali, E. & M.S. Ip. 2008. Obstructive sleep apnea and metabolic syndrome: alterations in glucose metabolism and inflammation. *Proc. Am. Thorac. Soc.* **5:** 207–217.

52. Barr, M.R.L., C.M. Sibigtroth & G.S. Mitchell. 2007. Daily acute intermittent hypoxia improves respiratory function in rats with chronic cervical spinal hemisection. *FASEB J.* **21:** 918.18, A1292.

53. Barr, M.R.L. *et al.* 2007. Daily acute intermittent hypoxia increases ipsilateral phrenic nerve output in rats with chronic cervical spinal hemisection. *Society for Neuroscience Meeting Abstract, 2007.* 600.23/BB19.

54. Satriotomo, I., E.A. Dale & G.S. Mitchell. 2007. Thrice weekly intermittent hypoxia increases expression of key proteins necessary for phrenic long-term facilitation: a possible mechanism of respiratory metaplasticity? *FASEB J.* **21:** 918.15, A1292.

55. Goshgarian, H.G. 2003. The crossed phrenic phenomenon: a model for plasticity in the respiratory pathways following spinal cord injury. *J. Appl. Physiol.* **94:** 795–810.

56. Golder, F.J. & G.S. Mitchell. 2005. Spinal synaptic enhancement with acute intermittent hypoxia improves respiratory function after chronic cervical spinal cord injury. *J. Neurosci.* **25:** 2925–2932.

57. Doperalski, N.J. & D.D. Fuller. 2006. Long-term facilitation of ipsilateral but not contralateral phrenic output after spinal cord hemisection. *Exp. Neurol.* **200:** 74–81.

58. Vinit, S. & G.S. Mitchell. 2009. dAIH restores phrenic long-term facilitation contralateral to cervical spinal injury. *FASEB J.* **23:** 784.5.

59. Fuller, D.D. *et al.* 2005. Cervical spinal cord injury upregulates ventral spinal 5-HT2A receptors. *J. Neurotrauma* **22:** 203–213.

60. Rymer, Z. *et al.* 2007. Effects of intermittent hypoxia on motor function in persons with incomplete SCI. *Society for Neuroscience Abstract* 82.18/LL2.

Ann. N.Y. Acad. Sci. ISSN 0077-8923

ANNALS OF THE NEW YORK ACADEMY OF SCIENCES
Issue: *Neurons and Networks in the Spinal Cord*

Protecting motor networks during perinatal ischemia: the case for delta-opioid receptors

Stephen M. Johnson and Sara M.F. Turner

Department of Comparative Biosciences, School of Veterinary Medicine, University of Wisconsin, Madison, Wisconsin

Address for correspondence: Stephen M. Johnson, Department of Comparative Biosciences, School of Veterinary Medicine, University of Wisconsin, 2015 Linden Drive, Madison, WI 53706. johnsons@svm.vetmed.wisc.edu

Perinatal ischemia is a common clinical problem with few successful therapies to prevent neuronal damage. Delta opioid receptor (DOR) activation is a versatile, evolutionarily conserved, endogenous neuroprotective mechanism that blocks several steps in the deleterious cascade of neurological events during ischemia. DOR activation prior to ischemia or severe hypoxia is neuroprotective in spinal motor networks, as well as cortical, cerebellar, and hippocampal neural networks. In addition to providing acute and long-lasting neuroprotection against ischemia, DOR activation appears to provide neuroprotection when given before, during, or following the onset of ischemia. Finally, DORs can be upregulated by several physiological and experimental perturbations. Potential adverse side effects affecting motor control, such as respiratory depression and seizures, are not well established in young mammals and may be mitigated by altering drug choice and method of drug administration. The unique features of DOR-dependent neuroprotection make it an attractive potential therapy that may be given to at-risk pregnant mothers shortly before delivery to provide long-lasting neuroprotection against unpredictable perinatal ischemic events.

Keywords: perinatal; ischemia; opioid; neuroprotection

Perinatal ischemia is a general term associated with the loss of blood flow to the CNS during the perinatal period; defined as the 20th week of gestation through the 28th postnatal day in humans.[1] Other diseases that occur in the perinatal period include hypoxic-ischemic encephalopathy (oxygen deficiency in the whole brain), perinatal asphyxia (lack of oxygen to the fetus during labor and delivery), and perinatal stroke (focal disruption of cerebral blood flow due to arterial or venous thrombosis). The net result of these pathological conditions is lack of oxygen (and glucose in some cases) to the brain and spinal cord, which initiates a cascade of events causing neuronal damage and cell death. Very few successful treatments exist for perinatal ischemia in humans despite the long list of successful neuroprotective drugs and treatments in animal preparations. This problem has raised the question as to whether neuroprotection in a clinical setting is possible. Thus, there is a compelling need for new strategies and ideas for treating perinatal ischemia (and related diseases). This review suggests that several factors favor the development

of successful treatments for perinatal ischemia, and that delta opioid receptor (DOR) activation may be a valuable mechanism for providing long-lasting neuroprotection during ischemia or hypoxia in the CNS and especially in motor networks.

Perinatal ischemia in the clinic

Perinatal ischemia is caused by a wide variety of clinical conditions, such as thrombosis,[2] perinatal ischemic stroke,[2] placental insufficiency,[3] respiratory or cardiac failure,[3] forceps application,[4] dysfunctional labor,[4] inappropriate use of maternal drugs causing pharmacologically induced fetal depression,[4] and birth asphyxia.[5] Perinatal stroke or birth asphyxia occur at rates of 1 per 2300–5000 and 9.4 per 1000 live births, respectively,[6–8] whereas hypoxic-ischemic encephalopathy occurs at a rate of 1.4 per 1000 live births.[8] Perinatal ischemia can lead to life-long conditions such as serious motor disabilities, seizure disorders, cerebral palsy, and respiratory difficulties.[3,9–11] In one study of 46 neonates with hypoxic-ischemic encephalopathy, 44% of

doi: 10.1111/j.1749-6632.2010.05434.x

surviving children had significantly delayed motor abilities.[11] A retrospective study of children with perinatal spinal cord injury suggests that ischemia accounts for ~23% of spinal cord injuries, but that spinal cord injury in the perinatal period is likely an underdiagnosed clinical condition.[12] Thus, perinatal ischemia can produce damage to central motor networks as well as cortical networks involved in higher cognitive functions. Hypothermia is the only treatment routinely used in term infants with moderate to severe encephalopathy to decrease excitatory neurotransmitter release, free radical production, edema, neutrophil infiltration, and cytokine release.[13] Hypothermic protection, however, depends on body size (smaller patients are more susceptible to overcooling) and cooling is tissue-dependent (cortex needs more cooling than deep gray matter).[14] Tailoring cooling treatment to each patient is a challenge and can only be used postnatally. Thus, no treatment for perinatal ischemia exists that is effective, standard, and readily administered throughout the entire perinatal period.

Ischemia-induced cascade

Reduced blood flow to the brain impairs delivery of oxygen and glucose, which reduces ATP availability, and initiates a harmful cascade of events (Fig. 1). Loss of ATP results in dysfunctional ATP-dependent ion channels and ion exchangers in the plasma membrane, such as the sodium–potassium pump. Deterioration of sodium and potassium gradients causes neurons to depolarize and release excessive amounts of neurotransmitters, especially excitatory amino acids such as glutamate and aspartate. During ischemia, extracellular glutamate concentrations can increase by 3–10-fold and cause increased influx of sodium and calcium ions via postsynaptic glutamate receptor activation.[15] Postsynaptic glutamate receptors differentially mediate ischemic injury in the perinatal brain.[15] Cortical injury is mediated mostly by NMDA receptors whereas brainstem injury is mainly AMPA receptor-dependent.[16] The influx of sodium and calcium ions produces further neuronal depolarization (positive feedback) and causes water to enter neurons to cause brain swelling. Also, excitotoxic injury is enhanced by impaired energy-dependent glutamate reuptake mechanisms. Along with glutamatergic excitotoxicity and calcium influx, there is free radical attack

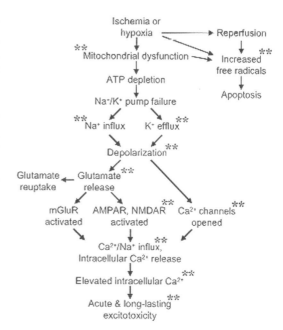

Figure 1. Ischemia or severe hypoxia reduces ATP production and initiates a cascade of events that leads to neuronal damage or death. Experimental evidence shows that DOR activation has the capacity to attenuate or block several steps in the cascade. **Indicates a step that is disrupted by DOR activation.

and prolonged seizure activity, which causes further neuronal damage.[17] Following the initial excitotoxic injury and loss of synaptic connectivity,[15] inflammation and apoptosis increase over hours to days and neurotrophic factors are downregulated,[17,18] hindering the neurons' ability to repair or regenerate.

Neuroprotection against perinatal ischemia

The ischemic cascade in the brain is well understood based on data from several mammalian models. However, translating animal model results to clinical practice has proven to be highly problematic.[19] In animal studies, neuroprotective drugs are typically given in healthy rats shortly after (or prior to) administering the ischemic insult (usually blood vessel occlusion) that results in a reproducible ischemic lesion. In contrast for human clinical trials, neuroprotective drugs are given at various times following strokes that produced highly variable brain lesions in aged humans who often have significant comorbidity. Also, brain reperfusion is usually well controlled in animal studies, whereas reperfusion in humans is left to chance (except for studies testing thrombolytic drugs). Similarly, it is difficult to attain therapeutic levels of neuroprotective agents within the poorly perfused brain tissue. Animal studies often use infarct volume as an outcome measure whereas human clinical trials focus on functional outcomes.[20] Finally, it is difficult to correlate ages of experimental animals to humans based on developmental neuronal landmarks and behaviors. For example, a detailed analysis of neurodevelopmental events suggests that a P14 rat corresponds most closely to a G211 human fetus, which represents the early third trimester.[21]

Accordingly, expectations and goals for neuroprotection research need to be adjusted to reflect these realities. Although ischemic events during the perinatal period are unpredictable, a woman in labor represents a clearly defined time when the mother and fetus are at risk for ischemic events that tend to occur during delivery and early postnatal life. Thus, it may be possible to prophylactically administer a drug combination to women to provide neuroprotection for the fetus before, during, and after parturition. Alternatively, a neuroprotective drug combination could be developed that would be available during an otherwise healthy delivery for use at the first sign of an ischemic event. The ideal neuroprotective agent against perinatal ischemia should be easy to administer, rapidly absorbed, and able to cross the placental and fetal blood–brain barriers with minimal or no adverse side effects. The ideal agent should also activate endogenous neuroprotective mechanisms, disrupt the ischemic cascade at multiple points, and provide long-lasting (>24 h) protection no matter if given before, during, or after an unexpected perinatal ischemic event.

DOR-dependent neuroprotection

DOR activation is a unique form of neuroprotection because it appears to be a highly conserved, inducible mechanism, which is used by vertebrate extremophiles (e.g., mammalian hibernators and hypoxia resistant vertebrates). Also, DOR-dependent protection is observed in various tissues other than brain, which makes it an attractive candidate for providing systemic protection during whole-body ischemia or hypoxia. The key features of DOR-dependent neuroprotection are discussed below.

DOR-dependent neuroprotection in extremophile vertebrates

Hibernating animals exemplify natural tolerance to oxygen, blood, or energy deprivation.[22] During hibernation, blood flow to the brain is severely reduced but central neurons remain viable[23] and cardiorespiratory function is still regulated during torpor.[24] Hibernation-induced neuroprotection is not simply due to colder brain temperatures, but appears to be due to increased resistance to ischemic conditions.[24] In summer active ground squirrels, intravenous infusion of DADLE (DOR agonist) induces hibernation.[25] Similarly, injections of Deltorphin-D$_{variant}$ (DOR agonist) as well as hibernating woodchuck plasma injected into mice induced neuroprotection prior to undergoing focal ischemia.[26] Similarly, hypoxia-resistant red-eared slider turtles can hold their breath for up to 48 h.[27] This ability is hypothesized, in part, to be due to endogenous DOR activation because hypoxia-resistant red eared slider turtles have greater DOR expression in the CNS compared to rats[28] and endogenous DOR activation protects against NMDA-dependent excitotoxicity in anoxic turtle cortical slices.[29]

DOR drugs disrupt several steps in the acute ischemic cascade

The goal of influencing multiple, complex, signaling pathways simultaneously over different time frames is unlikely to be achieved by a single drug. Thus, some argue for the introduction of pleiotropic drugs (i.e., single drugs that produce multiple effects) for the treatment of ischemia-reperfusion damage.[30] DOR agonist drugs are pleiotropic because they disrupt several steps in the acute phases of the ischemic cascade (see asterisks in Fig. 1) via different mechanisms (Table 1). For example, DOR activation decreases Na^+ and Ca^{2+} influx and decreases neuronal depolarization,[31–34] which attenuates a key part of the acute ischemic positive feedback loop shown in Figure 1. DOR activation also decreases K^+ efflux from ischemic cortical neurons,[33,35] which protects local network from further K^+-dependent depolarization due to excessive K^+ ions in the extracellular space. It is hypothesized that the gain from protecting the local neuronal network via decreased K^+ efflux overrides the advantage of having individual neurons undergo protective hyperpolarization via K^+ efflux.[33,35] Further down in the

Table 1. Potential mechanisms underlying DOR-dependent neuroprotection

Ischemic cascade event	DOR-dependent action	Key features	References
Mitochondrial depolarization	K_{ATP} channel activation	Protects cultured cortical neurons against sodium azide-induced mitochondrial respiratory chain injury and maintains DOR levels.	38
Na^+ influx	Decreases Na^+ influx	Blocks voltage-gated Na^+ channels and reduces Na^+ influx via NMDA channels in cortical slices exposed to anoxia.	31, 32
K^+ efflux	Decreases K^+ efflux	Attenuates K^+ efflux from cortical slices exposed to anoxia or OGD via PKC-dependent, PKA-independent pathway.	33, 35
		Inhibition of Ca^{2+} influx reduces activation of Ca^{2+}-activated K^+ (BK) channels in cortical slices exposed to anoxia.	33
Ca^{2+} influx	Decreases Ca^{2+} influx	Indirect evidence of reduced Ca^{2+} influx cortical slices exposed to anoxia.	33
		Hypoxia-induced Ca^{2+} influx reduced in adrenal medulla cells by decreasing voltage-gated Ca^{2+} currents.	34
Increased glutamate release	Inhibits glutamate release presynaptically	Decreased amplitude of AMPA EPSCs/EPSPs in lamina II of lumbar spinal cord slices without altering responses to pressure-ejected AMPA.	36
		Decreased frequency, but not amplitude, of mEPSCs in amygdala slices.	37
Increased AMPA and NMDA receptor activation	Decreases NMDA-dependent currents	Reduces Na^+ influx via NMDA channels in cortical slices exposed to anoxia.	32
		Reduces NMDA currents during anoxia in turtle cortical slices.	29
Increased free radical production	Decreases free radical release or impact	Hypoxic preconditioning attenuates decrease in antioxidant scavengers and increase in oxidant proteins via DOR-dependent mechanism in retinal cells.	39
		DOR agonist drug acts as free radical scavenger.	40
		DOR agonist and plasma from hibernating woodchuck reduces nitric oxide release in microglia cell culture via DOR mechanism.	26

ischemic cascade, DOR decreases excitatory synaptic transmission via presynaptic mechanisms,[36,37] postsynaptic mechanisms,[29,32] and reduction of Na^+ and Ca^{2+} influx.[31–34] Finally, DOR activation maintains intracellular homeostasis by decreasing mitochondrial respiratory chain injury (induced by sodium azide)[38] and decreasing intracellular free radical generation.[26,39,40] Although some mechanistic features may be tissue-specific and species-specific, Table 1 illustrates DOR agonists' capacity to attenuate multiple deleterious ischemic events at several membrane and intracellular sites. During clinical perinatal ischemic events, DOR agonists will likely need to be used in combination with other drugs that complement DOR-activation's beneficial effects.

Role of DOR in neuroprotective preconditioning treatments

Animals or tissues that are exposed to sublethal ischemic challenges become resistant to subsequent severe ischemic exposures due to a process referred to as preconditioning. Ischemic preconditioning in the brain represents a form of endogenous neuroprotection that can be triggered by numerous factors and involves several signaling pathways.[41,42] Although DOR activation is required for the expression of ischemic preconditioning in the heart,[43] there are currently no examples of DOR activation involvement in neuronal ischemic preconditioning. On the other hand, DORs are involved in hypoxic preconditioning where animal or tissue hypoxia is used to induce neuroprotection against lethal challenges. For example, hypoxia (1% O_2 for 30 min) applied 30 min before glutamate-induced excitotoxicity attenuates neuronal damage in cultured cortical neurons, an effect that is blocked by prior application of a DOR antagonist.[44] Also, hypoxic preconditioning (5% O_2 for 6 h) in cultured cortical neurons increased DOR expression and reduced damage to sustained hypoxic exposures.[45] Finally, hypoxia-induced preconditioning in rat retinal cells requires the increased expression and activation of DORs for neuroprotection against later ischemia.[39] Thus, hypoxic preconditioning in neurons induces a DOR-dependent neuroprotection.

DOR activation provides long-lasting neuroprotection

In addition to protecting against acute excitotoxicity during ischemia, DOR activation attenuates signaling pathways that continue for hours to days after the initial ischemic event. For example, Tan-67 (DOR agonist) administration 24 h prior to OGD solution (ischemia-like solutions that lack oxygen and glucose) application reduces cell death in organotypic hippocampal cell cultures.[46] Similarly, Tan-67 administration 24 h prior to right middle cerebral artery occlusion reduces infarct size and improves functional outcome.[46] Thus, DOR activation can induce neuroprotection lasting for at least one day.

DORs are expressed in developing mammals

DORs are expressed in neonatal rat spinal cord[47] and DOR-dependent neuroprotection is demonstrated in neonatal rat spinal cord (see below). Binding affinities for DOR in the rat brain or spinal cord are constant or increase from the first postnatal day[47–49] and DOR expression is postulated to increase 40-fold between neonates and adults.[50] The location of DORs in the neonatal rat spinal cord is not known, but DOR immunoreactivity is located in the ventral horn of adult rat spinal cords.[51] Thus, the substrate for DOR-dependent neuroprotection is present in the neonatal spinal cord, and may be located both pre- and postsynaptically in the ventral horn throughout development. Unfortunately, very little is known about the density or location of DOR expression in perinatal human brain and spinal cord. For example, radioligand binding studies show that DOR (and MOR) binding sites appear in the gray matter of human spinal cord at 14 weeks gestation and increase in density with maturation.[52] In cerebellum from human infants (gestational age 28–38 weeks) that died within 1 h to 19 days after birth, DORs are 7.8 more abundant compared to DORs from adult human cerebellum.[53] These data suggest that DORs are expressed in human infant brain and spinal cord, and potentially at high levels during the perinatal period in some parts of the brain. It's also important to note that these studies measured DORs using radioligand binding techniques because the anti-DOR antibodies used in immunocytochemical studies likely cross-react with an unidentified molecule instead of DORs.[54]

DOR agonist drugs cross the blood–brain and placental barriers

Any DOR agonist that proves to be neuroprotective has to reach its target tissues in the brain and spinal cord. For peptidergic DOR agonists, the placental and fetal blood–brain barriers represent significant obstacles to cross before activating central DORs. However, the peptidergic DOR agonist DPDPE, crosses the blood–brain barrier in rats via a carrier-mediated mechanism,[55] and DPDPE crosses the placental barrier via a paracellular route based on studies in cultured cells.[56] Alternatively, nonpeptidergic synthetic DOR agonists, such as SNC80, Tan-67 and BW373U86, easily cross these barriers and have increased systemic distribution. Thus, lipophilic DOR agonists administered to pregnant mothers or newborn infants will likely reach their target tissues in the CNS.

DOR-dependent neuroprotection in motor networks

Because cortical and hippocampal tissues are highly sensitive to ischemia, most information on DOR-dependent neuroprotection is derived from studies on these tissues. With respect to motor networks, a robust literature on spinal cord ischemia in adults exists due to the problem of spinal cord ischemia occurring during surgical aortic aneurysm repair. Several studies show that ischemic preconditioning is expressed in the spinal cord, but the involvement of DORs is not clear. However, DOR activation alone without hypoxia or ischemia is neuroprotective in the adult spinal cord. For example, intrathecal SNC80 (DOR agonist; 40 mM) protects against spinal cord ischemia when administered 9 min later in adult rat lumbar spinal cord.[57] Forty-eight hours afterwards, hind limb motor function is improved and significantly more neurons are uninjured compared to sham rats.[57] Although DOR activation is neuroprotective in mature spinal cords, it is important to understand how ischemia alters motor network function in younger mammals because perinatal ischemia causes significant morbidity with respect to motor function.

In isolated *in vitro* neonatal rat (P4-P6) preparations, electrically evoked responses in spinal motoneurons are rapidly depressed and abolished within 30 min when exposed to OGD solution.[58] The potential role of DOR activation in providing neuroprotection in the neonatal spinal cord during exposure to OGD solutions is not known. To address this question in our laboratory, the neuroprotective effects of DOR activation on spinal respiratory motor circuits were studied in neonatal rat brainstem-spinal cord preparations.[59] Instead of electrically evoking spinal motoneurons responses, we examined the effects of spinal OGD solutions on spontaneously produced, quantifiable respiratory motor output on cervical and thoracic spinal ventral roots. We tested whether cervical and thoracic respiratory motor output are equally sensitive to OGD, and whether neuroprotection is provided in the following conditions: (1) sustained spinal DOR activation prior to and during spinal OGD, (2) brief spinal DOR activation several minutes prior to spinal OGD (i.e., a form of neuroplasticity), and (3) spinal DOR activation following the onset of OGD exposure. Preliminary data show that cervical and thoracic motoneurons pools are equally sensitive to OGD exposure, and that DOR activation before, during, and after OGD onset prolongs spontaneous respiratory motor output. Thus, DOR-dependent neuroprotection induced in neonatal rat spinal cord protects motor networks controlling breathing.

Potential side effects of DOR activation

There are reports of DOR activation being associated with respiratory depression and seizures, but there is a wide range of conflicting data in the literature that is likely due to differences in species, drug specificity, dosage, method (bolus vs. infusion) and route (intravenous vs. intracerebroventricular) of drug administration, and animal state (awake vs. anesthetized). There is no clear consensus that most DOR agonist drugs cause respiratory depression and seizures in either the mother or offspring during the perinatal period. Even if mild side effects are present following DOR activation, the potential benefits of DOR-dependent neuroprotection during perinatal ischemia are likely to outweigh the consequences. Also, there may be several ways to overcome negative side effects, such as administering the safest and most effective DOR agonists over time in low dosages, or by combining the DOR agonist with other drugs that attenuate or block the side effects.

For respiratory depression in adult mammals, several DOR agonist drugs used in early experiments lacked specificity for DOR and crossed over to activate mu-opioid receptors (which typically depress breathing in mammals).[60] Despite the development of DOR selective drugs, there is still a large variability in respiratory responses to DOR activation. For example, intracerebroventricular injection of DPDPE does not alter respiration rate or blood gases in adult rabbits[61] and decreases arterial pH by only 0.05 pH units in adult rats.[62] Also, BW373U86 (DOR agonist) has no effect on pCO$_2$ levels in awake rats.[63] In pregnant ewes, an intravenous bolus (0.3 mg/kg) of DPDPE (0.3 mg/kg), deltorphin I (DOR agonist), or SNC80 causes respiratory depression in the ewes that lasts for only 15 min and resolves within 30–60 min.[64,65] Thus, the bulk of the evidence suggests that selective DOR activation causes only transient mild respiratory depression in adult mammals.

With respect to younger mammals, studies performed on neonatal rat and fetal sheep have strikingly different results. DPDPE injections (0.1 mg/kg, intraperitoneally) do not cause respiratory depression in P1 neonatal rats, but older pups (P17) have decreased breath amplitude and frequency.[66] Likewise, bath-applied DPDPE does not alter spinal respiratory motor output or bulbospinal respiratory neuronal discharge in neonatal rat (P0–P4) brainstem-spinal cord preparations.[66–68] In contrast, intracerebroventricular infusion of DPDPE or [D-Ala^2]deltorphin I (DOR agonist) in third-trimester fetal lambs increases breath frequency in a dose-dependent manner.[69–71] Thus, DOR activation appears to stimulate breathing movements *in utero*, have little or no effect on breathing in newborns, and cause mild respiratory depression during maturation in juveniles. Testing this hypothesis in several mammalian species, including primates, will be an important step toward understanding how DOR activation alters breathing during early development.

A second adverse side effect attributed to DOR activation is increased neuronal activity, which can lead to seizures or spasticity. In fetal lambs, intracerebroventricular administration of DPDPE stimulates EEG activity, but there were also reports of seizures.[69,70,72] In adult rhesus monkeys, SNC80 administration (10 mg/kg, intramuscular) at doses 3–10-fold greater than that required to produce behavioral effects produced convulsions and EEG seizures in only one of four monkeys.[73] A repeat challenge at the same dosage in the same monkey one year later had no effect. The authors concluded that the 10 mg/kg dosage of SNC80 was, at worst, a threshold dosage for inducing seizures in rhesus monkeys. The only other negative study showed that intrathecal administration of DPDPE in adult rats 30 min after spinal ischemia caused increased spasticity during the 30–60 min period following spinal

ischemia.[74] Although DOR activation increases cortical and spinal activity, the DOR agonist drug dosage that causes significant seizure activity probably depends on species, drug, dosage, and rate/route of drug administration. Thus, it is possible that DOR agonist drug dosages required to provide neuroprotection will be low enough to prevent induction of seizure activity.

Future directions

DOR-dependent neuroprotection holds promise for attenuating ischemic injury to the CNS throughout the perinatal period. Considerable work, however, is required to adequately test this hypothesis and produce meaningful results. One of the most important problems to consider is the choice of animal model and how the ischemic event is experimentally performed. Rodent models are valuable because they are inexpensive and readily available for high throughput studies. Progression to other species, such as sheep and nonhuman primates, should proceed only after careful assessment of the rodent data. For example, it is too laborious and time-consuming to run dose–response curves for several DOR agonist drugs in fetal lambs. The age of the rodent used in high throughput studies, however, is highly critical because newborn rats are not developmentally equivalent to newborn humans. The age of the rodents should be determined after careful consideration of the experimental question and the region of interest to be studied (e.g., cortex vs. spinal cord) because different parts of the CNS mature at different rates. The model of ischemia is also important depending on the experimental question: artery clamping or occlusion mimics stroke, clamping the umbilical artery mimics placental and umbilical cord pathologies, systemic hypoxia can mimic cardiac shunt and asphyxia.

As discussed above, drawing solid conclusions from studies that use a wide range of drugs and drug administration protocols is difficult. The choice of drug (peptide vs. nonpeptidergic synthetic), route of administration (intravenous vs. central), dosage, and timing are all critical to producing the most neuroprotection with the least side effects. Timing is particularly important because clinical conditions that cause perinatal ischemia are highly unpredictable. DOR agonists appear to provide substantial protection whether they are administered before or after the ischemic event, and likely have the ability to induce long-lasting neuroprotection (i.e., neuroplasticity). Therefore, DOR agonists might be administered in low dosages (to minimize side effects) intermittently to elicit long-lasting neuroprotection.

Assessment of neuroprotection needs to shift from morphological to functional experimental approaches. A large portion of the DOR-dependent neuroprotection literature to date has measured the number of live vs. dead cells, or the amount of lactate dehydrogenase released by damaged cells. More recent studies are quantifying behavior, motor function, ion shifts, electrophysiological responses, breathing, and EEG to better understand DOR-dependent effects on intact network function and system physiology.

Finally, a unique promise of the DOR system is the capacity to physiologically upregulate DOR expression and provide greater neuroprotection. Various physiological mechanisms to induce greater DOR expression should be explored and tested. For example, a single bout or several short bouts of mild hypoxia may greatly upregulate DOR expression within hours and last for several days, and thereby allow lower dosages of DOR agonist drugs to be effective. Ideally, such maneuvers may also enhance endogenous DOR-dependent neuroprotection, an area well explored for cardiac muscle, but only recently tested in central neural networks.

Acknowledgment

This work was supported by the National Institute of Neurological Disorders and Stroke (NS-051580).

Conflicts of interest

The authors declare no conflicts of interest; NIH funded.

References

1. Raju, T.N., K.B. Nelson, D. Ferriero, *et al.* 2007. NICHD-NINDS perinatal stroke workshop participants: ischemic perinatal stroke: summary of a workshop sponsored by the National Institute of Neurological Disorders and Stroke. *Pediatrics* **120:** 609–616.

2. Nelson, K.B. 2007. Perinatal ischemic stroke. *Stroke* **38:** 742–745.

3. Badr, L.K. & I. Purdy. 2006. Brain injury in the infant: the old, the new and the uncertain. *J. Perinat. Neonat. Nurs.* **20:** 163–175.

4. Volpe, J.J. 1994. Brain injury in the premature infant–current concepts. *Prev. Med.* **23:** 638–645.

5. Whitelaw, A. & M. Thoresen. 2002. Clinical trials of treatments after perinatal asphyxia. *Curr. Opin. Pediatr.* **14:** 664–668.

6. Legido, A., C.D. Katsetos, O.P. Mishra, *et al.* 2000. Perinatal hypoxic ischemic encephalopathy: current and future treatments. *Intl. Ped.* **15:** 143–151.

7. Laugesaar, R., A. Kolk, T. Tomberg, *et al.* 2007. Acutely and retrospectively diagnosed perinatal stroke: a population-based study. *Stroke* **38:** 2234–2240.

8. Palsdottir, K., A. Dagbjartsson, T. Thorkelsson, *et al.* 2007. Birth asphyxia and hypoxic ischemic encephalopathy, incidence and obstertric risk. *Laeknabladid* **93:** 595–601.

9. Volpe, J.J. 2001. Perinatal brain injury: from pathogenesis to neuroprotection. *Ment. Retard. Dev. Disabil. Res. Rev.* **7:** 56–64.

10. Sotero de Menezes, M., & D.W.W. Shaw. 2006. Hypoxic-ischemic brain injury in the newborn. *eMedicine* April, 1–39.

11. van Schie, P.E.M., J.G. Becher, A.J. Dallmeijer, *et al.* 2007. Motor outcome at the age of one after perinatal hypoxic-ischemic encephalopathy. *Neuropediatrics* **38:** 71–77.

12. Ruggieri, M., A. Smarason & M. Pike. 1999. Spinal cord insults in the prenatal, perinatal, and neonatal periods. *Dev. Med. & Child Neurol.* **41:** 311–317.

13. Barnette, A.R. & T.E. Inder. 2009. Evaluation and management of stroke in the neonate. *Clin. Perinatol.* **36:** 125–136.

14. Robertson, N.J. & O. Iwata. 2007. Bench to bedside strategies for optimizing neuroprotection following perinatal hypoxia-ischemia in high and low resource settings. *Early Hum. Dev.* **83:** 801–811.

15. Sanders, R.D., H.J. Manning, D. Ma, *et al.* 2007. Perinatal neuroprotection. *Curr. Anaesth. Crit. Care* **18:** 215–224.

16. Johnston, M.W. 2005. Excitotoxicity in perinatal brain injury. *Brain Pathol.* **15:** 234–240.

17. Hagberg, H., K. Blomgren & C. Mallard. 2001. Neuroprotection of the fetal and neonatal brain. In *Fetal and Neonatal Neurology and Neurosurgery*. M.I. Levene, F.A. Cherenak, M. Whittle, Eds.: 505–520. 3rd ed. Churchill Livingstone. London.

18. van Bel, F. & F. Groenendaal. 2008. Long-term pharmacologic neuroprotection after birth asphyxia: where do we stand? *Neonatology* **94:** 203–210.

19. Röther, J. 2008. Neuroprotection does not work! *Stroke* **39:** 523–524.

20. Hussain, M.S. & A. Shuaib. 2008. Research into neuro-protection must continue … but with a different approach. *Stroke* **39:** 521–522.

21. Clancy, B., B. Kersh, J. Hyde, *et al.* 2007. Web-based method for translating neurodevelopment from laboratory species to humans. *Neuroinformatics* **5:** 79–94.

22. Borlongan, C.V., Y. Wang & T.P. Su. 2004. Delta opioid peptide [D-Ala2 D-Leu5] enkephalin: linking hibernation and neuroprotection. *Frontiers Biosci.* **9:** 3392–3398.

23. Drew, K.L., M.E. Rice, T.B. Kuhn, *et al.* 2001. Neuroprotective adaptations in hibernation: therapeutic implications for ischemia-reperfusion, traumatic brain injury and neurodegenerative diseases. *Free Radic. Biol. Med.* **31:** 563–573.

24. Drew, K.L., C.L. Buck, B.M. Barnes, *et al.* 2007. Central nervous system regulation of mammalian hibernation: implications for metabolic suppression and ischemia tolerance. *J. Neurochem.* **102:** 1713–1726.

25. Oeltgen, P.R., S.P. Nilekani, P.A. Nuchols, *et al.* 1988. Further studies on opioids and hibernation: delta opioid receptor ligand selectively induced hibernation in summer-active ground squirrels. *Life Sci.* **43:** 1565–1574.

26. Govindaswami, M., S.A. Brown, J. Yu, *et al.* 2008. Delta 2-specific opioid receptor agonist and hibernating woodchuck plasma fraction provide ischemic neuroprotection. *Acad. Emerg. Med.* **15:** 265–266.

27. Musacchia, X. 1959. The viability of Chrysemys picta submerged at various temperatures. *Physiol. Zool.* **32:** 47–50.

28. Xia, Y. & G.G. Haddad. 2001. Major difference in the expression of delta- and mu-opioid receptors between turtle and rat brain. *J. Comp. Neurol.* **436:** 202–210.

29. Pamenter, M.E. & L.T. Buck. 2008. delta-Opioid receptor antagonism induces NMDA receptor-dependent excitotoxicity in anoxic turtle cortex. *J. Exp. Biol.* **211:** 3512–3517.

30. Menger, M.D. & B. Vollmar. 2007. Pathomechanisms of ischemia-reperfusion injury as the basis for novel preventive strategies: is it time for the introduction of pleiotropic compounds? *Transplant Proc.* **39:** 485–488.

31. Chao, D., A. Bazzy-Asaad, G. Balboni, *et al.* 2008. Activation of DOR attenuates anoxic K^+ derangement via inhibition of Na^+ entry in mouse cortex. *Cereb. Cortex.* **18:** 2217–2227.

32. Chao, D., G. Balboni, L.H. Lazarus, *et al.* 2009. Na^+ mechanism of delta-opioid receptor induced protection from anoxic K^+ leakage in the cortex. *Cell Mol. Life Sci.* **66:** 1105–1115.

33. Chao, D., A. Bazzy-Asaad, G. Balboni, *et al.* 2007. delta-, but not mu-, opioid receptor stabilizes $K^{(+)}$ homeostasis

by reducing $Ca(2^+)$ influx in the cortex during acute hypoxia. *J. Cell Physiol.* **212:** 60–67.

34. Keating, D.J., G.Y. Rychkov, M.B. Adams, *et al.* 2004. Opioid receptor stimulation suppresses the adrenal medulla hypoxic response in sheep by actions on $Ca(2^+)$ and $K^{(+)}$ channels. *J. Physiol.* **555:** 489–502.

35. Chao, D., D.F. Donnelly, Y. Feng, *et al.* 2007. Cortical delta-opioid receptors potentiate K+ homeostasis during anoxia and oxygen-glucose deprivation. *J. Cereb. Blood Flow Metab.* **27:** 356–368.

36. Glaum, S.R., R.J. Miller & D.L. Hammond. 1994. Inhibitory actions of delta 1-, delta 2-, and mu-opioid receptor agonists on excitatory transmission in lamina II neurons of adult rat spinal cord. *J. Neurosci.* **14:** 4965–4971.

37. Bie, B., W. Zhu & Z.Z. Pan. 2009. Rewarding morphine-induced synaptic function of delta-opioid receptors on central glutamate synapses. *J. Pharmacol. Exp. Ther.* **329:** 290–296.

38. Zhu, M., M.W. Li, X.S. Tian, *et al.* 2009. Neuroprotective role of delta-opioid receptors against mitochondrial respiratory chain injury. *Brain Res.* **1252:** 183–191.

39. Peng, P.H., H.S. Huang, Y.J. Lee, *et al.* 2009. Novel role for the delta-opioid receptor in hypoxic preconditioning in rat retinas. *J. Neurochem.* **108:** 741–754.

40. Tsao, L.I., B. Ladenheim, A.M. Andrews, *et al.* 1998. Delta opioid peptide [D-Ala2,D-leu5]enkephalin blocks the long-term loss of dopamine transporters induced by multiple administrations of methamphetamine: involvement of opioid receptors and reactive oxygen species. *J. Pharmacol. Exp. Ther.* **287:** 322–331.

41. Davis, D.P. & P.M. Patel. 2003. Ischemic preconditioning in the brain. *Curr. Opin. Anaesthesiol.* **16:** 447–452.

42. Dirnagl, U., R.P. Simon & J.M. Hallenbeck. 2003. Ischemic tolerance and endogenous neuroprotection. *Trends Neurosci.* **26:** 248–254.

43. Gross, G.J. 2003. Role of opioids in acute and delayed preconditioning. *J. Mol. Cell. Cardiol.* **35:** 709–718.

44. Zhang, J., H. Qian, P. Zhao, *et al.* 2006. Rapid hypoxia preconditioning protects cortical neurons from glutamate toxicity through delta-opioid receptor. *Stroke* **37:** 1094–1099.

45. Ma, M.C., H. Qian, F. Ghassemi, *et al.* 2005. Oxygen-sensitive {delta}-opioid receptor-regulated survival and death signals: novel insights into neuronal preconditioning and protection. *J. Biol. Chem.* **280:** 16208–16218.

46. Zhao, P., Y. Huang & Z. Zuo. 2006. Opioid preconditioning induces opioid receptor-dependent delayed neuroprotection against ischemia in rats. *J. Neuropathol. Exp. Neurol.* **65:** 945–952.

47. Attali, B., D. Saya & Z. Vogel. 1990. Pre- and postnatal development of opiate receptor subtypes in rat spinal cord. *Brain Res. Dev. Brain Res.* **53:** 97–102.

48. McDowell, J. & I. Kitchen. 1986. Ontogenesis of delta-opioid receptors in rat brain using [3H][D-Pen2, D-Pen5]enkephalin as a binding ligand. *Eur. J. Pharmacol.* **128:** 287–289.

49. Szucs, M. & C.J. Coscia. 1990. Evidence for delta-opioid binding and GTP-regulatory proteins in 5-day-old rat brain membranes. *J. Neurochem.* **54:** 1419–1425.

50. Milligan, G., R.A. Streaty, P. Gierschik, *et al.* 1987. Development of opiate receptors and GTP-binding regulatory proteins in neonatal rat brain. *J. Biol. Chem.* **262:** 8626–8630.

51. Mailly, P., M. Gastard, A. Cupo. 1999. Subcellular distribution of delta-opioid receptors in the rat spinal cord: an approach using a three-dimensional reconstruction of confocal series of immunolabelled neurons. *J. Neurosci. Methods* **87:** 17–24.

52. Sales, N., Y. Charnay, J.M. Zajac, *et al.* 1989. Ontogeny of mu and delata opioid receptors and of neutral endopeptidase in human spinal cord: an autoradiographic study. *J. Chem. Neuroanat.* **2:** 179–188.

53. Zagon, I.S., D.M. Gibo & P.J. McLaughlin. 1990. Adult and developing human cerebella exhibit different profiles of opioid binding sites. *Brain Res.* **523:** 62–68.

54. Scherrer, G., N. Imamachi, & Y.Q. Cao, *et al.* 2009. Dissociation of the opioid receptor mechanisms that control mechanical and heat pain. *Cell* **137:** 1148–1159.

55. Williams, S.A., T.J. Abbruscato, V.J. Hruby, *et al.* 1996. Passage of a delta-opioid receptor selective enkephalin, [D-penicillamine2,5] enkephalin, across the blood-brain and the blood-cerebrospinal fluid barriers. *J. Neurochem.* **66:** 1289–1299.

56. Ampasavate, C., G.A. Chandorkar, D.G. Vande Velde, *et al.* 2002. Transport and metabolism of opioid peptides across BeWo cells, an *in vitro* model of the placental barrier. *Int. J. Pharm.* **233:** 85–98.

57. Horiuchi, T., M. Kawaguchi, T. Sakamoto, *et al.* 2004. The effects of the delta-opioid agonist SNC80 on hind-limb motor function and neuronal injury after spinal cord ischemia in rats. *Anesth. Analg.* **99:** 235–240.

58. Jha, A., S. Das Gupta & S.B. Deshpande. 2003. Deprenyl blocks the aglycemia-induced depression of the synaptic transmission but not the ischemia-induced depression in neonatal rat spinal cord *in vitro. Neurosci. Res.* **47:** 23–29.

59. Freiberg, S.M. & S.M. Johnson. 2008. Delta-opioid receptor (DOR) activation provides neuroprotection against oxygen-glucose deprivation (OGD) in neonatal spinal respiratory motor circuits *in vitro. Soc. Neurosci. Abst.* 152.2.

60. Shook, J.E., W.D. Watkins & E.M. Camporesi. 1990. Differential roles of opioid receptors in respiration, respiratory disease, and opiate-induced respiratory depression. *Am. Rev. Respir. Dis.* **142:** 895–909.

61. May, C.N., M.R. Dashwood, C.J. Whitehead, *et al.* 1989. Differential cardiovascular and respiratory responses to central administration of selective opioid agonists in conscious rabbits: correlation with receptor distribution. *Br. J. Pharmacol.* **98:** 903–913.

62. Kiritsy-Roy, J.A., L. Marson & G.R. van Loon. 1989. Sympathoadrenal, cardiovascular and blood gas responses to highly selective Mu and Delta opioid peptides. *J. Pharmacol. Exp. Ther.* **251:** 1096–1103.

63. Su, Y.F., R. McNutt & K.J. Chang. 1998. Delta-opioid ligand reverses alfentanil-induced respiratory depression not antinociception. *J. Pharmacol. Exp. Ther.* **287:** 815–823.

64. Clapp, J.F., A. Kett, N. Olariu, *et al.* 1997. Cardiovascular and metabolic responses to two receptor-selective opioid agonists in pregnant sheep. *Am. J. Obstet. Gynecol.* **178:** 397–401.

65. Szeto, H.H., Y. Soong, D. Wu, *et al.* 1999. Respiratory depression after intravenous administration of δ-selective opioid peptide analogs. *Peptides* **20:** 101–105.

66. Greer, J.J., J.E. Carter & Z. al-Zubaidy. 1995. Opioid depression of respiration in neonatal rats. *J. Physiol.* **485:** 845–855.

67. Takita, K., E.A. Herlenius, S.G. Lindahl, *et al.* 1997. Actions of opioids on respiratory activity via activation of brainstem mu-, delta-, and kappa-receptors; an in-vitro study. *Brain Res.* **778:** 233–241.

68. Takeda, S., L.I. Eriksson, Y. Yamamoto, *et al.* 2001. Opioid action on respiratory neuron activity of the isolated respiratory network in newborn rats. *Anesthesiology* **95:** 740–749.

69. Cheng, P.Y., D.L. Wu, J. Decena, *et al.* 1993. Opioid-induced stimulation of fetal respiratory activity by [D-Ala^2]deltorphin I. *Eur. J. Pharmacol.* **230:** 85–88.

70. Cheng, P.Y., D.L. Wu, Y. Soong, *et al.* 1993. Role of μ1 and δ-opioid receptors in modulation of fetal EEG and respiratory activity. *Am. J. Physiol.* **265:** R433–R438.

71. Szeto, H.H., P.Y. Cheng, Y. Soong, *et al.* 1995. Lack of relationship between opioid-induced changes in fetal breathing and plasma glucose levels. *Am. J. Physiol.* **269:** R702–R707.

72. Szeto, H.H., P.Y. Cheng, D.L. Wu, *et al.* 1994. Effects of the delta-opioid agonist, [D-Pen2, D-Pen5]-enkephalin, on fetal lamb EEG. *Pharmacol. Biochem. Behav.* **49:** 795–800.

73. Danielsson, I., M. Gasior, G.W. Stevenson, *et al.* 2006. Electroencephalographic and convulsant effects of the delta opioid agonist SNC80 in rhesus monkeys. *Pharmacol. Biochem. Behav.* **85:** 428–434.

74. Kakinohana, M., S. Nakamura, T. Fuchigami, *et al.* 2006. Mu and delta, but not kappa, opioid agonists induce spastic paraparesis after a short period of spinal cord ischaemia in rats. *Br. J. Anaesth.* **96:** 88–94.

Ann. N.Y. Acad. Sci. ISSN 0077-8923

Immune response by microglia in the spinal cord

Julie K. Olson

Department of Neurological Surgery, School of Medicine and Public Health, University of Wisconsin, Madison, Wisconsin

Address for correspondence: Dr. Julie K. Olson, Department of Neurological Surgery, University of Wisconsin, 1300 University Avenue, Madison, WI 53706. j.olson@neurosurg.wisc.edu

Microglia are the resident immune cells of the central nervous system (CNS) and share many immunological characteristics with peripheral macrophage. Microglia exist in a quiescent state in the healthy CNS, however, upon injury or infection, microglia become activated immune cells. Microglia have been implicated in playing an important role in several neurological diseases that affect the spinal cord, especially multiple sclerosis (MS) and neuropathic pain. However, most studies, which examined the immune response by microglia have been conducted using microglia cultures generated from brain microglia. Therefore, our studies examined the immune response by microglia in the spinal cord compared to the immune response by microglia in the brain. Microglia in the spinal cord of mice expressed higher levels of surface immune molecules than microglia in the brain, and upon virus infection, microglia in the spinal cord expressed higher levels of immune molecules than microglia in the brain. These studies suggest that microglia in the spinal cord may have different immune reactivity than microglia in the brain, which may contribute to spinal cord diseases.

Keywords: microglia; rodent; neuroimmunology; virus infection

Introduction

Microglia are the resident central nervous system (CNS) immune cells. Microglia originate from the myeloid lineage and infiltrate into the CNS during embryonic development. Microglia play an important role as phagocytes during development and then continue to reside in the developed CNS as quiescent cells. Microglia are continually surveying their CNS environment and can be quickly activated following injury or infection. Microglia share many functional and phenotypic similarities to peripheral macrophage due to their common myeloid lineage. Microglia and macrophage express similar surface molecules, which makes it difficult to distinguish the two populations of cells in the CNS during an immune response. Microglia and macrophage both express surface integrin (CD11b), and the common leukocyte antigen (CD45). However, the microglia can be distinguished from macrophage by the intermediate expression level of CD45 compared to the high expression level of CD45 on macrophage.

Microglia in the healthy CNS have several fine, branched processes that are highly mobile and monitor the local environment without disturbing neuronal networks.[1,2] Microglia monitor the local environment for signs of infection or injury. Microglia participate in the innate immune response, which is the initial immune response following infection or injury. Microglia express innate immune receptors, such as the Toll like receptors (TLRs) that recognize pathogen associated molecular patterns or damage associated molecular patterns. Microglia express all the identified TLRs allowing them to sense infecting pathogens or damaged cells.[3] Microglia become activated immune cells following TLR engagement and express proinflammatory cytokines, such as TNFα and IL-6, chemokines for directing cell trafficking, and effector molecules, such as nitric oxide. Microglia in the healthy CNS do not express antigen presenting cell molecules such as MHC class II or costimulatory molecules, CD80, CD86, and CD40, which are involved in antigen presentation to CD4[+] T cells as part of the specific immune response or adaptive immune response to infection. Professional antigen presenting cells, such as macrophage, continually express MHC class II and costimulatory molecules and present antigens to CD4[+] T cells.

doi: 10.1111/j.1749-6632.2010.05536.x

However, upon activation, microglia can increase the expression of MHC class II and costimulatory molecules, which enables them to present antigen to CD4[+] T cells and participate in the adaptive immune response.[4] Therefore, microglia can sense an injury or infection in the CNS using innate immune receptors, which activate them to participate in the innate and adaptive immune response.

Microglia also have an important role in neural development and repair. Microglia enter the CNS during early neurogenesis and function as phagocytes for cells undergoing apoptosis during normal development.[5] Microglia have also been suggested to play a role in synaptic pruning of excess synapses during development.[6,7] Microglia have more recently been suggested to promote CNS repair following damage through regulation of neural progenitor stem cells. Microglia have been shown to secrete factors that promote neurogenesis of neural progenitor cells isolated from the subventricular zone.[8] Furthermore, microglia have been shown to promote neuronal differentiation from neural progenitor stem cells and to secrete chemokines that direct migration of neural progenitor stem cells.[9] On the other side, the neuronal environment may be influencing the immune functions of microglia. Microglia have different immune functions compared to peripheral macrophage, including reduced antigen presenting cell functions and reduced inflammatory responses. The healthy CNS lacks serum proteins, which are activators of macrophage. The healthy CNS also has detectable levels of cytokines such as TGFβ and prostaglandin E_2 that downregulate macrophage functions.[10] Interestingly, microglia in the healthy CNS express inhibitory receptors such as CD200R, CD172a/SIRPa, and TREM2, which bind to ligands found in the CNS, including CD200 expressed on neurons.[11–13] These inhibitory receptors have been shown to downregulate inflammatory immune functions. Therefore, the neural environment may be turning down the immune functions of microglia in the CNS to protect from damage, which can be associated with an inflammatory response. Overall, microglia are specialized CNS resident cells that have important functions during neuronal development and during the immune response.

Microglia rapidly respond to infection or injury in the CNS and have been identified as critical cells in several neurological diseases. Microglia in the spinal cord have been suggested to play an important role during demyelinating disease, during spinal cord injury, and during neuropathic pain. Many previous studies have examined the immune functions of microglia using microglia derived from the brain. However, microglia in the spinal cord may react differently than microglia in the brain during pathological conditions due to the differing regions of the CNS. Therefore, we isolated microglia from the spinal cord and from the brain of mice during a pathological condition, virus infection, and then we compared the immune reactivity of these cells. Our studies show that microglia in the spinal cord have a more reactive immune response than microglia in the brain. These results suggest that microglia in the spinal cord may contribute differently to the pathology of diseases than microglia in the brain. Most importantly, the immune responses by microglia in the spinal cord may directly affect the initiation and/or exacerbation of spinal cord diseases.

Results

Microglia are the immunocompetent resident cells of the CNS, which have been suggested to play an important role in infection and disease in the spinal cord. Many studies have examined the immune response by microglia using microglia derived from the brain, however, microglia in the spinal cord may have different immune reactivity than microglia in the brain. Therefore, we wanted to examine the immune response by microglia in the spinal cord compared to microglia in the brain during a pathological event, such as a virus infection. Theiler's murine encephalomyelitis virus (TMEV) is a natural mouse pathogen that is neurotropic infecting CNS cells in both the brain and spinal cord.[14,15] TMEV infection of mice results in a persistent infection of the CNS, which leads to the development of demyelinating disease around 40 days postinfection. We have previously shown that microglia can be persistently infected with TMEV.[4] Most importantly, microglia infected with TMEV *in vitro* become activated innate immune cells that secrete cytokines, chemokines, and effector molecules and become activated antigen presenting cells that present antigen to CD4[+] T cells.[4] Therefore, infection of mice with TMEV will affect microglia in the brain and in the spinal cord allowing for the comparison of the immune

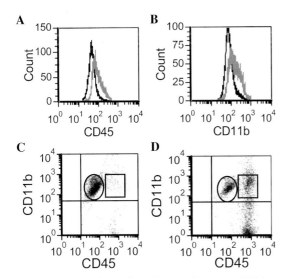

Figure 1. Microglia in the spinal cord expressed higher levels of CD45 and CD11b than microglia in the brain. Microglia were isolated from naïve SJL mice (six mice per group) and stained with fluorescently labeled antibodies for CD11b and CD45. Microglia were analyzed by flow cytometry. The florescent intensities (X-axis) (log scale) versus cell count (Y-axis) are shown for CD45 (**A**) and CD11b (**B**) staining of microglia in the brain (*black line*) and in the spinal cord (*gray line*). Microglia were gated based on living cells that stained CD11b$^+$CD45 intermediate, shown in the circle, in naïve mice (**C**) and TMEV-infected mice (**D**), compared to macrophage CD11b$^+$CD45 high, shown in the square. Florescent intensity is shown for CD11b on the Y-axis (log scale) and CD45 on the X-axis (log scale).

response by microglia in the different regions of the CNS.

Microglia express similar cell surface molecules as macrophage due to their common myeloid lineage, however, microglia express CD45 at an intermediate level compared to macrophage, which express CD45 at a high level. Microglia are the predominate myeloid cell in the CNS of naïve mice (Fig. 1C). However, macrophage infiltrate into the CNS during an immune response, therefore, microglia, CD11b$^+$CD45 intermediate cells, can be distinguished from the CNS infiltrating macrophage, CD11b$^+$CD45 high cells (Fig. 1D). First, the expression of CD45 and CD11b on the surface of microglia was compared between microglia in the brain and microglia in the spinal cord (Fig. 1). Microglia were isolated from the brain and

spinal cord of naïve SJL/J mice and stained with antibodies for flow cytometry. In brief, the brain and spinal cord were removed from the mice (six mice per group). The brains and spinal cords were minced and digested with collagenase type IV (Invitrogen) and DNAse (Invitrogen). The organs were then dissociated by passing through a 70 μm filter, and the cells were separated on a 70/30 percoll gradient from which the mononuclear cells are isolated from the interface. The isolated mononuclear cells were incubated with fluorescently labeled antibodies for CD45 and CD11b. The microglia were examined by flow cytometry on a FACSCaliber (BD Biosciences, San Jose, California) and analyzed using Cell Quest software (BD Biosciences). Microglia were identified by CD11b$^+$CD45 intermediate expression. Interestingly, microglia in the spinal cord expressed higher levels of CD45 and CD11b than microglia in the brain (Figs. 1A and 1B). Furthermore, microglia in the brain and in the spinal cord were similar in size (data not shown). These results show that microglia in the spinal cord express a higher level of CD45 than microglia in the brain, however, the CD45 expression level is still less than the high CD45 expression level on macrophage.

Based on the difference in expression of CD45 and CD11b on microglia in the brain and in the spinal cord of naïve mice, we wanted to determine whether the expression of these molecules was increased during virus infection. SJL/J mice (5–6 weeks old) were infected with the BeAn strain of TMEV or mock-infected by intracranial injection. On day 3 postinfection, the brain and spinal cord were removed from mice (six mice per group), and the mononuclear cells were isolated. The cells were stained with fluorescently labeled antibodies for CD45 and CD11b and analyzed by flow cytometry. Microglia were sorted based on CD11b$^+$CD45 intermediate expression. The microglia from the brain and from the spinal cord were compared for expression of CD11b and CD45. Microglia in the brain during TMEV infection increased the expression of CD45 and CD11b compared to microglia in the brain during mock-infection (Figs. 2A and 2B). Microglia in the spinal cord during TMEV infection also increased the expression of CD45 and CD11b compared to microglia in the spinal cord during mock-infection (Figs. 2C and 2D). Interestingly, the expression of CD45 and CD11b on microglia in the spinal cord was still slightly

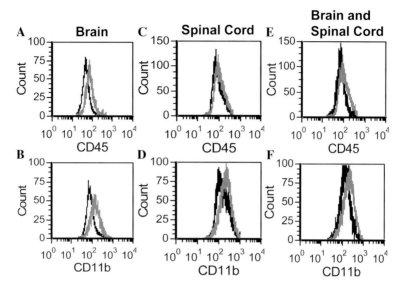

Figure 2. Microglia in the brain and in the spinal cord were activated to increase expression of CD45 and CD11b during virus infection. Mice were infected with TMEV or mock-infected. At 3 days postinfection, microglia were isolated from the brain and spinal cord of the mice (six mice per group). Microglia were stained with fluorescently labeled antibodies for CD45 and CD11b and analyzed by flow cytometry. Microglia were gated based on live cells and CD45 intermediate staining. The florescent intensities (X-axis) (log scale) versus cell count (Y-axis) are shown for CD45 and CD11b. The microglia in the brain (**A, B**) were analyzed for expression of CD45 and CD11b for mock-infected (*black line*) and TMEV-infected (*gray line*) mice. The microglia in the spinal cord (**C, D**) were analyzed for expression of CD45 and CD11b for mock-infected (*black line*) and TMEV-infected (*gray line*) mice. Microglia in the brain (*black line*) and in the spinal cord (*gray line*) of TMEV-infected mice (**E, F**) were compared for expression of CD45 and CD11b.

higher than the expression of CD45 and CD11b on microglia in the brain during TMEV infection (Figs. 2E and 2F). These results suggest that virus infection increases the expression of CD45 and CD11b on microglia in the brain and in the spinal cord, however, microglia in the spinal cord continue to express higher levels CD45 and CD11b. Furthermore, the size of microglia in the brain and in the spinal cord of TMEV-infected mice were slightly increased compared to mock-infected mice leading to similar size of microglia in both the brain and spinal cord of TMEV-infected mice (data not shown).

Next, we wanted to determine whether the immune activation of microglia in the spinal cord was different than microglia in the brain during virus infection. Mice were infected with TMEV or mock-infected. On day 3 postinfection, the brain and spinal cord were removed from the mice (6 mice per group), and mononuclear cells were isolated. The cells were stained with fluorescently labeled an-

tibodies for CD45, CD11b, and CD40, CD80, CD86, or MHC class II (IA^s) and analyzed by flow cytometry. Microglia were sorted based on CD11b$^+$CD45 intermediate cells, and then analyzed for expression of costimulatory molecules, CD80, CD86, and CD40, and for the expression of MHC class II (IA^s) during virus infection. Microglia in the brain and spinal cord did not express CD40 but expressed low levels of CD80 and CD86 when mock-infected (Figs. 3G–3I). These results are similar to microglia from naïve mice, which did not express CD40 and expressed very low levels of CD80 and CD86 (data not shown). Microglia in the brain did not express CD40 during TMEV infection but microglia in the spinal cord expressed CD40 during TMEV infection (Figs. 3A and 3D). Microglia in the brain during TMEV infection did not increase the expression of CD80 but increased the expression of CD86 compared to microglia from mock-infected mice (Figs. 3B and 3C). Microglia in the spinal cord of TMEV-infected mice increased the expression of

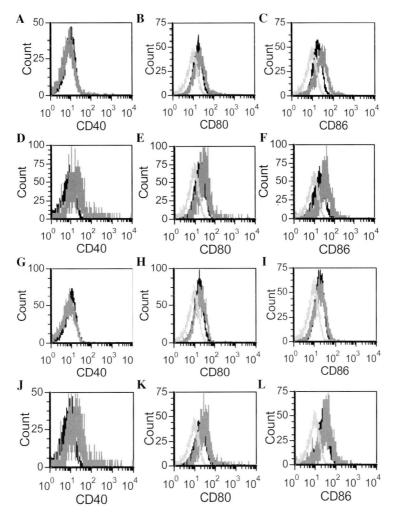

Figure 3. Microglia in the spinal cord were activated to express higher levels of immune molecules than microglia in the brain following virus infection. Mice were infected with TMEV or mock-infected. At 3 days postinfection, microglia were isolated from the brain and spinal cord of mice (six mice per group). Microglia were stained with fluorescently labeled antibodies for CD45 and CD11b and CD40, CD80, or CD86 and analyzed by flow cytometry. The florescent intensities (X-axis) (log scale) versus cell count (Y-axis) are shown for each molecule. Microglia were gated on CD45 intermediate CD11b$^+$ staining. Microglia in the brain of TMEV-infected mice (*gray line*) and mock-infected mice (*black line*) were analyzed for expression of CD40 (**A**), CD80 (**B**), and CD86 (**C**) compared to antibody isotype control (*silver line*). Microglia in the spinal cord of TMEV-infected mice (*gray line*) and mock-infected mice (*black line*) were analyzed for expression of CD40 (**D**), CD80 (**E**), and CD86 (**F**) compared to antibody isotype control (*silver line*). Microglia in the brain (*black line*) and in the spinal cord of mock-infected mice (*gray line*) were compared for expression of CD40 (**G**), CD80 (**H**), and CD86 (**I**) with isotype control (*silver line*). Microglia in the brain (*black line*) and spinal cord (*gray line*) of TMEV-infected mice were compared for the expression of CD40 (**J**), CD80 (**K**), and CD86 (**L**) with isotype control (*silver line*).

both CD80 and CD86 compared to microglia from mock-infected mice (Figs. 3E and 3F). Most interestingly, microglia in the spinal cord expressed higher levels of CD80 and CD86 during virus infection than microglia in the brain (Figs. 3K and 3L). These results are also shown in Table 1 with the mean florescence intensity calculated using Cell Quest Pro software for each immune molecule. The MFI for the

Table 1. Expression of immune molecules on microglia

	Mock brain	Mock spinal cord	TMEV brain	TMEV spinal cord
CD45	49.56 ± 1.21	$90.68 \pm 1.41^\wedge$	$76.58 \pm 1.09^*$	$107.96 \pm 1.11^{*\wedge}$
CD11b	83.86 ± 1.99	$152.98 \pm 2.58^\wedge$	$142.59 \pm 2.15^*$	$208.25 \pm 2.36^{*\wedge}$
CD40	8.52 ± 0.43	8.65 ± 0.29	8.15 ± 0.37	$16.30 \pm 0.84^{*\wedge}$
CD80	16.25 ± 0.68	$18.11 \pm 0.53^\wedge$	$19.63 \pm 0.73^*$	$24.90 \pm 0.83^{*\wedge}$
CD86	16.74 ± 0.53	17.25 ± 0.32	$24.39 \pm 0.88^*$	$30.63 \pm 1.04^{*\wedge}$
IA^s	6.87 ± 0.31	6.87 ± 0.22	$7.59 \pm 0.28^*$	$8.18 \pm 0.29^*$

Mice were infected with TMEV or mock-infected. At 3 days postinfection, microglia were isolated from the brain and spinal cord of mice (six mice per group). Microglia were stained with fluorescently labeled antibodies for CD45 and CD11b and CD40, CD80, or CD86 and analyzed by flow cytometry. Microglia were gated on CD45 intermediate CD11b$^+$ staining. The mean florescent intensity (MFI) for each antibody was determined by Cell Quest Pro software with the MFI for the isotype control antibody subtracted for each specific antibody. Significant difference ($P < 0.05$) was determined using the independent sample Student's t-test between mock-infected and TMEV-infected ($*$) and between brain and spinal cord ($\wedge$). The results shown are from three experiments.

isotype control for each antibody was subtracted to determine the final MFI for each immune molecule. The significant difference ($P < 0.05$) was determined using the Student's t-test. Microglia in the brain and microglia in the spinal cord expressed low levels of MHC class II during TMEV infection with microglia in the spinal cord expressing slightly more than microglia in the brain (Table 1). Therefore, microglia in the brain increased expression of one costimulatory molecule, CD86, and MHC class II following TMEV infection, however, microglia in the spinal cord increased expression of several costimulatory molecules, CD80, CD86, and CD40, and MHC class II following TMEV infection. These results show that microglia in the spinal cord are activated to express higher levels of immune molecules following TMEV infection than microglia in the brain. These results suggest that microglia in the spinal cord may be more immune reactive than microglia in the brain.

Conclusion

Microglia play an important role in the immune response in the spinal cord, which may be important in protecting the CNS during injury or infection. However, microglia have also been suggested to contribute to the development and/or exacerbation of spinal cord diseases. Microglia have been suggested to play an important role in the pathogenesis of multiple sclerosis (MS). MS is an inflammatory demyelinating disease of the central nervous system. Activated microglia expressing costimulatory molecules and MHC class II have been identified in active demyelinating lesions in the spinal cord of MS patients.[16] MS has been associated with activation of autoreactive, myelin-specific CD4$^+$ T cells, thus, microglia may be presenting myelin antigen to autoreactive T cells in the CNS contributing to demyelination. Further studies have suggested a role for microglia in the effecter stages of myelin destruction via production of inflammatory cytokines and other inflammatory effecter molecules.[17] Most significantly, recent studies have identified activated microglia in preactive MS lesions in the absence of infiltrating immune cells.[18] These studies suggest that microglia may be involved in the very early pathogenesis of MS by possibly responding to oligodendrocyte abnormalities in the preactive lesions. Therefore, microglia may be involved in initiation as well as exacerbation of the inflammatory response associated with demyelination during MS. However, studies have also suggested a role for microglia in protecting the CNS during MS.[19] Microglia are phagocytic cells that may be clearing the apoptotic cells and debris at the lesion site to promote remyelination and repair. Microglia may be secreting cytokines, chemokines, and effector molecules that reduce the inflammatory response and promote remyelination. Finally, microglia have been shown to promote neurogenesis as well as oligodendrogenesis required for remyelination and repair during MS.[20]

Microglia have also been suggested to contribute to neuropathic pain following peripheral nerve injury as wells as chronic pain following spinal cord injury. Microglia are activated and express MHC class II following spinal cord injury at the site of the lesion as well as in the surrounding areas.[21] Spinal cord injury can also activate microglia in the lumbar dorsal horn, which contributes to neuronal hyper-responsiveness and alterations in the pain thresholds. The sensitized neurons can release molecules that activate microglia. Thus, activation of microglia after spinal cord injury can result in a continual feedback loop of activation of microglia and neurons, which leads to the development of chronic pain.[22] Microglia also become activated following peripheral nerve injury. Microglia cluster around the cell bodies of injured motor neurons in the ventral horn of the spinal cord and around the central terminals of injured sensory nerve filbers in the dorsal horn.[23,24] The activated microglia secrete cytokines that may modulate dorsal horn neuron responsiveness leading to development of neuropathic pain.[25,26] Further, microglia activated by ATP through the purinergic receptors following peripheral nerve injury can release brain-derived neurotropic factor (BDNF). BDNF produces a depolarizing shift in the anion reversal potential of dorsal horn lamina I neurons that contribute to neuropathic pain.[27] Therefore, activation of microglia can modulate neuronal activity that can lead to chronic pain or neuropathic pain.

Microglia infiltrate into the CNS during early neuronal development and establish a resident immune cell population in the CNS. Microglia play an important role during neural development and have also been suggested to play a role in neurogenesis. However, microglia are the CNS resident immune cells that play an important role in protecting the CNS following injury or infection. The blood–brain barrier restricts the infiltration of peripheral immune cells under healthy conditions, thus microglia are the first cells to respond to injury or infection of the CNS. Our results demonstrate that microglia have low or no expression of immune molecules in the healthy CNS. However, microglia in the spinal cord of healthy mice expressed higher levels of immune molecules than microglia in the brain. The low expression of immune molecules on microglia in the healthy CNS may be due to the expression of inhibitory molecules, such as CD200, on neurons

and oligodendrocytes. Microglia have been shown to express CD200R that binds to CD200 and leads to the suppression of microglial immune functions.[11] Most importantly, our results showed that microglia in the spinal cord become more activated than microglia in the brain during pathological condition by expressing higher levels of immune molecules. Interestingly, during CNS diseases such as MS, CD200 expression is decreased in the areas of MS lesions that are associated with activated microglia.[28] Thus, one possible explanation for the variation in immune molecule expression on microglia in the brain and spinal cord may be due to the level of CD200 expressed on cells in the different areas of the CNS. Microglia in areas of the CNS expressing higher levels of CD200 may be functionally more suppressed than in areas of the CNS with lower CD200 expression.

Overall, these studies demonstrate that microglia in the spinal cord have different immune reactivity than microglia in the brain. Microglia in the spinal cord had an increased immune response compared to microglia in the brain, which may be more protective to injury or infection in the spinal cord. However, the increased immune reactivity of microglia in the spinal cord compared to microglia in the brain may contribute to the development and/or progression of diseases in the spinal cord. Activated microglia have been shown to mediate neuropathic pain following peripheral nerve injury and chronic pain after spinal cord injury. The higher immune reactivity of microglia in the spinal cord may contribute to the continual activation of microglia following spinal cord injury or peripheral nerve injury, which leads to chronic pain or neuropathic pain. Activated microglia have also been shown to be present in preactive lesions in MS patients as well as in active lesions, thus, immune activation of microglia in the spinal cord may be contributing to the development and exacerbation of MS. Finally, these studies demonstrate that microglia in different regions of the CNS may have different immune reactivity, therefore, the immune response by region-specific microglia may be important during CNS diseases.

Acknowledgment

This work was supported by grants from the National Multiple Sclerosis Society RG3625.

Conflicts of interest

The author declares no conflicts of interest.

References

1. Davalos, D. *et al.* 2005. ATP mediates rapid microglial response to local brain injury in vivo. *Nat. Neurosci.* **8:** 752–758.

2. Nimmerjahn, A., F. Kirchhoff & F. Helmchen. 2005. Resting microglial cells are highly dynamic surveillants of brain parenchyma in vivo. *Science* **308:** 1314–1318.

3. Olson, J.K. & S.D. Miller. 2004. Microglia initiate central nervous system innate and adaptive immune responses through multiple TLRs. *J. Immunol.* **173:** 3916–3924.

4. Olson, J.K., A.M. Girvin & S.D. Miller. 2001. Direct activation of innate and antigen presenting functions of microglia following infection with Theiler's virus. *J. Virol.* **75:** 9780–9789.

5. Streit, W.J. 2001. Microglia and macrophages in the developing CNS. *Neurotoxicology* **22:** 619–624.

6. Fourgeaud, L. & L.M. Boulanger. 2007. Synapse remodeling, compliments of the complement system. *Cell* **131:** 1034–1036.

7. Stevens, B. *et al.* 2007. The classical complement cascade mediates CNS synapse elimination. *Cell* **131:** 1164–1178.

8. Walton, N.M. *et al.* 2006. Microglia instruct subventricular zone neurogenesis. *Glia* **54:** 815–825.

9. Aarum, J., K. Sandberg, S.L. Haeberlein & M.A. Persson. 2003. Migration and differentiation of neural precursor cells can be directed by microglia. *Proc. Natl. Acad. Sci. USA* **100:** 15983–15988.

10. Adams, R.A. *et al.* 2007. The fibrin-derived gamma377–395 peptide inhibits microglia activation and suppresses relapsing paralysis in central nervous system autoimmune disease. *J. Exp. Med.* **204:** 571–582.

11. Hoek, R.M. *et al.* 2000. Down-regulation of the macrophage lineage through interaction with OX2 (CD200). *Science* **290:** 1768–1771.

12. van Beek, E.M., F. Cochrane, A.N. Barclay & T.K. Van Den Berg. 2005. Signal regulatory proteins in the immune system. *J. Immunol.* **175:** 7781–7787.

13. Takahashi, K. *et al.* 2007. TREM2-transduced myeloid precursors mediate nervous tissue debris clearance and facilitate recovery in an animal model of multiple sclerosis. *PLoS Med.* **4:** e124.

14. Lipton, H.L. 1975. Theiler's virus infection in mice: an unusual biphasic disease process leading to demyelination. *Infect. Immun.* **11:** 1147–1155.

15. Lipton, H.L., G. Twaddle & M.L. Jelachich. 1995. The predominant virus antigen burden is present in macrophages in Theiler's murine encephalomyelitis virus-induced demyelinating disease. *J. Virol.* **69:** 2525–2533.

16. Desimone, R. *et al.* 1995. The costimulatory molecule B7 is expressed on human microglia in culture and in multiple sclerosis acute lesions. *J. Neuropathol. Exp. Neurol.* **54:** 175–187.

17. Aloisi, F. 2001. Immune function of microglia. *Glia* **36:** 165–179.

18. Van Der Valk, P. & S. Amor. 2009. Preactive lesions in multiple sclerosis. *Curr. Opin. Neurol.* **22:** 207–213.

19. Napoli, I. & H. Neumann. 2009. Protective effects of microglia in multiple sclerosis. *Exp. Neurol.* doi: 10.1016/j.expneurol.2009.04.024.

20. Butovsky, O. *et al.* 2006. Induction and blockage of oligodendrogenesis by differently activated microglia in an animal model of multiple sclerosis. *J. Clin. Invest.* **116:** 905–915.

21. Popovich, P.G., P. Wei & B.T. Stokes. 1997. Cellular inflammatory response after spinal cord injury in Sprague-Dawley and Lewis rats. *J. Comp. Neurol.* **377:** 443–464.

22. Hains, B.C. & S.G. Waxman. 2006. Activated microglia contribute to the maintenance of chronic pain after spinal cord injury. *J. Neurosci.* **26:** 4308–4317.

23. Hu, P., A.L. Bembrick, K.A. Keay & E.M. McLachlan. 2007. Immune cell involvement in dorsal root ganglia and spinal cord after chronic constriction or transection of the rat sciatic nerve. *Brain Behav. Immun.* **21:** 599–616.

24. Beggs, S. & M.W. Salter. 2007. Stereological and somatotopic analysis of the spinal microglial response to peripheral nerve injury. *Brain Behav. Immun.* **21:** 624–633.

25. Winkelstein, B.A. *et al.* 2001. Nerve injury proximal or distal to the DRG induces similar spinal glial activation and selective cytokine expression but differential behavioral responses to pharmacologic treatment. *J. Comp. Neurol.* **439:** 127–139.

26. Scholz, J. & C.J. Woolf. 2007. The neuropathic pain triad: neurons, immune cells and glia. *Nat. Neurosci.* **10:** 1361–1368.

27. Coull, J.A. *et al.* 2005. BDNF from microglia causes the shift in neuronal anion gradient underlying neuropathic pain. *Nature* **438:** 1017–1021.

28. Koning, N., D.F. Swaab, R.M. Hoek & I. Huitinga. 2009. Distribution of the immune inhibitory molecules CD200 and CD200R in the normal central nervous system and multiple sclerosis lesions suggests neuron-glia and glia-glia interactions. *J. Neuropathol. Exp. Neurol.* **68:** 159–167.

Ann. N.Y. Acad. Sci. ISSN 0077-8923

ANNALS OF THE NEW YORK ACADEMY OF SCIENCES
Issue. *Neurons and Networks in the Spinal Cord*

How spinalized rats can walk: biomechanics, cortex, and hindlimb muscle scaling—implications for rehabilitation

Simon F. Giszter, Greg Hockensmith, Arun Ramakrishnan, and Ubong Ime Udoekwere

Neurobiology and Anatomy, School of Bioengineering, Drexel University College of Medicine, Philadelphia, Pennsylvania

Address for correspondence: Simon F. Giszter, Drexel Uinversity College of Medicine – Neurobiology, 2900 Queen Lane Philadelphia, PA 19129. sgiszter@drexelmed.edu

Neonatal spinalized (NST) rats can achieve autonomous weight-supported locomotion never seen after adult injury. Mechanisms that support function in NST rats include increased importance of cortical trunk control and altered biomechanical control strategies for stance and locomotion. Hindlimbs are isolated from perturbations in quiet stance and act in opposition to forelimbs in locomotion in NST rats. Control of roll and yaw of the hindlimbs is crucial in their locomotion. The biomechanics of the hind limbs of NST rats are also likely crucial. We present new data showing the whole leg musculature scales proportional to normal rat musculature in NST rats, regardless of function. This scaling is a prerequisite for the NST rats to most effectively use pattern generation mechanisms and motor patterns that are similar to those present in intact rats. Pattern generation may be built into the lumbar spinal cord by evolution and matched to the limb biomechanics, so preserved muscle scaling may be essential to the NST function observed.

Keywords: cortex; spinal transection; muscle scaling; pattern generation; locomotion

Introduction

The mechanisms of plasticity that operate in the locomotion of intact rats may also contribute to recovery after injury.[1–3] However, following injury, the control problems are much more severe. Injury alters motor organization: some pathways are lost and sprouting may add novel and unusual connections.[4] Neural plasticity and motor learning mechanisms must adapt this novel and reduced neural system structure to best restore function.[5–7] How does developmental reorganization, motor learning, and plasticity achieve function after injury?[8,9] A particularly interesting and informative example occurs in complete spinal cord injury (SCI) in very young rats or kittens.[5,7,10–17]

Paralysis of adult spinal transection animals is always complete, but some neonatal spinal transection animals walk

Adult mammals are very severely paralyzed after complete spinal transection (ST). Only perineal stimulation, epidural stimulation,[18] or drug delivery therapies[19–21] can initiate stepping. Rehabilitation training[19,22–25] and/or therapeutic interventions improve such stepping, but do not restore autonomy.[26] However, in stark contrast to this limited recovery, some neonatal spinal transected (NST) rats, or cats develop autonomous weight-supported stepping as adults.[5,7,10–17]

How do neonatal spinalized rats walk? Understanding this may be a roadmap to improve animal model therapies. The results of research on rehabilitating quadrupeds may translate to significant but lesser gains in man.[27,28]

In this paper, we review studies of the biomechanics and control operating in weight-supporting neonatal spinalized (WSNST) rats, compared to nonweight-supporting neonatal spinalized (NWSNST) rats, and intact control rats. We then describe new data on muscle scaling's role in these rats' function.

A definition of functional walking

Spinal cord contains the circuitry to organize complex movements using pattern generators and reflexes local to spinal cord.[29] Most postnatal day 1 (P1) to 5 (P5) NST rats can, as adults, generate stepping motions on a treadmill without additional stimuli. A subset of ~20% of NST rats also achieve what we term *independent or autonomous weight support* as adults.[5−7,14,17,30,31] We define *independent or autonomous weight-supported stepping* using a "sumo-wrestling" like criterion for a weight-supported step. It involves ground contact of nothing except some part of the feet through the full progression of swing and stance. We then measure the percentage of such steps in locomotion. In NST rats the distribution of this measure of function is bimodal[14] with peaks centered on ~20% and 75% allowing the division of NST rats into two groups, of weight-supporting rats (WSNST, with BBB[32] 12–16) and nonweight-supporting rats (NWSNST, BBB <8). WSNST rats all have better than 50% of their steps classified as weight-supported steps. The WSNST rats recover from falls and can balance the majority of steps.

How might function be achieved through the integration of two autonomous pieces of CNS connected to the same body? A model of function.

The NST rat has two autonomous pieces of CNS controlling its body: (1) the brain and cervical spinal system and (2) the lumbosacral spinal enlargement. These two pieces of CNS cannot directly communicate with one another in NST rats. They develop separately, although they control a single mechanical system, the rat's body, in a piecemeal fashion. From this piecemeal control, some rats develop a cooperative process that supports autonomous weight-supported stepping. The closest intuitive analogies to the problem that the transected rat faces may be children's wheelbarrow races, and the "pantomime horse" used in musical theater. In the former, as two children form a "wheelbarrow," the arms of the front child and legs of the rear child must be coordinated and balanced while the front child's body is supported cooperatively by both. In the pantomime horse, two actors form the front and rear of the horse. The rear actor has no vision, and only knows how to step through the mechanical actions and communications of the front actor. The NST rat is an amalgam of these: the lumbar CNS is "blinded" and lacks vestibular information, and all commu-

nication is through the mechanical coupling of the body parts, mediated primarily through the trunk. The thoracic axial musculature is partly shared by both. A natural hypothesis is thus that trunk control will play a central role in the function of these rats, as do the mechanical couplings and coordinations used in the wheelbarrow race and pantomime horse. To what extent are these ideas validated experimentally?

Sites of possible plasticity and compensation in the neonatal model of SCI

There are many points of plasticity in NST rats. Compensations may involve the cortex,[13,30,31,33–38] in cooperation with cerebellum and basal ganglia, the spinal central pattern generators,[2,8,24] primary afferents, autonomic pathways, the trunk, and the hindlimb biomechanical plant.[39–45] Development in NST rats occurs without many normal targets and inputs, and the functional and task contexts differ. Spinal cord development occurs without the normal descending neuromodulation from above the lesion.[46] Spinal pattern generation develops separated from its usual coordinating neural inputs, and in an unusual mechanical context.[47] Differing development of limb muscles could also contribute.[40–45] Mechanical and muscle changes can follow change in neural systems, drive patterns, or use of very different kinematic and kinetic behaviors.[40–45]

What is the rat cortex like after neonatal spinalization?

Trunk motor representations in relation to function

Trunk cortex changes after SCI. The motor representation of hindlimb and lumbar axial musculature in intact rats is in an area caudal to bregma and within 2.5 mm of the midline. This area also contains a sensory representation of trunk and hindlimbs: a sensorimotor amalgam.[48–50] Both these motor and sensory representations are vulnerable to SCI.[5,13,30,31,36] P1/P2 injuries occur before various critical periods in cortical organization. Sensory representations develop in this region in all P1/P2 rats but are lost in rats with ST after these critical periods.[36] The NST sensory representations can be enhanced with exercise: Kao *et al.*[13] showed that exercise increased both responses and the percentage of responding sensory cells in the hindlimb SI area in response to stimulation of dermatomes rostral to the transection.

Extensive trunk motor changes also occur in NST rats (Fig. 1).[30,31] There is no cortical hindlimb representation in WSNST rats. However, all WSNST rats developed low trunk motor representations. NWSNST rats lack them. All WSNST rats' motor cortex had a representation of mid to low trunk, and these matched 1:1 with achievement of autonomous weight support, i.e., rats with good weight support *all* possessed caudal trunk motor representations and vice versa.

How do spinalized rats walk: stance, locomotion, or both?

Usually, adult spinalized cats trained to walk do not stand well, and those that are trained to stand do not walk well.[8,22,24] However, with special efforts, spinalized cats may accomplish both, without autonomous weight support.[40] Cats and rats that are spinalized as neonates [10–12,15–17] can sometimes perform both autonomous locomotion and stance tasks competently as adults.[43] We trained WSNST rats to both walk on a treadmill and to stand quietly for rewards. They successfully managed both, and this allowed us to explore the biomechanics of fully spinalized rats that accomplish both tasks.[5,7]

Control of quadrupedal stance in spinalized rats

Our biomechanical testing for stance was similar to the mutual jostling of rats in cages.[5] We examined how stresses applied at the torso using a robot "saddle" were resisted, how the applied stress was distributed to the limbs, and how the stance center of pressure (CoP) was controlled. Both normal and WSNST rats adapted to the predictable occurence of perturbations. Each moved its resting CoP to produce a more even load distribution between fore- and hindlimbs during perturbation testing. The CoP for the normal rats was shifted forward, while the CoP for the WSNST rats moved caudally, actually increasing the load borne by the hindlimbs.

The robot interaction forces were examined for perturbations in eight directions.[5,51] During perturbations the robot applied force to the rats that rose smoothly to a plateau and the rats actively opposed this. In normal rats, during rostral perturbations, the opposing horizontal forces were larger in the forelimbs, and during caudal perturbations, the opposing horizontal forces were larger in the hindlimbs. In contrast, in WSNST rats the distinction between rostral and caudal perturbations was largely absent. Forelimb forces changed in all directions while hindlimb forces were little different from initial resting forces (Fig. 2). The way in which normal and WSNST rats compensated for perturbation forces thus differed. WSNST rats isolated the hindlimbs from the perturbation as much as possible.

Conceivably, the local lumbar circuitry and resistance reflexes could provide some additional useful hindlimb responses after initial loading. When perturbations were routine WSNST rats adjusted the resting CoP and the hindlimbs became more loaded than before perturbations. Why were the hindlimbs in WSNST rats not used dynamically? We believe that the strategy of minimizing transmission of perturbation forces to the hindlimbs reduced the likelihood of inappropriate stepping or reflex motions. Autonomous local pattern generators and reflexes may play a central role in weight-supported locomotion in spinally injured rats (see next section). However, their spurious activations could disrupt quiet stance.

Control of locomotion in spinalized rats

Stepping in WSNST rats is likely initiated through reflexes and through the available mechanical and reflex couplings and controlled voluntarily via trunk. To explore this we next compared kinetic features of locomotion in intact and WSNST rats.[7] WSNST rats exhibited a gait that was too variable to allow standard gait analysis, which requires averaging of many cycles of constant velocity locomotion.[52–58] WSNST gait was rarely if ever constant velocity. To compare statistically between normal and WSNST rats we examined and compared unconstrained locomotion on a runway. Although rats crossed the runway at various speeds, there were significant statistical differences in limb force coordination, net force and CoP between WSNST and normal rats tested in this way.

Normal rats crossed the runway with a diagonal trot, with 45% body weight on hindlimbs 55% on forelimbs. Forelimbs and hindlimb acted synergistically both limb pairs generated similar

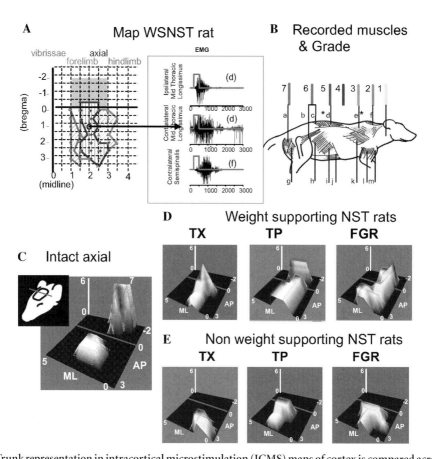

Figure 1. Trunk representation in intracortical microstimulation (ICMS) maps of cortex is compared across function and intervention in NST rats. Note the orientation of the maps indicated by the cartoon on the left in (C). (A) Cortical microstimulation example from rats transected as neonates with weight support, along with sample EMGs from their mapping. Rats with weight support all showed mid to low trunk motor representations (in *blue* regions) when mapped using 50 microAmps current pulses in 300 ms trains. In intact rats these representations would in general occur caudal to bregma (in the *gray* shaded regions in A, and see C). The midthoracic ipsilateral and contralateral latissimus dorsi and contralateral suprspinatus were activated at the site circled. (B) Muscle diagram. To create microstimulation maps and assess trunk control at different segmental levels the following muscles were recorded: (a) semitendinosus, (b) iliopsoas, (c) multifidus, (d) longissimus, (e) trapezius, (f) supraspinatus, (g) biceps femoris, (h) external oblique, (i) internal oblique, (j) rectus abdominis, (k) latissimus, (l) triceps brachii, (m) biceps brachii. Leg muscles (a, g) were never recruited in spinalized rats. Mid to low trunk muscles (c, d and i, j, k and very rarely b) could cause observable pelvic motion either directly or through reflex and mechanical couplings. Trunk or hind-leg segmental level found in ICMS maps was scored from 1 to 7 as shown in (1 upper cervical, 2 upper back, 3 upper shoulder/thorax, 4 mid back, 5 mid to low back, 6 low back/lumbar, 7 legs). The scored values for trunk alone were represented in panels C, D, and E in the figure in two ways: they were used as the height parameter for the surface and a false color mesh was applied to the surface with color related to height. The values were interpolated across the ICMS map so as to construct a continuous surface in which height represents the segmental level score and thus the caudal extent of motor recruitment of trunk from each site in the map. In the false color mesh *red* represents low trunk (color assignments as shown). (C) For the normal rat hindlimb recruitment (level 7) is achieved in the caudal region of the map behind bregma (AP coordinate 0 and purple line in each map, *gray* shaded region in Panel A). (D) In WSNST spinalized rats the maximum height was always 6 or less. Weight-supporting spinalized rats show peaks at level 5–6 but in TX (spinal transection alone, NST) rats these peaks are rostral to bregma, while in TP (fetal transplant repair NST) and FGR (fibrin glue repair NST) rats these are behind bregma, in the normal intact rats location.

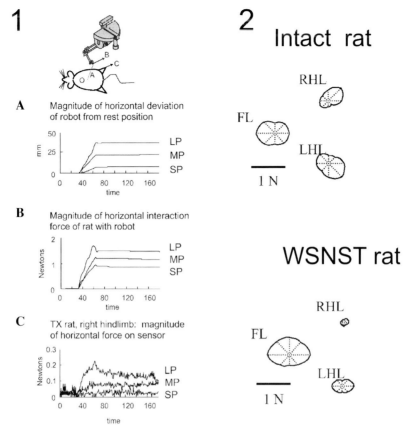

Figure 2. Panel (1): Plots of the responses in perturbation trials for a single direction perturbation applied to an operate rat's stance using the robot and saddle (cartoon above). Shown are: (**A**) the distance over time of the position of the phantom tip from rest, (**B**) the magnitude of the horizontal plane interaction force between an operate rat and the Phantom, and (**C**) the magnitude of the horizontal plane ground reaction force at the right hindlimb force-plate sensor. Rats picked a strategy for how to distribute horizontal ("shear") forces among the individual leg's ground reaction forces. Data is shown for a WSNST rat (indicated TX in figure). Data are plotted during each size perturbation, all in directions. Note the small hindlimb force responses in panel (**C**) relative to the applied force in panel (**B**) in this rat. Panel (2): Polar plots of tuning curves of the magnitude of the horizontal response forces for different directions of perturbations in the forelimbs and hindlimbs. The polar plots are centered on the compass center. Notice the much reduced hindlimb responses in the WSNST rat. Figure redrawn and rearranged from figures in Giszter *et al.*[5]

decelerative and propulsive rostrocaudal forces (Fig. 3, panel 1). These forces averaged about 15% of the antigravity forces. Occasional maximums were about 50% of body weight. Normal rats thus expended substantially less effort on control of forward progression than on weight support. The peak absolute mediolateral forces were substantially smaller than the other force components, averaging only 3–4% of antigravity forces. CoP progressed in jumps along a straight line. Mean lateral deviations of CoP were <1 cm. The normal rats were very well balanced.

Reproduced from Giszter *et al.*[31] (E) Nonweight-supported rats are unresponsive to microstimulation in the area behind bregma and the purple line regardless of intervention and show low axial scores of 3–4 (indicated by low hill peaks). Figure redrawn and rearranged from Fig. 6 in Giszter *et al.*[31]

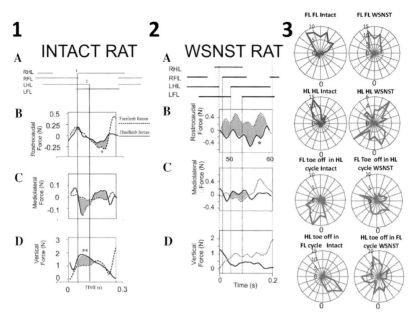

Figure 3. Forces when a rat spanned two force plates during locomotion, allowing separation of forelimb and hindlimb contributions. (1) Normal rat. Forelimb and hindlimb force contributions to propulsion, stabilization, and weight support. *Top*: stance phase of limbs during transition across plates. (A) Gait pattern. (B) Synergistic decelerative and then propulsive actions of forelimbs (*dotted line*) and hindlimbs (*solid line*) is shown by overlapping and similarly directed forces. Rostrocaudal forces correlate well. Individual peak contributions (∼0.25 N) of forelimbs or hindlimbs are under 10% of body weight (2.7 N). In the trial shown forelimbs play a larger part in acceleration (shaded and *). This is within the range of variability from the normal pattern observed in our runway task in which speed was not tightly controlled. (C) Lateral forces: most mediolateral force (∼0.15 N peak, ∼5% body weight) is exerted in hindlimbs (*solid line*). Difference of forelimb and hindlimb contributions is shaded. (D) Antigravity forces: hindlimbs (*solid line*) carry about 60% more body weight than forelimbs (*dotted line*). The difference is shaded, and indicated by **. Lines 1 and 2 indicate RHL foot strike and LHL lift. Panel redrawn and rearranged from Figure in Giszter *et al.*[7] (2) NWS ST rats. Forelimb and hindlimb propulsive forces are coordinated in opposition in injured rats. Phase II forces are shown and differences shaded. *Top*: stance phase of limbs during transition across plates. (A) Gait pattern. (B) Antagonistic decelerative actions of forelimbs (*dotted line*) and propulsive forces from the hindlimbs (*solid line*). Rostrocaudal forces correlate negatively and in a manner significantly different from normal. Individual peak contributions (∼0.5 N) of forelimbs or hindlimbs are ∼25% of body weight (<2 N). The forces show several peaks per cycle. Not all can be related to stance transitions, e.g., peak at *. (C) Lateral forces: mediolateral force (∼0.4 N peak) is exerted in both forelimbs (*dotted line*) and hindlimbs (*solid line*). (D) Antigravity forces: forelimbs (*dotted line*) carry about 60% of total body weight here, close to the typical mean of our ST rats, and significantly more than normal rats. Panel redrawn and rearranged from Figure in Giszter *et al.*[7] (3) Phase relations in gait of WSNST rats. Examples of phase distributions of swing onsets calculated for each girdle, and for hindlimb and forelimb on the same side. (FL FL: forelimb swing onset phase in contralateral forelimb cycle. HL HL: hindlimb swing onset phase in contralateral hindlimb cycle. FL in HL: forelimb swing onset phase in ipsilateral hindlimb cycle. HL in FL: hindlimb swing onset phase in ipsilateral forelimb cycle.) Intact rats are in left column of panel (3), WSNST rats are in right column of panel (3). FL FL phase is less variable in WSNST rats, while other phases show more unusual relationships. Note that the phase plotted may be associated with "winding numbers" of one or more for WSNST data, while this was never true in intact rats, i.e., the rat may show multiple steps of one limb, before the measured limb phase is expressed by its toe-off motion. The average gait ratio was around 7:3 forelimb to hindlimb stepping, but there is more phase patterning in the WSNST stepping than this ratio might suggest. New analysis using data from runway experiments shown in panels (1) and (2).

WSNST rats' hindlimbs bore significantly less weight than intact rats' hindlimbs (37% body weight on hindlimbs, 63% on forelimbs). WSNST rats showed similar mean rostrocaudal forces, but had significantly larger maximum fluctuations ranging up to 80% of body weight ($P < 0.05$). Joint force-plate recordings showed that in WSNST rats the forelimbs and hindlimb rostrocaudal forces acted in opposition, rather than synergistically, differing significantly from intact rats ($P < 0.05$) (Fig. 3, panel 2). Mediolateral forces (∼20% of body weight), were significantly larger than normal rats ($P < 0.05$). WSNST CoP zig-zagged, with mean lateral deviations of ∼2 cm (double those of intact rats), and a significantly larger range ($P < 0.05$). The WSNST rats' gait was highly variable, near a 7 to 3 stepping ratio (forelimbs to hindlimbs). WSNST rats had much more variable forelimb–hindlimb and hindlimb–hindlimb phasing (see Fig. 3, panel 3) but slightly more precise forelimb–forelimb step phasing. The haunches rolled much more than normal rats. The locomotor strategy of WSNST rats, using fore and hindlimbs in opposition, was inefficient but their complex gait was statically stable. Because forelimbs and hindlimbs acted in opposition, the trunk was held compressed. Injured rats contrasted strongly with normal rats in gait, control of ground reaction forces, and motion of the CoP.

These observations fit with the notion of the forelimbs and trunk acting as brakes and/or initiators and stabilizers for the hindlimb generated forces, and movements driven by pattern generation in the injured rats. Trunk control from cortex could be critical to manage, couple and direct the hindlimb generated forces.

The role of cortex in trunk control and SCI

Some trunk muscles physically span the lesioned segments, and these may have distributed motor pools spanning the lesion. Trunk muscles may be coordinated across a lesion by reflex chaining, in which mechanical interactions through the trunk elicit reflexes below the lesion, which coordinate the muscle contraction patterns that occur below the lesion. For example, emetic responses remain coordinated and effective in thoracic spinalized cats, with segmental trunk muscles both above and below the lesion contracting in concert.[59] Cortical motor control of trunk may thus provide several ways of interacting with the autonomous lumbar stepping. The trunk cortex might help coordinate forelimb–hindlimb mechanical transmissions, and thus shape the mechanical environment in which lumbar stepping occurs. Such mechanical shaping is known to play a role in pattern generator function after SCI.[1,8,16,24,25,41,43,60]

Cortical motor representations of mid/low trunk only occur in WSNST rats with high weight support as noted,[30] and Kao *et al.*'s study[13] of S1 showed exercise altered cortex representations in NST rats. Motor cortex might be engaged differently in locomotion developed by the WSNST rats because they were injured preceding critical periods in cortical and cerebellar wiring. However, alternatively, perhaps the trunk cortex motor representations were an outcome of function rather than the cause. To test the role of trunk cortex in WSNST rats, we used intracranial microstimulation to guide focal lesions placed in the trunk area of cortex.[31] We lesioned the normal hindlimb/trunk area in all rats, i.e., the area representing low trunk and hindlimb in normal rats. Injured rats could vary in their prelesion weight-support level, depending on their body weight.

In four intact control rats, lesions of hindlimb/trunk cortex caused no treadmill deficits. However, all NST rats lesioned in trunk cortex lost an average of ∼40% of their weight support, which did not recover. Although the role of hindlimb/trunk motor cortex in intact rats may be modest in normal locomotion, cortex must have become more significant after spinalization in NST rats. Trunk cortex became an essential participant in the weight-supporting locomotion of these rats.

WSNST joint angle ranges were comparable to intact rats on the treadmill and to published data.[61] WSNST hindlimb kinematic and joint parameters were also not significantly different pre- and postlesion (Fig. 4). However, the frequency of high roll (i.e., >45°) events in the haunches was increased substantially by lesions, and more than doubled. A prelesion probability per step of high roll of 0.1 increased postlesion to 0.25 (statistically significant, *t*-test, $P < 0.005$). Roll event probability correlated negatively with the percentage weight support measures (regression $r^2 = 0.81$, $P < 0.0001$), and correlated positively with the number of nonweight-supporting step cycles (regression $r^2 = 0.83$,

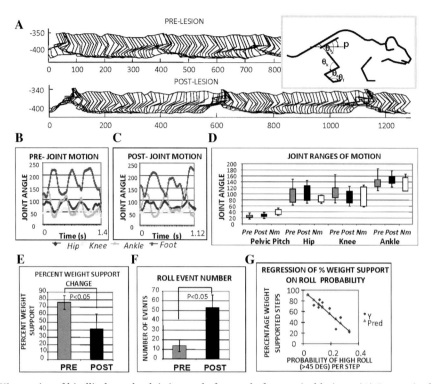

Figure 4. Kinematics of hindlimbs and pelvis in rats before and after cortical lesions. (**A**) Parasagittal stick figure motion was digitized for multiple step cycles before and after lesion. An example of data from one rat is shown. The measured internal angles are displayed to the right. (**B**) Prelesion and (**C**) postlesion joint angles. Pelvic pitch orientation and joint angles of hip, knee, ankle, and foot were measured from the captured stick figures pre- and postlesion. (**D**) Range of motion for each angle's time-series was compared pre–post for 8 WSNST rats (pre, post) and for normal rats (Nm). Ranges for data from B/C are shown, together with normal intact rat ranges measured similarly. The maximum and minimum joint angles and their standard deviations in the group of eight rats tested in detail for pre- and postlesion data were compared. In the NST eight rats tested, statistical comparisons of the kinematic features measured in the parasagittal plane were not significantly different. Neither the ranges of motion, the basic pattern of coordination among joints, nor the period of the hindlimb stepping were significantly altered by the cortical lesions ($n = 8$, $P > 0.1$). (**E**) After lesions, the group percent weight support decreased significantly (paired *t*-test, $P < 0.05$). (**F**) After lesion there were increased numbers of pelvic roll events where roll clearly exceeded 45° (paired *t*-test, $P < 0.05$). The probability of 45° roll for each step was calculated from these data and more than doubled postlesion (paired *t*-test, $P < 0.05$). The number of nonweight-supporting steps in rats was also linearly related to the number of roll events ($r^2 = 0.83$, slope coefficient ~2 and significance $P < 0.0005$). (**G**) The percentage of weight-supported steps in rats was negatively correlated to the probability of roll per step ($r^2 = 0.81$, slope coefficient significance $P < 0.0001$). Thus hindlimb kinematics were not altered significantly, but pelvic roll was increased and related to quality of weight support. Reworked from Fig. 6 in Giszter *et al.*[31]

$P < 0.0005$). The hindlimb/trunk cortex lesions thus disrupted aspects of the control of roll, pelvic balance, and the integration of forelimbs and hindlimb mechanics. The data support a significant role of trunk cortex in locomotion after complete neonatal spinalization.

Muscle masses, the biomechanics of pattern generation and their intimate relationships in effective locomotion

How much do altered limb muscle balances contribute to the autonomous weight-bearing of NST rats? The muscle balances in the WSNST and

NWSNST rats have not previously been explored. From first principles in biomechanics, it can be shown that if the limb's muscle masses differ in their proportions, then effects of identical pattern generation and reflex synergies will be mechanically different. This is because the relative scaling of joint torques by coactive muscles will differ. As a result, the force magnitude and direction at the foot will necessarily be different following the transformation of differently scaled torques into force, through the limb linkage.[6,62,63] In contrast, if muscles were scaled similarly, even after some atrophy, then similar motor patterns would cause similar balances of force and torque in the limb, and similar force directions at the foot, though more weakly. Human limbs in individuals of very different physical power and size are nonetheless similarly scaled.[64,65] Do muscle proportions that occur in the hindlimbs in WSNST and NWSNST rats permit the "normal" limb use? We set out to test this.

Muscle mass comparison methods

Muscle experiments were conducted with IACUC oversight according to PHS and USDA guidelines. Animals were spinalized as described in Giszter *et al.* (1998).[30] We examined both NST and normal rats: 9 normal rats, 11 NWSNST rats, and 10 WSNST rats. Rats were treadmill trained three times weekly as described by Giszter,[5,7,31] similarly to the NST rats described in preceding sections. To compare masses among the groups 11 muscles were excised from each perfused rat and weighed: biceps femoris, vastus lateralis, rectus femoris, gracilis, semimembranosus, semitendinosus, gastrocnemius group, tibialis anterior, iliopsoas, forelimb triceps, and biceps brachii. We combined medial and lateral gastrocnemius (the gastrocnemius group). We did not examine soleus or plantaris, which were difficult to dissect accurately in the perfused NST rats. In a separate analysis of nine NST and four normal rats we confirmed general symmetry of muscle masses measured bilaterally, between the limbs in these rats. Their mean difference in matched muscle mass measurements between the two sides was under 5%.

Estimated muscle cross-section areas. Cross-sectional area (CSA) and physiological cross-sectional area (PCSA) predict force producing capacity of muscle. CSA is a significant contributor

to PCSA. We estimated CSA of muscles from their muscle mass. We calculated CSA as mass raised to the 2/3 power, as used in allometric scaling.[66,67] We then tested this algorithm as a relative PCSA estimate by using data in the literature where both mass and PCSA, (which includes pennation angle, and sarcomere length) were measured in muscles after SCI.[44] We found that the regression coefficient between published PCSA measures and our estimate of CSA from our algorithm was >0.96 for all muscles reported.

Scaling measures. What is important in muscle scaling in NST rats and normal? Neonatal spinalized NST rats are often lighter than intact littermates. We thus examined several scalings. To compare scaling of muscles of interest we used raw data and also normalized to: (1) total body mass, (2) combined leg muscle mass, and (3) combined estimated muscle area. Normalizations 2 and 3 relate an individual muscle to the rest of the ensemble of hindlimb muscles within the leg, ignoring overall rat mass.

Scaling statistical tests. To test differences in scaling we used ANOVA, principal components analyses (PCA), regression and *post hoc* statistical *t*-tests. These were performed in the MINITAB statistical package, Excel, or Statview. Earlier work in this area examined smaller numbers of muscles, where *t*-tests were appropriate, so here we also examined results of *post hoc t*-test comparisons, with and without the Bonferroni correction, although such unadjusted *t*-tests may *overestimate* differences.

Muscle scaling results

Masses were always largest in normal and smallest in NWSNST rats. Mean body mass in Normals was 251 g, WSNST rats 194.6 g, and NWSNST rats 167.6 g. However, WSNST and NWSNST rats body weight did not differ significantly (*t*-test, $P = 0.513$), while both NST groups and the normal rats differed (all *t*-tests $P < 0.001$). Leg masses differed between all 3 groups (*t*-test comparing NWSNST and WSNST groups, $P < 10^{-5}$). Total mass of muscles mattered: In a subset of five WSNST rats, with total measured muscle mass >4.5 g, we found that percent weight support showed a positive relationship to leg muscle mass (adjusted linear regression coefficient 0.952, slope significant at $P < 0.005$, $N = 5$).

Table 1. Repeated measures ANOVAS of raw muscle masses and muscle measures scaled to the other muscles

	ANOVA					
Source of variation	SS	df	MS	*F*	*P*-value	*F* crit
(A) Raw hind leg muscle masses						
Function level/group	1.386384	2	0.693192	75.98011	2.51E-21	3.080388
Muscle	21.08176	8	2.63522	288.844	3.15E-69	2.025246
Interaction	1.49519	16	0.093449	10.2429	3.06E-15	1.738002
Within	0.98532	108	0.009123			
Total	24.94865	134				
(B) Muscle masses normalized to measured hind leg muscle mass						
Function level/group	0.001304	2	0.000652	1.857689	0.158826	3.042963
Muscle	0.973129	7	0.139018	396.0888	1.9E-110	2.057533
Interaction	0.005978	14	0.000427	1.216509	0.265868	1.743594
Within	0.067388	192	0.000351			
Total	1.047799	215				
(C) Hind leg muscle ratios (without iliopsoas)						
Function level/group	5.672938	2	2.836469	4.36662	0.013056	3.009127
Muscle pair ratio	1691.575	27	62.65091	96.44835	1.1E-210	1.502368
Interaction	47.53946	54	0.88036	1.355276	0.050322	1.356053
Within	436.5177	672	0.64958			
Total	2181.305	755				

All these significant differences held for estimated CSAs.

A two-way fixed effects ANOVA of raw muscle masses showed significant effects of level of function, muscle and their interaction (Table 1, section A). The masses of most individual muscles differed significantly ($P < 0.05$) between each NST rat group and normal, excepting forelimb biceps and triceps, Figure 5A. Spinalization thus reduced muscle mass in the hindlimbs but not the forelimbs compared to normal. *Post hoc* tests (Bonferroni correction) showed that vastus lateralis, semitendinosus and tibialis anterior also differed significantly between WSNST and NWSNST groups (*t*-tests, $P < 0.05$). Thus, weight support in NST rats apparently correlated with increased limb mass, and significant differences in a subset of individual muscles.

We next normalized the muscle masses to body mass, assessing muscle scaling with the whole body. All NWSNST and normal muscles were again significantly different. However, these differences all disappeared when we examined *within limb scaling*.

Muscle masses normalized to leg mass

We examined muscle masses normalized as percentages of total muscle mass measured within the leg (Fig. 6A). Scaling to limb muscle mass examines local scaling within the limb. It is unaffected by fat, or bone density changes in the body or limbs. After the normalization to leg mass, *none of the muscle masses were significantly different among the groups*. We first performed an ANOVA of normalized data (Table 1, section B). *There were no significant effects of group or interaction in the* ANOVA *with this normalization. In 27 post hoc t-test comparisons (3 groups × 9 muscles) with the Bonferroni correction, none were significant.* Variances relative to mean values in the data were decreased, not increased, as a result of normalization (compare Figs. 5 and 6). Thus we cannot attribute the absence of significant differences to an increased variance of the data sets. Including a forelimb muscle in the ANOVA, it alone showed significant effects, showing the normalization had power to detect variations. Unsurprisingly, results were unaltered by a transformation of muscle mass to a cross-section area estimate (Fig. 5B). Within leg muscle scaling was thus preserved between all three groups. This

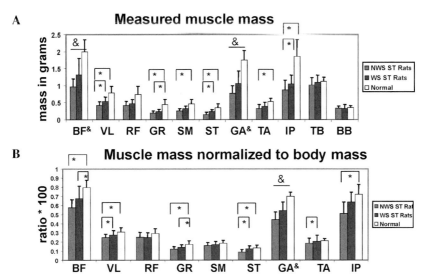

Figure 5. (A) Measured muscle masses by weight-support group. NWS ST group (*gray*), WS ST group (*black*), N normal group (*white*). Muscles: (**1**) BF biceps femoris, (**2**) VL vastus lateralis, (**3**) RF rectus femoris, (**4**) GR gracilis, (**5**) SM semimembranosus, (**6**) ST semitendinosus, (**7**) GA gastrocnemius, (**8**) TA tibialis anterior, (**9**) IP iliopsoas, (**10**) TB forelimb triceps, and (**11**) BB biceps brachii. Vertical bars: standard deviations. Bars and asterisks indicate significant differences in muscle masses (*t*-tests $P < 0.05$). Ampersands on bars indicate all three comparisons were significant. (B) Muscle masses of leg normalized to body weight. NWS ST group (*gray*), WS ST group (*black*), N normal group (*white*). Muscles labeled as in A. Vertical bars: standard deviations. Bars and asterisks indicate significant differences in muscle masses (*t*-tests $P < 0.05$). Ampersands on bars indicate all three comparisons were significant. Data not previously published.

was surprising given the different levels of function and loading conditions in the three groups. However, note that this scaling provides the necessary mechanical basis for similar pattern generation to generate similar mechanics.[63]

Muscle mass and area ratio matrices are similar

To further test the proportionality of muscles, we calculated the 9 × 9 diagonally symmetric matrices of the ratios of muscle masses (and also ratios of area estimates) for each rat. We then compared these data among tested muscles in each rat group. These ratios did not involve any normalization steps; they were simply raw mass ratios. We tested statistically whether the balances among the ratios of any of the muscles differed significantly among the groups. We again used a two factor ANOVA of groups (NWS, WS, normal, Table 1, section C) using the 27 muscle ratios (we omitted iliopsoas ratios with only partial data), with a *post hoc* Bonferroni/Dunn correction, testing at the 0.05 significance level. In the ratiometric analysis there was a significant ef-

fect of function/group. However, most variance was captured due to choice of muscle ratio (78%), and the function/treatment group provided only 0.2%. Interaction of treatment group and ratio combined provided 3%, with residual noise of 18.8%. Only two muscle ratios differed significantly among groups in *post hoc* tests with the Bonferroni correction: (1) the ratio of semimembranosus and gastrocnemius differed between normal and NWS, and (2) the ratio of tibialis and gastrocnemius ratio differed between NWS and normal. The simple ratiometric analysis thus also supports the idea of a largely uniform scaling of limb muscle mass regardless of function, with the possible exception of ankle spanning muscles.

Principal components analysis shows muscle masses covary strongly among rats

Principal components analysis (PCA) examines the variance structure of data without any preconceived reference. The dimensionality of the overall muscle scaling was thus assessed more directly. The preceding analyses suggest the major source of variance in muscle masses, is simply whole limb mass

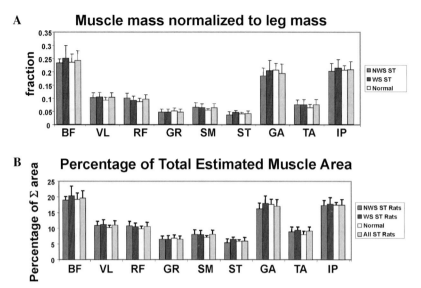

Figure 6. (A) Muscle masses of the leg normalized to leg total muscle mass. NWS ST group (*dark gray*), WS ST group (*black*), N normal group (*white*), All ST rats (*light gray*). Muscles: (**1**) BF biceps femoris, (**2**) VL vastus lateralis, (**3**) RF rectus femoris, (**4**) GR gracilis, (**5**) SM semimembranosus, (**6**) ST semitendinosus, (**7**) GA gastrocnemius, (**8**) TA tibialis anterior, (**9**) IP iliopsoas, (**10**) TB forelimb triceps, and (**11**) BB biceps brachii. Vertical bars: standard deviations. There were no significant differences in *post hoc t*-tests with Bonferroni corrections. Note lowered standard deviations and increased similarities compared to Figure 5. (B) Percentage of estimated muscle area as a fraction of summed leg muscle estimated areas, obtained applying a nonlinear scaling. NWS ST group (*dark gray*), WS ST group (*black*), N normal group (*white*), All ST rats (*light gray*). All spinalized combined (*cyan*). Muscles labeled as in A. Vertical bars: standard deviations. Note similarity across groups and the reduced variance after these normalizations and scalings compared to Figure 5. Data not previously published.

scaling. If true, PCA should capture most variance in the first component. We thus combined all three groups' data and applied PCA. For measured mass, the first principal component captured 89.8% of variance with the second component capturing 3% and the third 2%. This result indicates that there was strong linear covariation of individual muscle masses between animals and groups.

The strong proportionality of muscles we found may be surprising given the differences in function of the rats. However, this scaling suggests that differences in the physical plant balance of muscles do not limit NWSNST rats, causing failure to achieve autonomous function. The balance of muscles significantly affects the extent to which similar central pattern generation, and feedback, can generate similar mechanics and stepping kinematics. Because muscle masses scale closely despite functional differences in the rats, biomechanical factors, and muscle interactions intrinsic to the rat limb (i.e., largely independent of weight support, akin to scaling *in utero*) may

cause and conserve the scaling. Similar proportionality across different individuals of greatly varying size, capacity, and activities have also been reported in man.[64,65] Many factors may be critical to weight support in NST rats. The preserved muscle scaling reported here is one of these contributing factors, with overall leg mass then determining power capability.

Conclusions: future questions, combined therapies, and future needs

Transection of the spinal cord is an unambiguous lesion. Plastic reorganization, novel strategies and altered control by cortex probably allow the greater development of function seen in neonatally lesioned rats. Preserved muscle scaling may permit similar pattern generation in both NST rats and normal. It is not yet clear if the same reorganization of control and movement strategies as are seen in NST rats are possible in adult spinalized rats. NST rats likely learn their motor strategies in critical periods in development. Whether injured adults can relearn these is an open question. However, the best experimental therapies may require this learning.[68] Any interventions that assist in training the trunk controls will likely help. Rehabilitation should maximize trunk integration and enable the adult injured rats to explore novel control strategies.

Acknowledgments

Supported by NIH (grants NS24707, NS44564, and NS54894).

Conflicts of interest

The authors declare no conflicts of interest.

References

1. Barbeau, H. & S. Rossignol. 1987. Recovery of locomotion after chronic spinalization in the adult cat. *Brain Res.* **412:** 84–95.

2. Bouyer, L.J., P.J. Whelan, K.G. Pearson & S. Rossignol. 2001. Adaptive locomotor plasticity in chronic spinal cats after ankle extensors neurectomy. *J. Neurosci.* **21:** 3531–3541.

3. Wolpaw, J.R. 2006. The education and re-education of the spinal cord. *Prog. Brain Res.* **157:** 261-280.

4. Donoghue, J.P. & J.N. Sanes. 1987. Peripheral nerve injury in developing rats reorganizes representation pattern in motor cortex. *PNAS* **84:** 1123–1126.

5. Giszter, S.F., M.R. Davies, V.G. Graziani. 2007a. Motor strategies used by rats spinalized at birth to maintain stance in response to imposed perturbations. *J. Neurophysiol.* **97:** 2663–2675.

6. Giszter, S.F., V. Patil & C.B. Hart. 2007b. Primitives, premotor drives and pattern generation: a combined computational and neuroethological perspective. *Prog. Brain Res.* **165:** 325–349

7. Giszter, S.F., M.R. Davies & V. Graziani. 2008a. Coordination strategies for limb forces during weight-bearing locomotion in normal rats, and in rats spinalized as neonates. *Exp. Brain Res.* **190:** 53–69. Epub 2008 Jul 9.

8. Hodgson, J.A., *et al.* 1994. Can the mammalian lumbar spinal cord learn a motor task? *Med. Sci. Sports Exercise* **26:** 1491–1497.

9. Rossignol, S. 2006. Plasticity of connections underlying locomotor recovery after central and/or peripheral lesions in the adult mammals. *Philos. Trans. R Soc. Lond. B Biol. Sci.* **361:** 1647–1671.

10. Forssberg, H., S. Grillner & A. Sjostrom. 1974. Tactile placing reactions in chronic spinal kittens. *Acta Physiol. Scand.* **92:** 114–120.

11. Howland, D.R., B.S. Bregman, A. Tessler & M.E. Goldberger. 1995a. Development of locomotor behavior in the spinal kitten. *Exp. Neurol.* **135:** 108–122.

12. Howland, D.R., B.S. Bregman, A. Tessler & M.E. Goldberger. 1995b. Transplants enhance locomotion in neonatal kittens whose spinal cords are transected. *Exp. Neurol.* **135:** 123–145.

13. Kao, T., J.S. Shumsky, M. Murray & K.A. Moxon. 2009. Exercise induces cortical plasticity after neonatal spinal cord injury in the rat. *J. Neurosci.* **29:** 7549–7557.

14. Miya, D. *et al.* 1997. Fetal transplants alter the development of function after spinal cord transection in newborn rats. *J. Neurosci.* **17:** 4856–4872.

15. Robinson, G.A. & M.E. Goldberger. 1986. The development and recovery of motor function in spinal cats. I. The infant lesion effect. *Exp. Brain Res.* **62:** 373–386.

16. Smith, J.L., L.A. Smith, F. Zernicke & M. Hoy. 1982. Locomotion in exercised and nonexercised cats cordotomized at two and twelve weeks of age. *Exp. Neurol.* **76:** 393–413.

17. Stelzner, D.J., W.B. Ershler & E.D. Weber. 1975. Effects of spinal transection in neonatal and weanling rats: survival of function. *Exp Neurol.* **46:** 156–177.

18. Gerasimenko, Y.P. *et al.* 2006. Spinal cord reflexes induced by epidural spinal cord stimulation in normal awake rats. *J. Neurosci. Methods* **157:** 253–263.

19. de Leon, R.D. & C.N. Acosta. 2006. Effect of robotic-assisted treadmill training and chronic quipazine treatment on hindlimb stepping in spinally transected rats. *J. Neurotrauma.* **23:** 1147–1163.

20. Orsal, D. *et al.* 2002. Locomotor recovery in chronic spinal rat: long-term pharmacological treatment or transplantation of embryonic neurons? *Prog. Brain Res.* **137:** 213–230.

21. Ribotta, M.G. *et al.* 2000. Activation of locomotion in adult chronic spinal rats is achieved by transplantation of embryonic raphe cells reinnervating a precise lumbar level. *J. Neurosci.* **20:** 5144–5152.

22. de Leon, R.D. *et al.* 1999. Hindlimb locomotor and postural training modulates glycinergic inhibition in the spinal cord of the adult spinal cat. *J. Neurophysiol.* **82:** 359–369.

23. De Leon, R.D., J.A. Hodgson, R.R. Roy & V.R. Edgerton. 1998. Full weight-bearing hindlimb standing following stand training in the adult spinal cat. *J. Neurophysiol.* **80:** 83–91.

24. Tillakaratne, N.J. *et al.* 2002. Use-dependent modulation of inhibitory capacity in the feline lumbar spinal cord. *J. Neurosci.* **22:** 3130–3143.

25. Timoszyk, W.K. *et al.* 2005. Hindlimb loading determines stepping quantity and quality following spinal cord transection. *Brain Res.* **1050:** 180–189.

26. Belanger, M., T. Drew, J. Provencher & S. Rossignol. 1996. A comparison of treadmill locomotion in adult cats before and after spinal transection. *J. Neurophysiol.* **76:** 471–491.

27. Dietz, V. 2002. Do human bipeds use quadrupedal coordination? *Trends Neurosci.* **25:** 462–467.

28. Dietz, V. & J. Michel. 2009. Human bipeds use quadrupedal coordination during locomotion. *Ann. N.Y. Acad. Sci.* **1164:** 97–103.

29. Grillner, S. 1975. Locomotion in vertebrates: central mechanisms and reflex interaction. *Physiol. Rev.* **55:** 247-304.

30. Giszter, S.F., W.J. Kargo, M. Davies & M. Shibayama. 1998. Fetal transplants rescue axial muscle representations in M1 cortex of neonatally transected rats that develop weight support. *J. Neurophysiol.* **80:** 3021–3030.

31. Giszter, S.F., *et al.* 2008b. Trunk sensorimotor cortex is essential for hindlimb weight-supported locomotion in adult rats spinalized as P1/P2 neonates. *J. Neurophysiol.* **100:** 839–851. Epub 2008 May 28.

32. Basso, D.M., M.S. Beattie & J.C. Bresnehan. 1995. A sensitive and reliable locomotor rating scale for open field testing in rats. *J. Neurotrauma* **12:** 1–21.

33. Chakrabarty, S. & J.H. Martin. 2005. Motor but not sensory representation in motor cortex depends on postsynaptic activity during development and in maturity. *J. Neurophysiol.* **94:** 3192–3198.

34. Friel, K.M. & J.H. Martin. 2005. Role of sensory-motor cortex activity in postnatal development of corticospinal axon terminals in the cat. *J. Comp. Neurol.* **485:** 43–56.

35. Friel, K.M., T. Drew & J.H. Martin. 2007. Differential activity-dependent development of corticospinal control of movement and final limb position during visually-guided locomotion. *J. Neurophysiol.* **97:** 3396–3406.

36. Jain, N., P.S. Diener, J.O. Coq & J.H. Kaas. 2003. Patterned activity via spinal dorsal quadrant inputs is necessary for the formation of organized somatosensory maps. *J. Neurosci.* **23:** 10321–10330.

37. Martin, J.H. 2005. The corticospinal system: from development to motor control. *Neuroscientist* **11:** 161–173.

38. Martin, J.H., M. Choy, S. Pullman & Z. Meng. 2004. Corticospinal system development depends on motor experience. *J. Neurosci.* **24:** 2122–2132.

39. Dupont-Versteegden, E.E., *et al.* 2000. Mechanisms leading to restoration of muscle size with exercise and transplantation after spinal cord injury. *Am. J. Physiol. Cell Physiol.* **279:** C1677–C1684.

40. Edgerton, V.R., R.R. Roy, D.L. Allen & R.J. Monti. 2002. Adaptations in skeletal muscle disuse or decreased-use atrophy. *Am. J. Phys. Med. Rehabil.* **81**(11 Suppl): S127–S147.

41. Ohira, Y. *et al.* 2000. Dependence of normal development of skeletal muscle in neonatal rats on load bearing. *J. Gravit. Physiol.* **7:** P27–P30.

42. Peterson, C.A., R.J. Murphy, E.E. Dupont-Versteegden, J.D. Houle. 2000. Cycling exercise and fetal spinal cord transplantation act synergistically on atrophied muscle following chronic spinal cord injury in rats. *Neurorehabil. Neural Repair* **14:** 85–91.

43. Roy, R.R. & L. Acosta, Jr. 1986. Fiber type and fiber size changes in selected thigh muscles six months after low thoracic spinal cord transection in adult cats: exercise effects. *Exp. Neurol.* **92:** 675–685.

44. Roy, R.R. *et al.* 1999. Differential response of fast hindlimb extensor and flexor muscles to exercise in adult spinalized cats. *Muscle Nerve.* **22:** 230–241.

45. Roy, R.R., H. Zhong, B. Siengthai & V.R. Edgerton. 2005. Activity-dependent influences are greater for fibers in rat medial gastrocnemius than tibialis anterior muscle. *Muscle Nerve* **32:** 473–482.

46. Vinay, L. *et al.* 2002. Development of posture and locomotion: an interplay of endogenously generated activities and neurotrophic actions by descending pathways. *Brain Res. Brain Res. Rev.* **40:** 118–129.

47. Westerga, J. & A. Gramsbergen. 1993. Development of locomotion in the rat: the significance of early movements. *Early Hum. Develop.* **34:** 89–100.

48. Donoghue, J.P. & J.N. Sanes. 1988. Organization of adult motor cortex representation patterns following neonatal forelimb nerve injury in rats. *J. Neurosci.* **8:** 3221–3232

49. Hall, R.D. & E.P. Lindholm. 1974. Organization of motor and sensory neocortex in the albino rat. *Brain Res.* **66:** 23–28.

50. Hummelsheim, H. & M. Wiesendanger. 1986. Is the hind-limb representation of the rat's cortex a sensorimotor amalgam? *Brain Res.* **346:** 75–81.

51. Udoekwere, U.I., L.T. Mbi, A. Ramakrishnan & S.F. Giszter. 2006. Robot applied elastic fields at the pelvis of the spinal transected rat: a tool for detailed assessment and rehabilitation. In *Proceedings of the IEEE/EMBC Conference*, New York, NY.

52. Clarke, K.A. 1995. Differential fore- and hindpaw force transmission in the walking rat. *Physiol. Behav.* **58:** 415–419.

53. Gregor, R.J., D.W. Smith & B.I. Prilutsky. 2006. Mechanics of slope walking in the cat: quantification of muscle load, length change, and ankle extensor EMG patterns. *J. Neurophysiol.* **95:** 1397–1409. Epub 2005 Oct 5.

54. Howard, C.S. *et al.* 2000. Functional assessment in the rat by ground reaction forces. *J. Biomech.* **33:** 751–757.

55. Kaya, M., T.R. Leonard & W. Herzog. 2006. Control of ground reaction forces by hindlimb muscles during cat locomotion. *J. Biomech.* **39:** 2752–2766. Epub 2005 Nov 28.

56. Lavoie, S., B. McFadyen & T. Drew. 1995. A kinematic and kinetic analysis of locomotion during voluntary gait modification in the cat. *Exp Brain Res.* **106:** 39–56.

57. Muir, G.D. & I.Q. Whishaw. 1999. Complete locomotor recovery following corticospinal tract lesions: measurement of ground reaction forces during overground locomotion in rats. *Behav. Brain Res.* **103:** 45–53.

58. Muir, G.D. & I.Q. Whishaw. 2000. Red nucleus lesions impair overground locomotion in rats: a kinetic analysis. *Eur. J. Neurosci.* **12:** 1113–1122.

59. Iscoe, S. 1998. Control of abdominal muscles. *Prog. Neurobiol.* **56:** 433–506

60. de Leon, R.D. *et al.* 2002a. Using robotics to teach the spinal cord to walk. *Brain Res. Brain Res. Rev.* **40:** 267–273.

61. Thota, A.K. *et al.* 2005. Neuromechanical control of locomotion in the rat. *J. Neurotrauma* **22:** 442–465.

62. Asada, H. & J-J. E. Slotine. 1986. *Robot Analysis and Control.* Wiley Interscience. New York.

63. Kargo, W.J. & S.F. Giszter. 2008. Individual premotor drive pulses, not time-varying synergies, are the units of adjustment for limb trajectories constructed in spinal-cord. *J. Neuroscience* **28:** 2409–2425.

64. Holzbaur, K.R., S.L. Delp, G.E. Gold & W.M. Murray. 2007. Moment-generating capacity of upper limb muscles in healthy adults. *J. Biomech.* **40:** 2442–2449.

65. Holzbaur, K.R., W.M. Murray, G.E. Gold & S.L. Delp. 2007. Upper limb muscle volumes in adult subjects. *J. Biomech.* **40:** 742–749. Epub 2007 Jan 22.

66. Lindstedt S. L. & P.J. Schaeffer. 2002. Use of allometry in predicting anatomical and physiological parameters of mammals. *Laboratory Animals* **36:** 1–19.

67. Payne, R.C. *et al.* 2006. Morphological analysis of the hindlimb in apes and humans. I. Muscle architecture. *J. Anat.* **208:** 709–724.

68. Giszter, S.F. 2008. Spinal cord injury: present and future therapeutic devices and prostheses. *Neurotherapeutics* **5:** 147–162.